Peritoneal Adhesions

Springer
Berlin
Heidelberg
New York
Barcelona
Budapest
Hong Kong
London
Milan
Paris
Santa Clara
Singapore
Tokyo

K.-H. Treutner   V. Schumpelick (Eds.)

Peritoneal Adhesions

With 139 Figures and 85 Tables

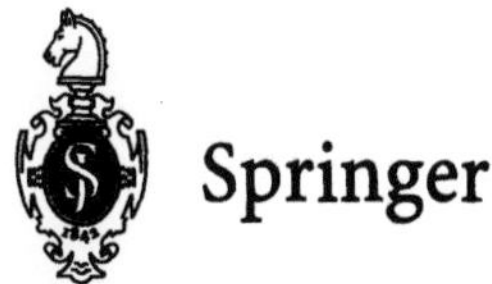

Springer

Dr. med. Karl-Heinz Treutner
Professor Dr. med. Volker Schumpelick

Chirurgische Universitätsklinik u. Poliklinik
Rheinische-Westfälische Technische Hochschule
Pauwelsstraße 30
52057 Aachen
Germany

ISBN-13:978-3-540-61192-9   e-ISBN-13:978-3-642-60433-1
DOI: 10.1007/978-3-642-60433-1

Library of Congress Cataloging-in-Publication Data. Peritoneal adhesions/K.-H. Treutner, V. Schumpelick
(Eds.). p.   cm. Includes bibliographical references and index. ISBN-13:978-3-540-61192-9(softcover; alk. paper)
1. Adhesions - Congresses. I. Treutner, K.-H. II. Schumpelick, V. (Volker) [DNLM 1. Peritoneal Diseases -
prevention & control - congresses. 2. Peritoneal Cavity - physiopathology - congresses. 3. Adhesions -
congresses. WI 575 P4453 1997] RD647.A3P47 1997 616.3′8-dc20 DNLM/DLC for Library of Congress 97-
28281

Cover design: Design & Production GmbH, Heidelberg

Typesetting: Scientific Publishing Services (P) Ltd, Madras

SPIN: 10531613   24/3135/SPS – 5 4 3 2 1 0 – Printed on acid-free paper

Preface

Adhesions and adhesion-related morbidity are common sequelae of surgical procedures. They are induced by the inevitable dissection and retraction of tissues and organs during the course of the operation. Additional microscopic lesions resulting from accidental trauma of the delicate mesothelial lining of the peritoneum are caused by the unavoidable use of retractors, towels and swabs, and tissue handling and drying out. Furthermore, infections, ischemia, and foreign body reactions to suture and mesh materials and glove powder can lead to the formation of peritoneal adhesions.

Uniform reaction of the peritoneum to these injuries is the release of a fibrinous exudate which forms transient adhesions. Due to a decreased fibrinolytic activity of the traumatized peritoneum, however, these fibrinous adhesions can be infiltrated by fibroblasts, become vascularized, and subsequently transformed to permanent strands of connective tissue. The nature and severity of possible symptoms is related to the extent and location of the adhesive bridges.

Adhesions are the cause of every second case of intestinal obstruction and the reason for about 1% of all admissions and 3% of all laparotomies in general surgery. Furthermore, adhesions make reoperations more time-consuming, difficult, and hazardous. Hereby they account for a significant morbidity and mortality, a large clinical workload, and a noteworthy socioeconomic impact. Within the scope of an increasing number of abdominal operations performed around the world and the need and feasability of repeated surgery increasing with longevity and medical progress the problem will even gain more relevance in the near future.

Gynecologists are facing adhesion-related problems of female infertility and failure of refertilization. Adhesions may interfere with local chemotherapy and peritoneal dialysis (CAPD). Beyond the abdominal cavity, cardiac surgeons are confronted with pericardial adhesions and thoracic surgeons with pleural adhesions. Adhesions play a crucial part in laparoscopic procedures. Minimal invasive surgery is advocated to reduce adhesion formation – extensive adhesions, however, can render the laparoscopic approach impossible.

Despite these well-known problems, there is still no clinical standard for any preventive measure, either surgical or pharmaceutical, to control the formation of postoperative adhesions. This prompted the idea of a congress that would bring together all who are involved in the research, diagnosis, and therapy of adhesions and adhesion-related problems, regardless of their original field in the medical profession.

A number of renowned specialists contributed their laboratory findings and clinical experience to the meeting at the Department of Surgery of the Rhenish-Westphalian Technical University in Aachen, October 5–7, 1995, and the publication of this volume. The topics range from basic science and animal experiments to clinical trials and observations in the fields of anatomy, pathology, radiology, general and cardiothoracic surgery, gynecology, oncology, and nephrology.

This wide array of approaches to the subject of adhesion formation, prevention, and treatment resulted in exciting lectures and lively discussions. Altogether the contributions reflect current knowledge in this field. Although the time has not yet come to recommend specific measures as a clinical standard for prophylaxis and therapy of adhesions, the results and statements presented may serve as a sound foundation for further research.

We wish to thank Stig Bengmark, Prof. em. of the Department of Surgery, Lund University, Sweden, for his initiative in bringing this meeting to Aachen in succession of previous meetings of the PAx (peritoneum and peritoneal access) Society. Thanks also to our colleague Dr. M. Rau who provided the cover illustration. And we thank Ms. Gabriele M. Schröder, Mr. Udo Schiller, and the staff of Springer-Verlag for their work in publishing this book.

K.-H. Treutner
V. Schumpelick

Contents

1   Basics on Adhesion Formation

1.1   Serous Membranes and Their Development, Structure,
and Topography
F. Thors and J. Drukker   3

1.2   New Aspects of Peritoneal Pathology
M. Morganti, L. Tietze, B. Amo-Takyi, K. Tory, D. Budianto,
U. Henze, and C. Mittermayer   14

1.3   The Role of Wound Healing
in the Formation of Peritoneal Adhesions
G.B. Köveker, S. Coerper, T. Gottwald, I. Flesch,
and H.-D. Becker   23

1.4   Pathophysiology and Classification of Adhesions
E.P.M. Lorenz, H.V. Zühlke, R. Lange, and V. Savvas   29

2   Animal Studies on Peritoneal Adhesions

2.1   Neoangiogenesis in Adhesion Formation
and Peritoneal Healing
G. Bigatti, W. Boeckx, L. Gruft, N. Segers, and I. Brosens   37

2.2   A Three-Dimensional Cell Culture Method
for Studying Peritoneal Adhesions
F. Bittinger, C.L. Klein, C. Skarke, C. Brochhausen, M. Otto,
H. Köhler, and C.J. Kirkpatrick   49

2.3   Zinc Induces Heat Shock Protein-70
and Metallothionein Expression in the Small Bowel
and Protects Against Ischemia
B. Klosterhalfen, C. Töns, H.M. Klein, L. Tietze,
C. Mittermayer, M. Anurov, B.S. Titkova, and A. Öttinger   64

2.4   Anti-interleukin-10: Effect on Postoperative Intraperitoneal
Adhesion Formation in a Murine Model
F.J. Montz, P.M. Cristoforoni, C. Holschneider, M. Punyasavatsut,
and E. Abed   72

2.5   A New Technique for Surgical Treatment
of Large Abdominal Wall Defects: An Experimental Study
A. Iuppa, M. Migliore, D. Santagati, G. Petralia, C. Sapienza,
A. Sciuto, and G. Romeo   80

2.6   Influence of Peritoneal Transplants in an Experimental Animal
      Model for the Study of Readhesion Formation
      M. Korell   86
2.7   Postoperative Adhesions – Laparoscopy Versus Laparotomy
      A. Tittel, E. Schippers, M. Anurov, K.-H. Treutner, A. Öttinger,
      and V. Schumpelick   91

3   Aetiology and Pathogenesis of Adhesions

3.1   Studies on the Aetiology and Consequences
      of Intra-abdominal Adhesions
      H. Ellis   99
3.2   Aetio-pathogenesis of Peritoneal Adhesions
      with Respect to Post-traumatic Fibrinolytic Activity
      D. Menzies 105
3.3   Role of Sutures and Suturing in the Formation
      of Postoperative Peritoneal Adhesions
      D.P. O'Leary 111
3.4   Cytokine Response to Elective Surgery: A Possible Mechanism
      for Intraperitoneal Adhesion Pathogenesis
      D.M. Scott-Coombes, J.M. Badia, S.A. Whawell,
      R.C.N. Williamson, and J.N. Thompson 121
3.5   Prostaglandin Synthesis of Human Mesothelial Cells
      In Vitro Is Regulated by Transforming Growth Factor-β_1,
      Tumor Necrosis Factor-α, and Interleukin-1β
      L. Tietze, T. Rütters, C. Schauerte, B. Amo-Takyi,
      B. Klosterhalfen, K.-H. Treutner, C. Mittermayer, and S. Handt .. 127
3.6   Peritoneal Fibrinolysis and Its Role in Adhesion Formation
      J.N. Thompson, S.A. Whawell, D.M. Scott-Coombes,
      and M.N. Vipond 138
3.7   Decreased Fibrinolytic Activity of Human Mesothelial Cells
      In Vitro Following Stimulation with Transforming
      Growth Factor-β_1, Interleukin-1β, and Tumor Necrosis Factor-α
      L. Tietze, S. Handt, A. Ellbrecht, B. Klosterhalfen, B. Amo-Takyi,
      K.-H. Treutner, and C. Mittermayer 146

4.   Diagnostic of Peritoneal Adhesions

4.1   Value of Ultrasonography in Diagnosis of Peritoneal Adhesions
      J. Conze, S. Truong, and V. Schumpelick 163
4.2   Conventional Radiography and Cross-sectional
      Imaging Modalities in the Diagnosis of Intestinal Adhesions
      H.M. Klein, B. Klosterhalfen, C. Töns, G. Steinau,
      and R.W. Günther 172

5 Complications of Peritoneal Adhesions

5.1 Adhesion Formation Following Incisional Hernia Repair:
A Randomized Porcine Model
P.M. Cristoforoni, Y.B. Kim, Z. Preys, R.Y. Lay, and F.J. Montz .. 181

5.2 The Role of Adhesion Formation in Gynecology
and Reproductive Surgery
W. Schröder and W. Rath 187

5.3 Causes of Intestinal Obstruction – A Retrospective Study
of 550 Surgical Cases
K.-H. Treutner, P. Bertram, G. Lätzsch, and V. Schumpelick 191

6 Peritonitis and Sepsis

6.1 The Peritoneal Cytokine Profile in Acute Peritonitis
J.M. Badia, S.A. Whawell, D.M. Scott-Coombes, A.J. Waghorn,
P.D. Abel, and J.N. Thompson 197

6.2 Peritoneum and Sepsis: The Role of Sepsis
in the Genesis of Peritoneal Adhesions
S. Bengmark 201

6.3 Stage-Related Surgical Therapy of General Peritonitis
G.J. Winkeltau, P. Bertram, K.-H. Treutner, and V. Schumpelick . 208

7 Peritoneal Drainage and Chemotherapy

7.1 Effects and Side Effects of Abdominal Drainage
V. Zumtobel, R. Ernst, and M. Senkal 219

7.2 Influence of Different Abdominal Drainages
on the Bioelectrical and Motor Activities of the Small Bowel
P. Klever, C. Töns, G. Arlt, A.P. Oettinger, and V. Schumpelick . 223

7.3 Problems and Future Directions of Intraperitoneal Therapy
with Antineoplastic Agents
W. Schröder 229

8 Pleura, Pericardium, and Peritoneal Dialysis

8.1 Indication, Technique, and Results of Therapeutic Pleurodesis:
Formation of Adhesions and Parallels to Abdominal Surgery
M. Hürtgen, A. Linder, and H. Toomes 235

8.2 Hazards and Prevention of Postsurgical Pericardial Adhesions
D.M. Wiseman 240

8.3 Intra-abdominal Complications in Peritoneal Dialysis
with Special Reference to Peritoneal Fibrosis
H. Schmitt, B. Hermanns, W. Boeckmann, S. Drube,
and H.G. Sieberth 255

9   Treatment of Peritoneal Adhesions

9.1   Indications and Therapeutic Strategy for Intestinal Obstruction
      Due to Intra-abdominal Adhesions
      U. Schöffel, W. Sendt, R. Häring, and E.H. Farthmann   271
9.2   CO$_2$ Laser Adhesiolysis
      B. Lehmann   278
9.3   Laparoscopic Treatment of Peritoneal Adhesions:
      A Clinical Study of 53 Patients
      M. Schnabel, W. Dietz, U. Malewski, and H. Feist   284
9.4   Efficiency of Laparoscopy in Treatment
      of Acute Small Bowel Obstruction Caused by Adhesions
      G. Federmann, J. Walenzyk, A. Schneider, C. Scheele,
      and G. Bauermeister   291
9.5   A New Probe Optimizes Closed Decompression
      and Temporary Intestinal Splinting in Small Intestine Ileus
      J. Ermisch   297
9.6   Benefit and Risk of Long Intestinal Tubes
      in Intestinal Obstruction
      J. Faß, S. Müller, M. Jansen, G. Ages, K.-H. Treutner,
      S. Truong, and V. Schumpelick   303

10   Prevention and Control of Adhesion Formation

10.1 The Management of Adhesive Disease
      C.L. Kowalczyk and M.P. Diamond   315
10.2 Adhesion Prophylaxis in Gynecology
      M. Korell   325
10.3 Prevention of Postoperative Formation and Reformation
      of Pelvic Adhesions
      B. Larsson   331
10.4 Immunomodulation of the Acute Postinjury Phase
      of Mesothelial Repair
      A. Steinleitner   335
10.5 Prevention of Adhesions in Rabbits
      by Intraabdominal Application of Lipid Compounds
      K.-H. Treutner, P. Bertram, M. Klimaszewski,
      and V. Schumpelick.   344
10.6 Two-Phase In Vivo Comparison Studies
      of the Tissue Response to Polypropylene, Polyester,
      and Expanded Polytetrafluoroethylene Grafts Used
      in the Repair of Abdominal Wall Defects
      K.A. LeBlanc.   352
10.7 Evaluation of Seprafilm Bioresorbable Membrane
      in a Rat Cecal Abrasion Model
      J.M. Burns, M.J. Colt, R.L. Carver, L. Burgess, and K.C. Skinner. .   363
10.8 Use of Adhesion Prevention Barriers in Gynecological Surgery
      M.H. Thornton, J.D. Campeau, and G.S. diZerega   370

List of Contributors

Abed, E.
Gynecologic Oncology Service, Department of Obstetrics and Gynecology,
UCLA Center for Health Sciences, Los Angeles, CA 90024, USA

Abel, P.D.
Department of Surgery, Royal Postgraduate Medical School,
Hammersmith Hospital, London W12 0NN, UK

Ages, G.
Department of Surgery, Technical University Aachen, 52057 Aachen, Germany

Amo-Takyi, B.
Institute of Pathology, Technical University Aachen, 52057 Aachen, Germany

Anurov, M.
Department of Physiology and Digestion, I. Medical Institute,
University of Moscow, Moscow 117347, Russia

Arlt, G.
Department of Surgery, Technical University Aachen, 52057 Aachen, Germany

Badia, J.M.
Department of Surgery, Royal Postgraduate Medical School,
Hammersmith Hospital, London W12 0NN, UK

Bauermeister, G.
Department of Surgery and Vascular Surgery, Quedlinburg District Hospital,
06484 Quedlinburg, Germany

Becker, H.-D.
Department of General and Transplant Surgery, University of Tübingen,
72076 Tübingen, Germany

Bengmark, S.
Ideon Research Center, Lund University, 22370 Lund, Sweden

Bertram, P.
Department of Surgery, Technical University Aachen, 52057 Aachen, Germany

Bigatti, G.
II. Department of Obstetric and Gynecology, University of Milan, 20122 Milan, Italy

Bittinger, F.
Institute of Pathology, Johannes Gutenberg-University, 55101 Mainz, Germany

Boeckmann, W.
Department of Urology, Technical University Aachen, 52057 Aachen, Germany

Boeckx, W.
Department of Plastic Surgery, University Hospital Gasthuisberg, 3000 Leuven, Belgium

Brochhausen, C.
Institute of Pathology, Johannes Gutenberg-University, 55101 Mainz, Germany

Brosens, I.
Department of Obstetric and Gynecology, University Hospital Gasthuisberg, 3000 Leuven, Belgium

Budianto, D.
Institute of Pathology, Technical University Aachen, 52057 Aachen, Germany

Burgess, L.
Genzyme Corporation, Cambridge, MA 02139, USA

Burns, J.M.
Genzyme Corporation, Cambridge, MA 02139, USA

Campeau, J.D.
Department of Obstetrics and Gynecology,
Livingston Reproductive Biology Laboratory, School of Medicine,
University of Southern California, Los Angeles, CA 90033, USA

Carver, R.L.
Genzyme Corporation, Cambridge, MA 02139, USA

Coerper, S.
Department of General and Transplant Surgery, University of Tübingen, 72076 Tübingen, Germany

Colt, M.J.
Genzyme Corporation, Cambridge, MA 02139, USA

Conze, J.
Department of Surgery, Technical University Aachen, 52057 Aachen, Germany

Cristoforoni, P.M.
Gynecologic Oncology Service, Department of Obstetrics and Gynecology,
UCLA Center for Health Sciences, Los Angeles, CA 90024, USA

Diamond, M.P.
Department of Reproductive Endocrinology and Infertility, Hutzel Hospital,
Wayne State University, Detroit, MI 48201, USA

Dietz, W.
Department of Surgery, Städtische Kliniken Delmenhorst, 27753 Delmenhorst,
Germany

DiZerega, G.S.
Department of Obstetrics and Gynecology, Livingston Reproductive Biology
Laboratory, School of Medicine, University of Southern California,
Los Angeles, CA 90033, USA

Drube, S.
Department of Internal Medicine II, Technical University Aachen,
52057 Aachen, Germany

Drukker, J.
Department of Anatomy and Embryology, Faculty of Medicine,
University of Limburg, 6200 Maastricht, The Netherlands

Ellbrecht, A.
Institute of Pathology, Technical University Aachen, 52057 Aachen, Germany

Ellis, H.
Division of Anatomy and Cell Biology, Guy's Hospital, London SE1 9RT, UK

Ermisch, J.
Department of Surgery, Grimma District Hospital, 04668 Grimma, Germany

Ernst, R.
Department of Surgery, St. Josef Hospital, Ruhr University, 44791 Bochum,
Germany

Farthmann, E.H.
Department of Surgery, University of Freiburg, 79106 Freiburg, Germany

Fass, J.
Department of Surgery, Technical University Aachen, 52057 Aachen,
Germany

Federmann, G.
Department of Surgery, Völkingen District Hospital, 66333 Völkingen,
Germany

Feist, H.
Department of Surgery, Städtische Kliniken Delmenhorst, 27753 Delmenhorst,
Germany

Flesch, I.
Department of General and Transplant Surgery, University of Tübingen,
72076 Tübingen, Germany

Gottwald, T.
Department of General and Transplant Surgery, University of Tübingen,
72076 Tübingen, Germany

Gruft, L.
II. Department of Obstetric and Gynecology, University of Milan, 20122 Milan,
Italy

Günther, R.W.
Department of Diagnostic Radiology, Technical University Aachen,
52057 Aachen, Germany

Häring, R.
Department of Surgery, University of Freiburg, 79106 Freiburg, Germany

Handt, S.
Institute of Pathology, Technical University Aachen, 52057 Aachen, Germany

Henze, U.
Institute of Pathology, Technical University Aachen, 52057 Aachen, Germany

Hermanns, B.
Institute of Pathology, Technical University Aachen, 52057 Aachen, Germany

Holschneider, C.
Gynecologic Oncology Service, Department of Obstetrics and Gynecology,
UCLA Center for Health Sciences, Los Angeles, CA 90024, USA

Hürtgen, M.
Department of Thoracic Surgery, Klinik Schillerhöhe, 70839 Gerlingen,
Germany

Iuppa, A.
Department of Surgery, Section of General and Oncological Surgery,
School of Medicine, University of Catania, 95124 Catania, Italy

Jansen, M.
Department of Surgery, Technical University Aachen, 52057 Aachen, Germany

Kim, Y.B.
Gynecologic Oncology Service, Department of Obstetrics and Gynecology,
UCLA Center for Health Sciences, Los Angeles, CA 90024, USA

Kirkpatrick, C.J.
Institute of Pathology, Johannes Gutenberg-University, 55101 Mainz, Germany

Klein, C.L.
Institute of Pathology, Johannes Gutenberg-University, 55101 Mainz, Germany

Klein, H.M.
Department of Diagnostic Radiology, Technical University Aachen,
52057 Aachen, Germany

Klever, P.
Department of Surgery, Technical University Aachen, 52057 Aachen, Germany

Klimaszewski, M.
Department of Surgery, Technical University Aachen, 52057 Aachen, Germany

Klosterhalfen, B.
Institute of Pathology, Technical University Aachen, 52057 Aachen, Germany

Köhler, M.O.H.
Institute of Pathology, Johannes Gutenberg-University, 55101 Mainz, Germany

Köveker, G.B.
Department of General and Transplant Surgery, University of Tübingen,
72076 Tübingen, Germany

Korell, M.
Department of Obstetrics and Gynecology, Klinikum Großhadern,
Ludwig Maximilian-University, 81366 München, Germany

Kowalczyk, C.L.
Department of Reproductive Endocrinology and Infertility, Hutzel Hospital,
Wayne State University, Detroit, MI 48201, USA

Lätzsch, G.
Department of Surgery, Technical University Aachen, 52057 Aachen, Germany

Larsson, B.
Department of Obstetrics and Gynecology, Karolinska Institute,
Danderyd Hospital, 18288 Danderyd, Sweden

Lay, R.Y.
Gynecologic Oncology Service, Department of Obstetrics and Gynecology,
UCLA Center for Health Sciences, Los Angeles, CA 90024, USA

LeBlanc, K.A.
Surgical Specialty Group, Medical Plaza, Baton Rouge, LA 70808, USA

Lehmann, B.
Department of Gynecology and Obstetrics, Heide District Hospital,
25748 Heide, Germany

Linder, A.
Department of Thoracic Surgery, Klinik Schillerhöhe, 70839 Gerlingen,
Germany

Lorenz, E.P.M.
Department of Surgery, Medical Center Benjamin Franklin,
Free University of Berlin, 12200 Berlin, Germany

Malewski, U.
Department of Surgery, Städtische Kliniken Delmenhorst, 27753 Delmenhorst,
Germany

Menzies, D.
Department of Surgery, Colchester General Hospital, Colchester,
Essex CO4 5JL, UK

Migliore, M.
Department of Surgery, Section of General and Oncological Surgery,
School of Medicine, University of Catania, 95124 Catania, Italy

Mittermayer, C.
Institute of Pathology, Technical University Aachen, 52057 Aachen, Germany

Montz, F.J.
Gynecologic Oncology Service, Department of Obstetrics and Gynecology,
UCLA Center for Health Sciences, Los Angeles, CA 90024, USA

Morganti, M.
Institute of Pathology, Technical University Aachen, 52057 Aachen, Germany

Müller, S.
Department of Surgery, Technical University Aachen, 52057 Aachen, Germany

Öttinger, A.
Department of Physiology and Digestion, I. Medical Institute,
University of Moscow, Moscow 117347, Russia

O'Leary, D.P.
Gloucestershire Royal Hospital, Gloucester GL1 3NN, UK

Petralia, G.
Department of Surgery, Section of General and Oncological Surgery,
School of Medicine, University of Catania, 95124 Catania, Italy

Preys, Z.
Gynecologic Oncology Service, Department of Obstetrics and Gynecology,
UCLA Center for Health Sciences, Los Angeles, CA 90024, USA

Punyasavatsut, M.
Gynecologic Oncology Service, Department of Obstetrics and Gynecology,
UCLA Center for Health Sciences, Los Angeles, CA 90024, USA

Rath, W.
Department of Gynecology and Obstetrics, Technical University Aachen,
52057 Aachen, Germany

Romeo, G.
Department of Surgery, Section of General and Oncological Surgery,
School of Medicine, University of Catania, 95124 Catania, Italy

Rütters, T.
Institute of Pathology, Technical University Aachen, 52057 Aachen, Germany

Santagati, D.
Institute of Pathology, School of Medicine, University of Catania,
95124 Catania, Italy

Sapienza, C.
Institute of Pathology, School of Medicine, University of Catania,
95124 Catania, Italy

Schauerte, C.
Institute of Pathology, Technical University Aachen, 52057 Aachen, Germany

Scheele, C.
Department of Surgery and Vascular Surgery, Goslar District Hospital,
38609 Goslar, Germany

Schippers, E.
Department of Surgery, Technical University Aachen, 52057 Aachen, Germany

Schmitt, H.
Department of Internal Medicine II, Technical University Aachen,
52057 Aachen, Germany

Schnabel, M.
Department of Surgery, Städtische Kliniken Delmenhorst, 27753 Delmenhorst,
Germany

Schneider, A.
Department of Surgery and Vascular Surgery, Goslar District Hospital,
38609 Goslar, Germany

Schöffel, U.
Department of Surgery, University of Freiburg, 79106 Freiburg, Germany

Schröder, W.
Department of Gynecology and Obstetrics, Technical University Aachen,
52057 Aachen, Germany

Schumpelick, V.
Department of Surgery, Technical University Aachen, 52057 Aachen, Germany

Sciuto, A.
Department of Surgery, Section of General and Oncological Surgery,
School of Medicine, University of Catania, 95124 Catania, Italy

Scott-Coombes, D.M.
Department of Surgery, Royal Postgraduate Medical School,
Hammersmith Hospital, London W12 0NN, UK

Segers, N.
Department of Plastic Surgery, University Hospital Gasthuisberg,
3000 Leuven, Belgium

Sendt, W.
Department of Surgery, University of Freiburg, 79106 Freiburg, Germany

Senkal, M.
Department of Surgery, St. Josef Hospital, Ruhr University, 44791 Bochum,
Germany

Sieberth, H.G.
Department of Internal Medicine II, Technical University Aachen,
52057 Aachen, Germany

Skarke, C.
Institute of Pathology, Johannes Gutenberg-University, 55101 Mainz, Germany

Skinner, K.C.
Genzyme Corporation, Cambridge, MA 02139, USA

Steinau, G.
Department of Surgery, Technical University Aachen, 52057 Aachen,
Germany

Steinleitner, A.
Astarte Fertility Center, San Francisco, CA 94108, USA

Thompson, J.N.
Department of Surgery, Royal Postgraduate Medical School,
Hammersmith Hospital, London W12 0NN, UK

Thornton, M.H.
Department of Obstetrics and Gynecology,
Livingston Reproductive Biology Laboratory, School of Medicine,
University of Southern California,
Los Angeles, CA 90033, USA

Thors, F.
Department of Anatomy and Embryology, Faculty of Medicine,
University of Limburg, 6200 Maastricht, The Netherlands

Tietze, L.
Institute of Pathology, Technical University Aachen, 52057 Aachen,
Germany

Titkova, B.S.
Department of Physiology and Digestion, I. Medical Institute,
University of Moscow, Moscow 117347, Russia

Tittel, A.
Department of Surgery, Technical University Aachen, 52057 Aachen, Germany

Töns, C.
Department of Surgery, Technical University Aachen, 52057 Aachen, Germany

Toomes, H.
Department of Thoracic Surgery, Klinik Schillerhöhe, 70839 Gerlingen,
Germany

Tory, K.
Institute of Pathology, Technical University Aachen, 52057 Aachen, Germany

Treutner, K.-H.
Department of Surgery, Technical University Aachen, 52057 Aachen, Germany

Truong, S.
Department of Surgery, Technical University Aachen, 52057 Aachen, Germany

Vipond, M.N.
Department of Surgery, Royal Postgraduate Medical School,
Hammersmith Hospital, London W12 0NN, UK

Waghorn, A.J.
Department of Surgery, Royal Postgraduate Medical School,
Hammersmith Hospital, London W12 0NN, UK

Walenzyk, J.
Department of Surgery and Vascular Surgery, Goslar District Hospital,
38609 Goslar, Germany

Whawell, S.A.
Department of Surgery, Royal Postgraduate Medical School,
Hammersmith Hospital, London W12 0NN, UK

Williamson, R.C.N.
Department of Surgery, Royal Postgraduate Medical School,
Hammersmith Hospital, London W12 0NN, UK

Winkeltau, G.J.
Department of Surgery, Technical University Aachen, 52057 Aachen, Germany

Wiseman, D.M.
SYNECHION, INC. 15775 Hillcrest Road, Suite 508, Dallas, TX 75248, USA

Zühlke, H.V.
Department of Surgery, Paul Gerhardt Stiftung, 06886 Lutherstadt-Wittenberg,
Germany

Zumtobel, V.
Department of Surgery, St. Josef Hospital, Ruhr University, 44791 Bochum,
Germany

1 Basics on Adhesion Formation

1.1 Serous Membranes and Their Development, Structure, and Topography

F. Thors and J. Drukker

Introduction

This review of normal development and morphology of pleura, pericard, and peritoneum is presented in order to contribute to a better understanding of several aspects of peritoneal adhesions. Developmental history explains some crucial situations in topographical anatomy. The development of the walls of the prospective body cavities is therefore specifically dealt with. The structure of the tissues, which constitute the serous membranes, define the limiting conditions of their ability to react by the formation of adhesions. Consequently, details regarding practical anatomy of the serous membranes are discussed.

Embryonal Development

At the end of week 3 (postconceptional age), the intraembryonic mesoderm on each side of the neural groove differentiates into a paraxial part, an intermediate part, and a lateral plate.

When intercellular clefts appear in the lateral mesoderm, the plates become divided into two layers: the somatic (wall-related) mesoderm layer (somatopleura) and the visceral (organ-related) one (visceropleura). The margins of these layers, formed by a continuous mesothelial membrane, border the coelom (body cavity) (Fig. 1) [6]. In later developmental stages, the visceropleura is locally firmly attached to the capsule of the adjoining organs. It is vascularized, innervated, and lymphatically drained via vessels and nerves that also supply these organs and can therefore be considered as a part of the underlying organ. For similar reasons, the somatic layer should be considered a part of the body wall. It is attached to a submesothelial layer of loose connective tissue, which in turn adheres to the deep general body fascia. Furthermore, the somatopleura is provided with nerves possessing thermo-, chemo-, and mechanoreceptors, whereas the nerves of the visceropleura do not possess such specialized receptors but instead form networks which respond to tension [7]. Between week 3 and the end of week 4, the coelom has communicating intra- and extraembryonic divisions. After this period, the visceral mesoderm layers from the left and the right side fuse in the midline as a consequence of latero-

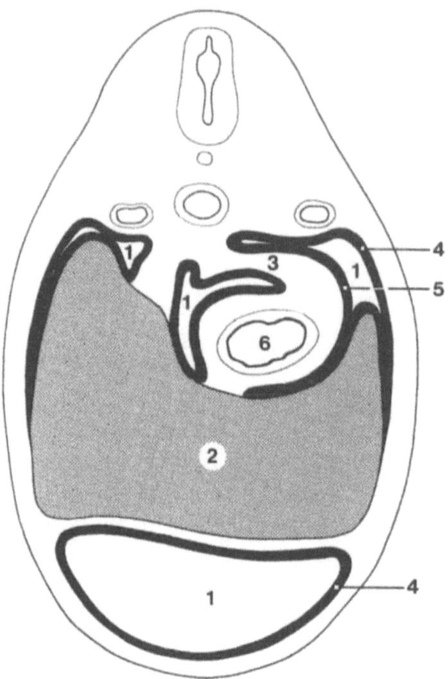

Fig. 1. Human embryo of about 5 weeks (postconceptional); transverse section of upper abdominal region. *1*, Coelom; *2*, future liver; *3*, future meso; *4*, somatopleura; *5*, visceropleura; *6*, future stomach. (Redrawn from [4])

lateral and craniocaudal embryonic folding. At abdominal levels, this ventral mesenterial mass for the greater part breaks down soon after its formation.

At approximately 5 weeks, there is still one, partly divided body cavity. The thoracic cavity remains temporarily in open communication with the abdominal cavity by means of two pericardio-peritoneal canals (the future pleural cavities). The body cavity is then subdivided during the following phases of development by processes of septation into a future pericardial cavity, two pleural cavities, and a peritoneal one. At about 7 weeks, the diaphragm, which is largely derived from the septum transversum and muscular components of the body wall, is eventually completed by fusion of two pleuroperitoneal folds and the mesenterial mass of the esophagus [6]. Closing defects lead to congenital diaphragmatic hernias.

In this phase of development, the mesothelial and submesothelial walls of the coelom are referred to as the pericardium, pleura, and peritoneum, respectively, and together as serous membranes. At the same time, the volume of the organs greatly increases.

This event occurs simultaneously with a kind of peeling process. In the course of this process, the majority of the organs are largely freed from the surrounding tissue. The contours of these organs seem to be carved out of the submesothelial mesenchyme (Figs. 1–3) [4].

The lungs and the heart thus become situated within the pleural and the pericardial cavities, respectively. In the abdomen, those organs which are subject to this developmental process become situated intraperitoneally, while the other organs remain in an extraperitoneal position.

The parts of the heart, lungs, and intraperitoneal organs which remain connected to the wall are generally the hilar regions. In the reflection around the hilus, the visceral part of the serous membrane is continuous with the parietal part. In between the mesothelial linings mesenchyme is still present to a greater or lesser extent. This mesenchyme is relatively broad in the younger stages, but diminishes in both a relative and an absolute sense (Figs. 1–3). With respect to the intraperitoneal organs it is referred to as "*meso*," bounded by mesothelial linings and containing vessels and nerves that supply the organ. (*Note:* The term "mesentery," strictly speaking, refers exclusively to the suspension system of the small intestine.)

Because of the relatively wide diameters of the vessels and bronchi, the hilar regions of the heart and lungs are correspondingly large. Therefore, a meso cannot be perceived. Some organs, e.g., the pancreas, which originally come to be situated intraperitoneally, later in development become positioned between the parietal peritoneum and the other parts of the body wall, which is known as a secondary extraperitoneal position (Figs. 2, 3). This phenomenon can be

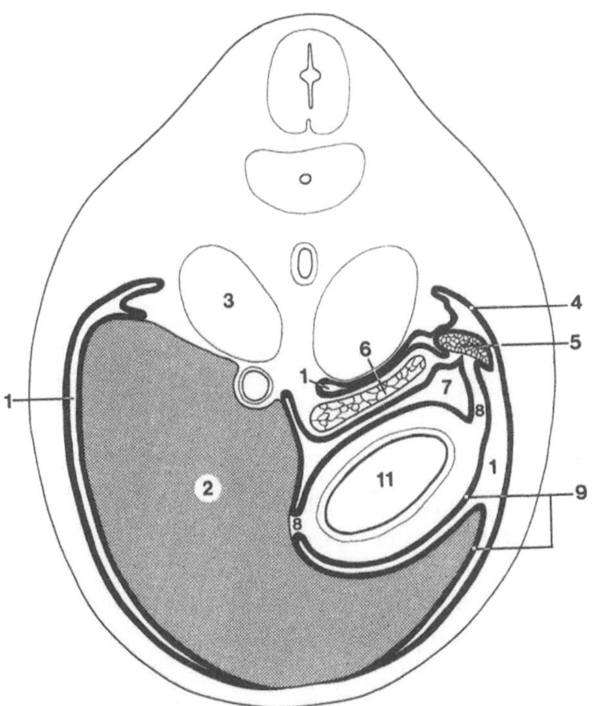

Fig. 2. Human embryo of about 7 weeks (postconceptional); transverse section of upper abdominal region. *1,* Peritoneal cavity; *2,* liver; *3,* right kidney; *4,* parietal peritoneum; *5,* spleen; *6,* pancreas; *7,* lesser sac of peritoneum; *8,* meso; *9,* visceral peritoneum; *11,* stomach. (Redrawn from [4])

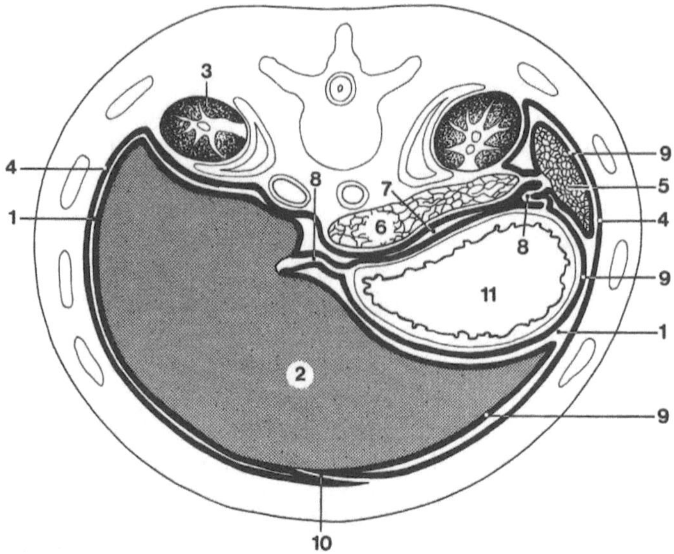

Fig. 3. Human embryo of about 16 weeks (postconceptional); transverse section of upper abdominal region. *1,* Peritoneal cavity; *2,* liver; *3,* right kidney; *4,* parietal peritoneum; *5,* spleen; *6,* pancreas; *7,* lesser sac of peritoneum; *8,* meso; *9,* visceral peritoneum; *10,* falciform ligament; *11,* stomach. (Redrawn from [4])

characterized as physiological adhesion of the peritoneal linings and suggests a natural tendency of serous linings to form adhesions.

Structure of the Serous Membranes

The pleura, serous pericardium, and the peritoneum consist of a single cell layer, supported by a basement membrane and an underlying sheet of connective tissue. The layer of flattened mesothelial cells which faces the cavity is smooth, with varying numbers of microvilli, and is kept moist by a thin film of serous fluid. The fluid and the microvilli function in the same way as lubricants and ball-bearings, thus reducing friction. This allows free movement between the organs and between the organs and the body wall, thus preventing adhesion.

As was mentioned above, the visceral layer of the serous membrane can be considered to be part of the wall of the underlying organ, whereas the properties of the parietal layer mean that it should be considered part of the body wall. The parietal layer is for the most part attached to a subserous layer of loose connective tissue, which varies in composition and thickness. This subserous layer in turn adheres to the deep general body fascia. Those parts of the parietal and visceral divisions of the submesothelial layer which consist of loose connective tissue are populated with abundant numbers of macrophages, eosinophils, and lymphocytes [1, 5].

Epithelium, mesothelium, and endothelium are often considered to be equivalent, because they all form a continuous sheet of covering cells. Their intrinsic properties are markedly different, however. The process of regeneration illustrates the relevance of this issue. The development of new epidermal cells is the result of mitotic cleavage of extant epidermal cells and their descendants; consequently, wound healing in the epidermis is initiated from the margins of the wound. In regenerative processes in serous membranes, on the other hand, mesothelial cells are not derived from fellow mesothelial cells, but directly from primitive mesenchymal cells or via transforming fibroblasts. As these cell types are present in the submesothelial layer, repair does not only take place at the rims of the defect, by migration of unaffected mesothelial cells, but also to a substantial degree in the center of the wound. Even free serosal cells floating in the serous fluid may contribute to wound healing. As a consequence, this form of regeneration takes considerably less time than epidermal repair.

Reconstruction of the smooth mesothelial surface, however, may easily be disturbed by morbid growth of mesenchyme or even the presence of fibers produced by fibroblasts [8]. These properties are likely to contribute to adhesion between adjoining surfaces. The pluripotent character of serous membrane tissue is illustrated by the fact that in surgery parts of peritoneal structures (i.e., greater omentum) are successfully used as a substitute, e.g., to replace an injured tendon sheath.

Pericard and Pleura and Their Cavities

The different compartments with their mesothelial coverings, derived from the lining of the coelom, are principally similar, due to the similar developmental history. In addition, the pericard develops an extra tissue layer on the outside, which is called fibrous pericard (Fig. 4). This part of the pericardium, which is a derivative of the mesenchyme in between parietal pleura and serous pericard, is very firm and thoroughly attached to the parietal layer of the serous pericardial membrane. It is continuous with the adventitia of the large vessels.

The hilus of the heart is dispersed, as it is composed of the arterial and venous poles, which themselves are extended. The reflections of serous pericard are situated at some distance from the heart on the vessel walls.

The thoracic cavities largely enclose the lungs. In the interlobar fissures, there is direct contact between two sections of visceral pleura of opposing lobar surfaces (Fig. 4). Some marginal parts of the pleural cavities, the recessus or sinus pleurae, do not contain lung tissue during expiration and are partly filled during inspiration. In these recesses there is direct contact between two divisions of parietal pleura, i.e., costal and diaphragmatic or costal and mediastinal pleura.

Examples of recesses include the costomediastinal recesses, between fibrous pericard and the dorsal aspect of the ventral thoracic wall, and the costodiaphragmatic recesses, between the diaphragm and ventral, lateral, and dorsal parts of the inner aspect of the thoracic wall. The dorsally situated division of

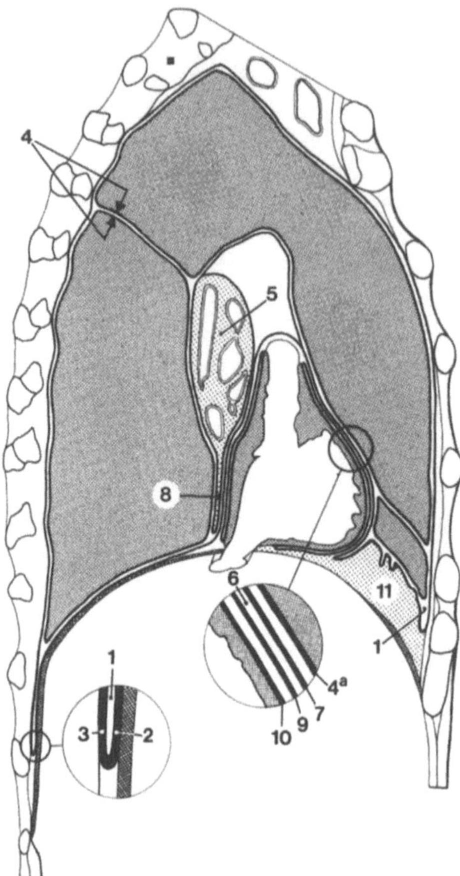

Fig. 4. Sagittal section through the right pulmonary hilum. *1*, costodiaphragmatic recess; *2*, parietal pleura, diaphragmatic division; *3*, parietal pleura, costal division; *4*, visceral pleura of superior and inferior lobe of right lung, bordering interlobar fissure; 4^a, visceral pleura; *5*, hilar region of right lung; *6*, fibrous pericard; *7*, parietal pleura, mediastinal division; *8*, pulmonary ligament; *9*, serous pericard, parietal layer; *10*, serous pericard, visceral layer; *11*, subpleural fat. (Redrawn from [10])

the costodiaphragmatic recess (on the left and right sides) includes the caudalmost extension (Fig. 4).

The reflection around the hilar region of the lung indicates the transitional site at which visceral becomes parietal pleura. The so-called pulmonary ligament is a caudal extension of this reflection. It defines the plane between middle and posterior mediastinum (Fig. 4). It should have become clear that the so-called pericardial and pleural cavities are nothing more than capillary clefts. This is also true of the peritoneal cavity.

Peritoneum and Peritoneal Cavity

The peritoneum is the largest and most complexly arranged serous membrane in the body. It is a vital organ with several important functions such as the capacity to synthesize, secrete, and absorb. The peritoneum also plays an important role in the immune defense system of the body and in the regulation of fluid movements between the peritoneal cavity and the bloodstream. Its surface area roughly equals that of the skin, i.e., about 2 m^2 in adults. The parietal peritoneum constitutes about 10% of this area, and the visceral peritoneum (including the mesenterial peritoneum) about 90% [1].

As for absorption, the peritoneum of the upper abdomen seems to possess the greatest absorbing capacity, most probably due to greater amounts of microvilli present and to respiratory movement, which accelerates absorption in this area [1, 7].

In males, the peritoneum constitutes a closed sac. In females, however, there are two tiny openings at the ampullae of the uterine tubes. Their fimbriae may be subject to peritoneal adhesions, leading to infertility. It should also be mentioned that in males a separate subdivision of peritoneum, called the tunica vaginalis testis, partly covers the testis.

It may be recalled that, as far as the position of abdominal and pelvic organs with regard to the peritoneal cavity are concerned, two extreme situations are possible:

1. The contours of all sides of an organ protrude clearly into the wall of the peritoneal sac, e.g., small intestine (Fig. 5).

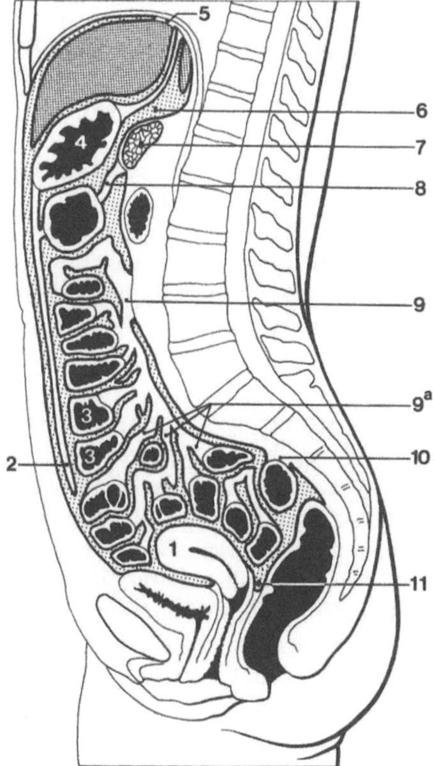

Fig. 5. Midsagittal section through abdominal and pelvic regions. The peritoneal cavity is *shaded*. *1*, Uterus; *2*, greater omentum; *3*, small intestine; *4*, stomach; *5*, bare area of liver; *6*, lesser sac; *7*, pancreas; *8*, transverse mesocolon; *9*, mesenterial root; *9ª*, mesentery; *10*, sigmoid mesocolon; *11*, pouch of Douglas. (Modified from [10])

2. The contact between an organ and the peritoneal lining does not affect all sides, but is only partial. This is due either to incomplete "peeling" or to secondary adhesion to the body wall, e.g., kidneys and pancreas, respectively (Fig. 5).

In the first case, the organ is situated intraperitoneally, whereas in the second case it is situated between the parietal peritoneum and the other parts of the body wall, known as retro- or subperitoneal taken together as extraperitoneal.

In most cases, intraperitoneally situated organs possess a so-called meso, a double-layered mesothelial sheet, containing connective tissue, fat, vessels, and nerves, by which the organ is connected to the body wall. These organs can move more freely than extraperitoneal ones, the extent of possible movement depending, among other factors, on the length of this meso.

In distinguishing extra- from intraperitoneal organs, the position with regard to the peritoneum is not the only criterion. The liver, for example, is partially in direct contact with the diaphragm (i.e., bare area), but is considered to be situated intraperitoneally. On the other hand, the uterus is largely covered by peritoneum, but is considered a subperitoneal organ (Fig. 5). In addition to the development of topographical relations, the distinction between the intra- and extraperitoneal situation is also based on the development of different innervation patterns in visceral and parietal peritoneum. The nerves supplying the visceral peritoneum form networks, with tension as the specific stimulus, whereas the nerves in the parietal peritoneum possess specialized receptors (see "Embryonal Development"). Because nerves of the latter type supply the peritoneal coverings of the uterus, this is considered a subperitoneal organ [7].

A very remarkable part of the peritoneum is the greater omentum (Fig. 5). It is a peritoneal structure, comparable with a curtain. It is often sited between the dorsal aspect of the ventral abdominal wall and the small intestine. It is variable in size and contains fatty tissue to a greater or lesser extent and free cells, including concentrations of macrophages and lymphocytes, which appear to the naked eye as milky spots. The absorbing capacity is lower than in other regions of peritoneum. Greater omentum is known for its capacity to delimit the spread of infection in the peritoneal cavity by walling off the inflammatory region [2, 3, 7].

Although the peritoneal cavity can be considered as a continuous cleft, several barriers exist. These include the falciform ligament between left and right upper abdomen, the transverse mesocolon between the upper and lower abdomen, and the mesenterial root between the upper right and lower left abdomen. Well-known pathways from the upper to lower abdomen are the paracolic gutters (Fig. 6). Fluid (e.g., pus) present in the cavity follows predictable pathways, dependent on the position of the body. In an upright body position, fluid eventually collects in the pouch of Douglas, the caudalmost part of the peritoneal cavity (Fig. 5). In the supine position, the hepatorenal recess is the deepest part of the peritoneal cavity (Fig. 6).

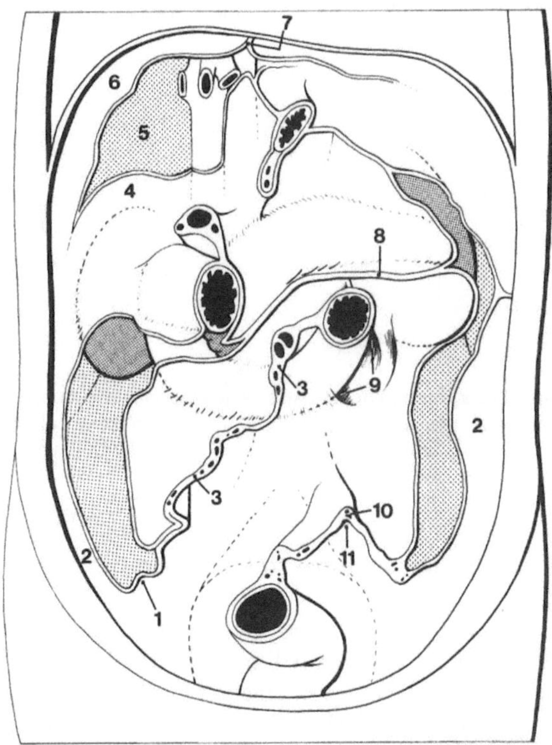

Fig. 6. Dorsal aspect of abdominal cavity; intraperitoneal organs and ascending and descending colon removed. *1,* Retrocaecal recess; *2,* paracolic gutters; *3,* mesenterial root; *4,* hepatorenal recess; *5,* division of diaphragm, corresponding with bare area of liver; *6,* subphrenic recess; *7,* falciform ligament; *8,* root of transverse mesocolon; *9,* duodenojejunal recesses; *10,* root of mesosigmoid; *11,* intersigmoid recess. (Modified from [9])

Pathological processes also spread more easily to and from retroperitoneal organs, because no peritoneal barriers are present. Two layers of peritoneum are present between adjacent intraperitoneal organs and between juxtaposed intraperitoneal and retroperitoneal organs (Fig. 7). These two peritoneal sheets, separated by a capillary cleft, act as a barrier which may impede the spread of pathological processes. However, in the case of peritoneal adhesions, ulcers and tumors do spread into adjacent organs. A peptic ulcer, for instance, may bridge over the adhered lesser sac walls and affect the pancreas (Fig. 5).

The aforementioned peeling process (see "Embryonal Development") leads to the formation of a number of recesses in the peritoneal sac, mainly at sites at which intraperitoneal divisions of the intestine become situated extraperitoneally (or vice versa). In such recesses, internal herniation can occur, which may lead to strangulation. The most common sites of this phenomenon are the lesser sac (via the foramen of Winslow), duodenojejunal recesses, the retrocecal recess, and the intersigmoid recess.

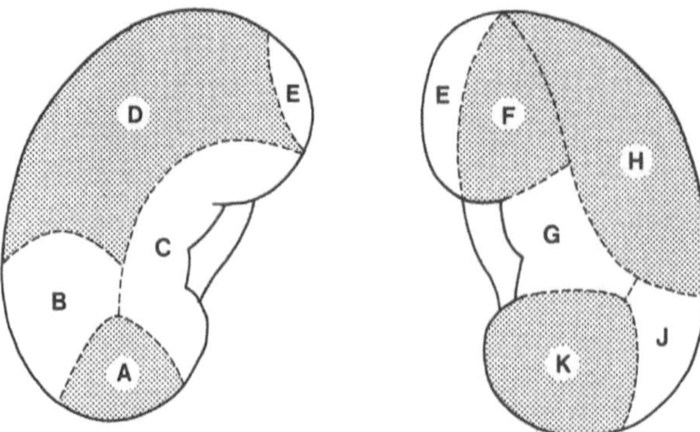

Fig. 7. Ventral aspect of right and left kidneys; contact sites with adjacent organs are indicated. Intraperitoneally situated organs are *shaded*. *A*, ileum; *B*, hepatic flexure of colon; *C*, duodenum; *D*, liver; *E*, suprarenal glands; *F*, stomach; *G*, pancreas; *H*, spleen; *J*, splenic flexure of colon; *K*, jejunum

A number of recesses also constitute preferred sites for abscesses, e.g., the lesser sac, subphrenic recesses, and the retrocecal recess (Figs. 5, 6) [2].

In conclusion, it can be stated that the name "peritoneal cavity" is inaccurate. In reality, the cavity is a very complicated, capillary cleft. This cleft-like configuration is a risk factor for the development of adhesions. Local irritation (e.g., surgical manipulation) in combination with relative local immobility substantially increase this risk.

Barriers of peritoneum do exist; however, they are only relative. Adhesions may easily decrease the efficiency of the barrier function, and spreading of pathological processes is thus promoted by adhesions. They may also cause ileus or infertility.

Summary

In the young human embryo, the originally undivided body cavity, which is lined by mesothelial tissue, becomes compartmentalized into the prospective, pericardial, pleural and peritoneal cavities. These, in reality, cleft-like cavities expand simultaneously with the growth of the spatially related organs. This gives the impression of growing embryonal organs, like heart, lungs and (parts of) the digestive tract, being freed by the coelomic mesothelium from the surrounding mesenchyme. Eventually, the organ is covered with the visceral part of the serous membrane, except for a hilar or mesenterial radix region. The parietal part of the serous membrane is the complementary part of the lining of the body cavity. The visceral part of the serous membrane is continuous with the parietal part in the reflection around the hilus, or via the mesenterium. These intimate connections are not only visible as a topographical relationship, but are also reflected in the vascular and nervous constellation.

Abdominal organs with a mesenterium are situated intraperitoneally, other organs extraperitoneally. Some organs, which were originally situated intraperitoneally, later in development become positioned between the parietal peritoneum and other parts of the body wall, which is known as secondary extraperitoneal. This phenomenon can be characterized as physiological adhesion of the peritoneal linings, and suggests a natural tendency of serous linings to form adhesions. These complex developmental events make great variability and a large number of congenital anomalies plausible.

In the adult, the serous membrane consists of a mesothelial lining resting on a basement membrane and an underlying layer of connective tissue. This single layer of flattened mesothelial cells is smooth, with varying numbers of microvilli, and is kept moist by a thin film of serous fluid. The submesothelial sheet consists of connective tissue with varying numbers of fat cells, macrophages, eosinophils and lymphocytes.

The close apposition of parietal and visceral parts of the serous membranes, together with the abundance of reactive cells, and the mode of regeneration of mesothelium taken into account, explain that adhesions may easily occur.

Predilection sites for such adhesions are those locations where visceral and visceral, visceral and parietal, parietal and parietal and mesenterial and visceral or parietal parts of serous membranes lie in close vicinity, in combination with relative local immobility (e.g., in fissures, other clefts, and recesses). External influences, such as inflammation or surgical intervention, may then easily act as promoting factors.

Acknowledgements. The authors wish to thank Mr. Hans Rensema for preparing the illustrations and Mrs. Greta Gerrits for her secretarial assistance.

References

1. Bengmark S (ed) (1989) The peritoneum and peritoneal access. Wright, London
2. Ellis H (1992) Clinical anatomy. Blackwell, London
3. Ger R, Abrahams P (1986) Essentials of clinical anatomy. Pitman, London
4. Hinrichsen KV (ed) (1993) Humanembryologie. Springer, Berlin Heidelberg New York
5. Kelley DE, Wood RL, Enders AC (1984) Bailey's textbook of microscopic anatomy. Williams and Wilkins, Baltimore
6. Sadler TW (1990) Langman's medical embryology. Williams and Wilkins, Baltimore
7. Williams PL, Warwick R, Dyson M, Bannister LH (eds) (1989) Gray's anatomy. Churchill Livingstone, Edinburgh
8. diZerega GS (1994) Contemporary adhesion prevention. Fertil Steril 61: 219–235
9. Feneis H (1980) Anatomisches Bildwörterbuch der internationalen Nomenkatur. Thieme, Stuttgart
10. Ferner H (1980) Brust, Bauch und Extremitäten, Bd. 2. In: Pernkopf E (ed) Atlas der topographischen und angewandten Anatomie des Menschen. Urban and Schwarzenberg, Munich

1.2 New Aspects of Peritoneal Pathology

M. Morganti, L. Tietze, B. Amo-Takyi, K. Tory, D. Budianto, U. Henze,
and C. Mittermayer

Introduction

The peritoneum is a membranous structure consisting of a single layer of
mesothelial cells and the subserosal stroma. The visceral peritoneum covers the
surface of various organs and continues to the abdominal wall as the parietal
peritoneum. This membrane creates a gliding surface, regulates the traffic of
molecules and fluid, and plays an important role in some pathological conditions, particularly formation of fibrous adhesions, peritonitis, and implantation of metastatic cancer. The fibrinolytic and antifibrinolytic properties
of mesothelial cells are partly regulated by cytokines. Tumor necrosis factor
(TNF)-α, transforming growth factor (TGF)-β_1, and interleukin (IL)-1β in
particular cause a shift toward antifibrinolytic activity. This may contribute to
the decreased fibrinolytic activity of serosal biopsies during peritonitis. This
observation and its relationship to formation of fibrous adhesion are discussed
in detail in Chap. 10 of this volume. The inflammatory response of this
membrane is regulated by expression of a variety of cytokines [1]. The cell–cell
interaction is partly mediated by expression of inducible and constitutive cell
adhesion molecules [2]. The early inflammatory response with edema, vasodilation, and hyperalgesia is probably augmented by mesothelial prostaglandin
production (see Chap. 12, this volume). In this chapter, we will focus on the
developmental and morphological aspects of the peritoneal membrane and
discuss pathological aspects of primary and secondary neoplasms of the
peritoneal cavity.

Embryology

During the third week of embryonic life, segmentation of the paraxial intraembryonic mesoderm commences, and the embryo enters the somite period
of development. At the same time, clefts appear in the lateral mesoderm plate
and gradually coalesce to form a U-shaped intraembryonic coelom. The arms
of the cavity lie within the lateral mesoderm plate and meet in the midline in
the cardiogenic area of mesoderm at the rostral border of the embryonic disc.
The cells that line the primitive coelom and its derivates – the peritoneal,
pleural, and pericardial cavities – constitute the mesothelium. Initially, they

have a cuboidal form, and later a basal lamina that separates the mesothelium from the underlying mesenchyme appears and the cells begin to change to squamous cells [3].

Structure

The peritoneum is covered by a monolayer of simple, squamous epithelial cells that cannot be morphologically distinguished from pleura, pericardium, and tunica vaginalis. By histochemical studies, Whitaker et al. [4] have demonstrated a substantial similarity in the various compartments of mesothelia, supporting the concept of the mesothelium as an entity. However, differences do exist: (a) the quality and quantity of the submesothelial tissues vary among the three serous cavities [3] and (b) the benign mesotheliomas that originate from peritoneum often have different morphological and cytochemical characteristics from pleural neoplasms (adenomatoid tumors occur exclusively in the peritoneum, in particular at the epididymis) [5]. Light microscopic examination of the peritoneum in perpendicular section shows a single layer of squamous cells overlying the connective tissue. Vertically, it appears as a regular carpet of round to oval-shaped cells with prominent central nuclei. The squamous form is typical of peritoneal cells, but in some regions cuboidal cells predominate. The epithelial layer covering the ovary is continuous with the squamous peritoneum at the mesovarium and shows some special features; histochemically, these cuboidal cells can be distinguished by their content of sulfuric acid and neutral mucopolysaccharides. Unlike other mesothelial cells, ovarian surface epithelial cells of the ovary have 17β-hydroxysteroid dehydrogenase activity. They also have estrogen and progesterone receptors [6]. These surface epithelial cells are immunoreactive for cytokeratin and vimentin, but not desmin [6]. Cuboidal mesothelial cells are also present in subdiaphragmatic peritoneum.

Immunohistochemistry

The intermediary filaments cytokeratins-8, -18, and -7, vimentin, and Desmin [7] were found by immunohistochemistry in cell cytoplasm and considered to participate in the formation of the cytoskeleton of mesothelial cells. The abundant expression of cytokeratins is considered a helpful feature in discriminating mesothelial cells from endothelial cell and fibroblasts. Other differential staining patterns have been reported, in comparison with endothelial cells (Table 1) [8].

These immunohistochemical characteristics are a useful tool in discriminating between primary and secondary malignant tumors which infiltrate the serosal surface, particularly in the distinction of primary malignant mesothelioma from tumor implants of adenocarcinoma. Furthermore, the immunohistochemical profile allows identification and characterization of mesothelial cells in vitro.

Table 1. Staining patterns in endothelial and mesothelial cells

	Endothelial Cells	Mesothelial cells
Pancytokeratin	–	++
Desmin	++	++
Vimentin	++	++
vWF	++	+/–
Uptake dil-acetyl LDL	++	++
t-PA	+	++
S-100	–	–
CD14	–	–
CD68	–	–
Leu M1	–	–

LDL, low-density lipoprotein; vWF, von Willebrand Factor; t-PA, tissue-type plasminogen activator. –, No staining; +/–, weakly positive; +, positive; ++, strongly positive.

Ultrastructure

Analyses with scanning electron microscopy show cells with a hexagonal profile; some show evidence of peripheral interdigitations, and others regions of cell overlap. A variable distribution of microvilli is found on the luminal cell surface. In some instances, the cell surface is covered with a homogeneous layer (Fig. 1), but in others the microvilli tend to be concentrated at the cell periphery, leaving a smooth supranuclear plasma membrane. Analyses with transmission electron microscopy display tight and gap junctions between the bodies of adjacent cells.

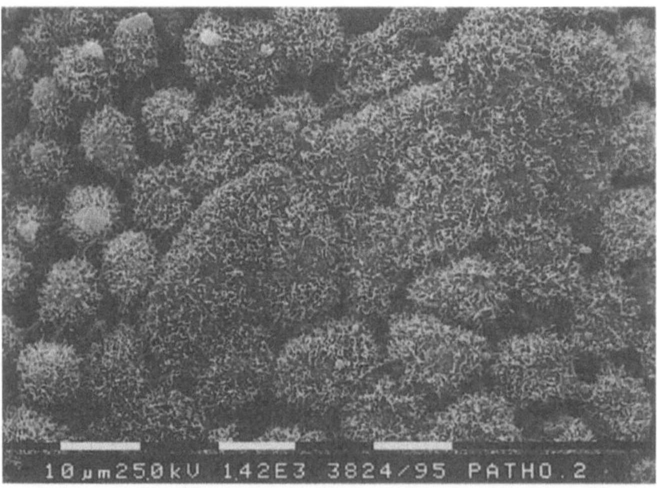

Fig. 1. Scanning electron micrograph showing the surface of flattened mesothelial cells covered with microvillous projections

Using a novel fixation procedure without aldehydes, Hills [9] demonstrated the presence of multiple (five to seven) osmiophilic layers apparently attached to the membrane. These structures seem to be made up of phospholipids (surface-active phospholipid, SAPL) with surfactant properties that are able to reduce the friction between the peritoneal surfaces. Dobbie et al. [10] demonstrated by means of transmission electron microscopy that mesothelial cells produce this surfactant in intracellular lamellar bodies. The nucleus of mesothelial cells has an irregular outline and lies centrally. The cytoplasm contains the normal complement of organelles, but pinocytic vesicles are frequently the dominant element. The vesicles are found along the luminal and opposing surfaces, giving credence to the transport role of the mesothelium. Dobbie et al. [11] described the structure of subperitoneal connective tissue as follows: a short distance beneath the basal lamina there is a discontinuous layer of elastic fibers through which bundles of collagen fibers run from the basal lamina to the deeper muscle layer. The subserosa contains fibroblasts and mast cells, while vascular and lymphatic elements are deeply placed.

Mesothelial Healing

The mesothelial healing after injury is a complex and partly unknown process. In attempting to explain this, at least four different hypothesis have been put forward:

1. Mature mesothelial cells from adjacent or opposing surfaces multiply, exfoliate, and repopulate the site of injury [12].
2. Free-floating serosal reserve cells settle on the wound and gradually differentiate into new mesothelium [13].
3. A two-stage process occurs with macrophages transiently occupying the wound and the new mesothelial cells eventually arising through "metaplasia" of a mesenchymal precursor [14].
4. The replenishing cells originate in the bone marrow [15].

Whitaker and Papadimitriou [4] proposed the following possible model of mesothelial healing: initially, macrophages occupy the surface of a wound on the injured visceral layer, while mesothelial proliferation proceeds at the edges of wound and the opposing parietal surface; fibrin is formed on the wound surface within 24 h. The presence of reserve cells in the subserosa which are able to differentiate as squamous cell is still under discussion, and it has not been proved that fibroblast-like cells or a similar type of cells can be the source of new mesothelial cells. Mesothelial ingrowth most probably begins with isolated cells migrating from the wound edges as well as from the serosal surface apposing the wound, where mesothelial cells are actively replicating. The cells slide over a bridge of fibrin and macrophages to form a new layer, which isolates the lesion and prevents the formation of fibrotic adherences.

Peritoneal Neoplasms

The neoplasms of the peritoneum can be subdivided into primary and secondary tumors. The primary neoplasms are rare and include diffuse malignant mesotheliomas, intra-abdominal desmoplastic, small, round cell tumors, and (very infrequently) benign tumors such as localized fibrous tumors, adenomatoid tumors, low-grade cystic mesotheliomas, inflammatory myofibroblastic tumors, and omental-mesenteric myxoid hamartoma [16]. More than 90% of peritoneal neoplasms are secondary [17].

Basically, all advanced-phase cancers can infiltrate the serous membranes *per continuitatem*, but peritoneal metastases most often result from tumor cell implantations from primary tumors arising in the abdomen or pelvis. The most common sources of tumor implants are metastasizing cancer of the ovary, colon, stomach, and pancreas. Despite its distance from the abdominal cavity, breast cancer also shows a marked tropism for peritoneum [18]. Metastatic spread to the peritoneum can follow three possible routes [1]:

1. Direct extension
2. Lymphatic spread
3. Transcoelomic dissemination

Transcoelomic dissemination has been the subject of numerous studies carried out to elucidate the possible interactions between tumoral cells and epithelial lining in metastatic development. Yoshioka et al. [19] investigated the morphological changes in the peritoneum of mice resulting from tumor cell dissemination by electron microscopy. From day 5 to day 7 after intraperitoneal transplantation of tumor cells, mesothelial cells began to swell, with the intercellular boundaries becoming distinct. Microvilli increased in numbers, forming a mesh-like structure that was sometimes found to be in direct contact with tumor cells. About 10 days after the tumor cell introduction, the mesothelium showed enlarged intercellular spaces, and tumor cells were seen to have adhered at these sites. After 11 days, the tumor cells started proliferating and infiltrating the muscle layer. The molecular events which mediate these morphological reactions of mesothelial cells are not known in detail, but there are some data about the molecules that may play a role in tumor cell adhesion. Cannistra et al. [20] demonstrated the presence of the adhesive molecule CD44H on the surface of ovarian cancer cells. Peritoneal cell membrane shows receptors for this protein. Suppression of CD44H with blocking antibodies inhibited tumor cell adhesion to mesothelial cells in culture, suggesting that binding of ovarian cancer cells to peritoneal mesothelium in vitro is partially mediated by CD44H. Morganti et al. [21, 22] demonstrated that colocarcinoma cell lines (HRT-18, RT-29, CX-2) are able to induce and enhance the production of von Willebrand factor (vWF) in endothelial cells in vitro. This molecule can facilitate cell–cell adhesion and seems to be involved in tumor cell attachment to endothelial cells [22].

Immunohistochemistry, enzyme-linked immunosorbent assay (ELISA), and polymerase chain reaction (PCR) have also revealed the presence of vWF in mesothelial cell cultures from human omentum majus, although the quantity

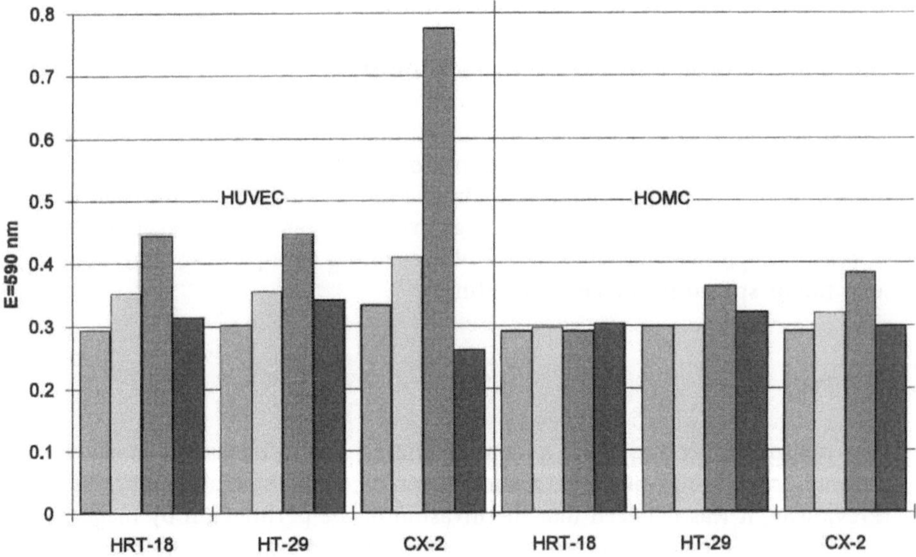

Fig. 2. Influence of von Willebrand factor (vWF) in adhesion assays of human colon neoplasms cell lines (HRT-18, HT-29, CX-2) on endothelial (human umbilical vein endothelia cells, *HUVEC*; *left*) or mesothelial (human omentum majus mesothelial cells, *HOMC*; *right*) cell cultures. The *first column* of each probe shows the colorimetric absorbance of HOMC or HUVEC monocultures. The *second column* indicates the colorimetric absorbance of HOMC or HUVEC plus the tumor cells (HRT-18, HT-29, CX-2) with adherence on the monocultures after 6 h. The *third* and *fourth columns* show the adhesion tests in the presence of vWF and vWF–blocking antibodies, respectively, both diluted 1: 100 in 1640 RPMI (GIBCO BRL, Life Technologies Inc., USA) medium. This molecule clearly facilitates cell–cell adhesion in vitro, whereas the presence of neutralizing antibodies against vWF decreased tumor cell adhesion on HUVEC and HOMC

was less than the amount produced by endothelial cells. This suggests a possible role of this protein in tumor cell adhesion to the mesothelium. Addition of vWF to cocultures of mesothelial cells and tumor cells (RT-29, CX-2) caused a small increase in tumor cell attachment (Fig. 2), whereas incubation with neutralizing antibodies against vWF decreased tumor cell adhesion on mesothelial cells. Asao et al. [23] suggested that the fucosyltransferase activity present in mice peritoneal cells is related to tumor cell adhesion, and the specific inhibition of this activity by oligosaccharides and glycoprotein resulted in a decreased adhesion of cancer cells. Following attachment, the tumor cells interact with the basement membrane, thus dissolving the basement components, probably via specific collagenases. Bosman et al. [24] reported that the peritoneal basement membrane infiltrated by ovarian tumor showed a reduction of type-4 collagen and laminin.

Mesothelial cells also seem to participate in tumor growth. In vitro tumor cell line HRT-18 is able to stimulate mesothelial cells to enhance the antifibrinolytic activity. Morganti [21, 22] indicated that, in cocultures of mesothelial cells/tumoral cells HRT-18, the plasminogen activator inhibitor-1

(PAI-1) concentration is strongly enhanced, whereas the tissue-type plasminogen activator (t-PA) concentration is unchanged. This may contribute to deposition of fibrin. Fibrin by itself may stimulate neoangiogenesis [25], an important secondary step in metastatic growth.

These studies prove that CD44H, vWF, fucosyltransferasy enzyme, t-PA, and PAI-1 are involved in each step of tumor implantation. However, the physiological relevance of these observations for the understanding of metastatic implantation in vivo remains unknown. Further analyses of the molecules involved in tumor cell implantation may eventually permit the development of specific antagonists that are capable of preventing or inhibiting intra-abdominal tumor spread in the clinical setting.

Summary

The peritoneum is frequently a focus of interest due to metastatic invasion by tumors originating from organs such as ovary, colon, stomach, pancreas etc. Previously, it was believed that the invasion of the peritoneum by metastases was the simple consequence of the passive diffusion of the tumor cells. However, it has been demonstrated recently that this is an active process that promotes interaction between tumor cells and mesothelial cell surfaces.

Our present contribution focuses on the morphological and biochemical modifications reported during the interaction between tumor cells and the mesothelial cells. Yoshioka et al. [19] reported that mesothelial cells react to the presence of tumor cells with an increase in the number of microvilli present on their surfaces, and that these structures help in the adherence of the tumor cells on the mesothelial surfaces. Cannistra et al. [20] demonstrated the presence of the adhesive molecule CD44H on the surface of ovarian cancer cells which bind selectively to mesothelial receptors. Another molecule, the von Willebrand factor, was also found to act as a bridge protein between mesothelial and colocarcinoma cells. Ovarian tumor cells also seem to interact with basement membrane, causing its dissolution through specific collagenases, thereby allowing free access to the tumor cells. Morganti et al. have also revealed that tumor cells increase the antifibrinolytic activity, thus allowing fibrin deposition. Fibrin is known to be a strong stimulator of tumor neoangiogenesis and growth.

All these data show the importance of many molecules in the development and sustenance of metastases, and it is possible that the use of specific antagonists may eventually be capable of slowing down peritoneal metastases.

Acknowledgements. The authors express their gratitude to Professor H.C.V. Schumpelick (Department of Surgery, Klinikum Aachen) and to Professor H.R. Willmen (Department of Surgery, Kreiskrankenhaus Grevenbroich) for their contributions and helpful comments.

References

1. Jonijc N, Peri G, Bernasconi S, Scacca FL, Calotta F, Pelicci PG, Lanfrancone L, Mantovani A (1992) Expression of adhesion molecules and chemotactic cytokines in cultured human mesothelial cells. J Exp Med 176: 1165–1174
2. Hinsberg VWM, Kooistra T, Scheffer A, van Bockel JH, Goos NP (1990) Characterization and fibrinolytic properties of human omental tissue mesothelial cells. Comparison with endothelial cells. Blood 75: 1490–1497
3. Thomas NW (1987) Embryology and structure of the mesothelium. In: Jones JSP (ed) Pathology of the mesothelium. Springer, Berlin Heidelberg New York
4. Whitaker D, Papadimitriou J (1985) Mesothelial healing: morphological and kinetic investigations. J Pathol 145: 159–175
5. Craig JR, Hart WR (1979) Extragenital adenomatoid tumor. Evidence for the mesothelial origin. Cancer 433: 1678–1679
6. Blaustein A, Lee H (1979) Surface cells of the ovary and pelvic peritoneum: a histochemical and ultrastructural comparison. Gynecol Oncol 8: 34–43
7. LaRocca P, Rheinwald JG (1984) Coexpression of simple epithelial keratins and vimentin by human mesothelium and mesothelioma in vivo and in culture. Cancer Res 44: 2991–2999
8. Pötzsch B, Grulich-Henn J, Rössing R, Wille D, Berghaus GM (1990) Identification of endothelial and mesothelial cells in human omental tissue and in omentum derived cultured cells by specific cell markers. Lab Invest 63: 841–852
9. Hills BA (1992) Graphite like lubrification of mesothelium by oligolamellar pleural surfactant. J Appl Phys 73: 1034–1039
10. Dobbie JW, Zaki M, Wilson L (1988) From philosopher to fish: the comparative anatomy of the peritoneal cavity as an excretory organ and its significance for peritoneal dialysis in man. Perit Dial Int 8-3
11. Dobbie JW, Zaki M, Wilson L (1981) Ultrastructural studies on the peritoneum with special reference to chronic ambultory peritoneal dialysis. Scott Med J 26: 223–231
12. Watters WB, Buck RC (1972) Scanning electron microscopy of mesothelial regeneration in rats. Lab Invest 26: 604–609
13. Ryan GB, Groberty J, Majno G (1973) Mesothelial injury and recovery. Am J Pathol 71: 93–102
14. Raftery AT (1973) Regeneration of parietal and visceral peritoneum: a light microscopical study. Br J Surg 60: 293–299
15. Wagner JC, Johnson NF, Brown DG, Wagner MMF (1982) Histology and ultrastructure of serially transplanted rat mesothelium and mesothelioma in vivo and in culture. Cancer Res 46: 294–299
16. Clement PB, Young H, Scully RE (1994) Peritoneum. In: Stemberg S (ed) Diagnostical surgical pathology. Raven, New York
17. Bercovici B, Gallily R (1978) The cytology of the human peritoneal fluid. Acta Cytol 22: 124
18. Von Haam E (1977) Cytology of transudates and exudates. Monogr Clin Cytol 5: 3–17
19. Yoshioka M, Yasuda M, Tahira K, Murae M, Nakabayshi Y, Fujiya S, Isonishi S, Terashima Y, Hachiya S (1986) Experimental study of the mechanism of peritoneal dissemination with special references to scanning electron microscopic observations. Nippon Sanka Fujinka Gakkai Zasshi 38: 1683–1691
20. Cannistra A, Kansa GS, Niloff J, DeFranzo B, Kim Y, Ottesmeier C (1993) Binding of ovarian cancer cells to peritoneal mesothelium in vitro is partly mediated by CD44H. Cancer Res 53: 3830–3838
21. Morganti M, Hauptmann S, Tietze L, Carpi A, Sagripanti A, Henze U, Mittermayer C (1995) Macrophages marker PGM1 and vWF expression by mesothelial cells in mixed cultures with neoplastic cell lines. Int J Med 3: 19–24
22. Morganti M, Hauptmann S, Budianto D, Carpi A, Sagripanti A, Henze U, Mittermayer C (1995) Expression of t-PA, PAI-1 and vWF in the supernatant of endothelial and mesothelial cultures in response to the seeding with HRT-18 tumor cells. XV European Congress of Pathology Poster, Falconer Center, Copenhagen, 3–8 Sept, 1995

23. Asao T, Nagamachi Y, Morinaga N, Tachenoshita S, Yazawa S (1995) Fucosyltransferase of peritoneum contributed to the adhesion of cancer cells to the mesothelium. Cancer 15: 1539–1544
24. Bosman FT, Havenith M, Cleutjens JP (1985) Basement membranes in cancer. Ultrastruct Pathol 8: 291–304
25. Nagy JA, Morgan H, Kemp T, Manseau J, Dvorak AM, Dvorak HF (1995) Pathogenesis of ascites tumor growth: angiogenesisis, vascular remodeling and stroma formation in the peritoneal lining. Cancer Res 55: 376–385

1.3 The Role of Wound Healing
in the Formation of Peritoneal Adhesions

G.B. Köveker, S. Coerper, T. Gottwald, I. Flesch, and H.-D. Becker

Wound healing represents a complex cascade of biochemical and cellular events designed to achieve regeneration or restoration of tissue integrity following injury. After a long-lasting lag phase, during the past decade substantial progress has been made towards the understanding of the cellular regulation of repair in health and disease [3]. Locally acting growth factors (cytokines) play a key role in the regulation of all phases of tissue repair. Tissue repair is not restricted to the skin, although much of the present knowledge is based on data generated from experimental and clinical skin wounds [4, 15].

Repair Versus Regeneration

The capacity for self-repair is an important attribute of organisms; however, the spectrum of repair may differ substantially depending on species, age, and the localization and extent of the defect. Regeneration is the preferential response to injury in the fetal stage, whereas in adults the same type of lesion is followed by repair with scar formation. Repair processes include not only restoration of deficient tissue, as is typical for chronic ulcers (venous, diabetic), but also hyperproliferative reactions, as can be observed in keloids and intimal hyperplasia following vascular interventions (Fig. 1).

Peritoneal Healing Differs

In a way peritoneal healing exhibits characteristics of "too much repair", although the healing mechanism following peritoneal injury differs substantially from that in the skin, as the entire peritoneal surface becomes reepithelialized, not only from the borders but also at the center of the defect. Regardless of the differences in reepithelialization, the formation of peritoneal adhesion displays many phenomena which can also be observed in other tissues [5].

The wound healing process can be divided into three phases: (1) inflammation, (2) proliferation, and (3) remodeling (maturation).

The inflammatory phase, from day 0 to about day 4, is characterized by activation of the coagulation system, the kinin system and the complement system. Following injury, when collagen is exposed to blood platelet aggregation occurs. Subsequent platelet degranulation growth factors and cytokines

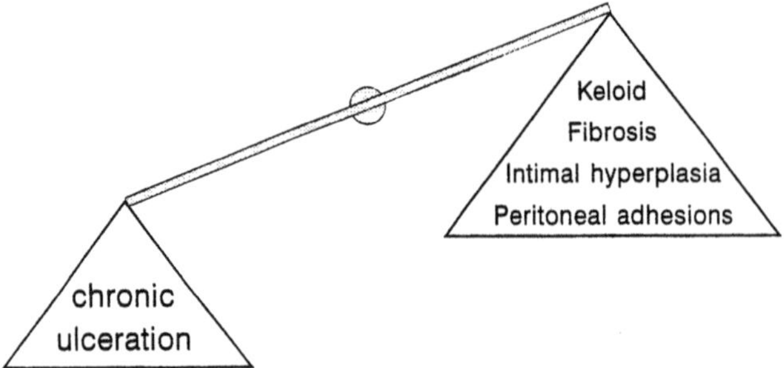

Fig. 1. Illustration of deficient and excessive healing responses

will accumulate at the site of injury. Generation of thrombin triggers the conversion of fibrinogen to fibrin. Kinins and prostaglandins induce vasodilatation and increase of capillary permeability. Polymorphonuclear cells (PMN) are the first cells to enter the wound site, reaching a maximum at 24–48 h post injury. Their main functions are related to phagocytosis of bacteria, removal of cell debris and control of wound infection. Like the neutrophils, monocytes extravasate from the blood to the wound site in response to chemoattractants such as bacterial products and activated complement factor C5a. Monocytes/macrophages initially participate in the process of inflammation and debridement. Thereafter, they play a regulatory role in the proliferative phase of wound healing through the release of biologic mediators (growth factors) [3].

The proliferation phase is characterized by the formation of granulation tissue starting at day 3 post injury. In contrast to normal uninjured tissue, in which fibroblasts are sparsely distributed and in a quiescent state, after injury fibroblasts are activated to migrate into the wound site. Fibroblast function in wound healing is controlled by a number of growth factors released from the blood and in later stages from wound cells themselves.

Accelerated production of collagen with subsequent crosslinking provides mechanical strength of the wound. Granulation is followed by the process of reepithelialization, starting at the edge of the lesion. Again this process is controlled by growth factors and may be limited by contact inhibition at the time when the lesion is completely covered with epithelium.

The maturation phase in normal wound healing starts between 8 and 10 days after injury and may last, depending on the type of tissue, for several months. It is characterized by redistribution and reorganization of collagen, which becomes aggregated into fibers. Parallel to the increase of crosslinkage the tensile strength of the wound increases and will be around 50% of normal at 4–6 weeks. Histologically this process is accompanied by a reduction of cellularity and vascularity. Following surgical injury to the peritoneum, macrophages harvested from the peritoneal cavity secrete substances to modulate growth of fibroblasts and other tissue repair cells.

The cellular events in tissue repair are regulated by growth factors, including migration, proliferation, and phenotype modulation of connective tissue cells, epithelial, and endothelial cells. Circulating platelets and inflammatory cells are the source of such endogenous growth factors controlling the normal process of wound healing [6]. In later stages of tissue repair, growth factors are released by tissue repair cells themselves and act in an autocrine or paracrine fashion. Distinct surface receptors for several growth factors have been identified. Binding of growth factors to specific cell membrane receptors activates tyrosine kinase activity and initiates intracellular signal transduction.

Growth factors can be classified as competence factors when acting in the G_1 phase of the cell cycle and as progression factors when acting in the G_2/S phase. The functions in humans of the many growth factors that have been identified during the past 10 years have not been fully evaluated. There is also some confusion about the nomenclature. This article will focus on platelet-derived growth factor (PDGF) and transforming growth factor β (TGFβ). Their role in tissue repair has been evaluated in a variety of in vitro and experimental animal models [7–9].

Platelet-derived Growth Factor

PDGF is a dimeric polypeptide consisting of α- and β-chains. In mammals there exist three forms: PDGF-AA, PDGF-BB and PDGF-AB. PDGF is not only synthesized and stored in platelets but also secreted by other cell types, such as activated macrophages, endothelial cells, fibroblasts, and smooth muscle cells [10]. PDGF is a potent mitogen for cells of mesenchymal origin, but it has no direct growth effect on epithelial and endothelial cells, since those cells do not express the specific PDGF receptors [13]. Like many other growth factors, the mode of action of PDGF is determined by the cytokine concentration. At low concentration PDGF acts as a chemotactic factor for monocytes and neutrophils. PDGF seems to play an important role in the early stages of repair when aggregating platelets release PDGF from their α-granules, initiating the process of chemotactic influx of inflammatory cells. The concentrations of PDGF needed for chemotaxis vary among neurophils, macrophages, and fibroblasts, possibly regulating the sequence of cellular infiltration. PDGF is a strong mitogen for fibroblasts and smooth muscle cells. It also enhances the synthesis of extracellular matrix components. Some data in the literature support the thesis that exogenous application of PDGF to experimental or clinical wounds may accelerate the healing of acute and chronic wounds [11].

As mentioned above, the thrombin-induced release of products from platelets includes substantial amounts of growth factors such as PDGF and TGFβ [6]. Thrombin has been applied locally to support the healing of several thousands of patients with diabetic foot ulcers. To date, however, the number of clinical trials of this approach is limited. Knighton et al. [6] demonstrated the therapeutic benefit of local platelet releasate treatment for patients with chronic diabetic foot ulcers in a prospective placebo-controlled study. In collaboration with other European institutions we are currently investigating the effect of homologous PDGF concentrate in patients with diabetic foot ulcers. In a similar therapeutic approach we applied autologous instead of homologous platelet releasate products for treatment of venous stasis ulcers. PDGF content did not influence the speed of healing, but there was a statistically significant correlation ($p < 0.05$) between the TGFβ content of the releasate and the time required for healing of 50% of the initial wound surface.

Recombinant PDGF-BB was investigated in a multicenter placebo-controlled trial in patients with diabetic foot ulcer. In the PDGF-BB group the healing rate was 46%, compared to 25% in the control group [16]. Beside the few clinical studies there are many data from experimental studies supporting the tissue inductive effect of PDGF and its isoforms [12].

Transforming Growth Factor Beta

TGFβ is a dimeric glycoprotein with three isoforms (TGFβ1, TGFβ2, and TGFβ3) existing in humans. TGFβ is released from thrombocytes, macrophages, fibroblasts, osteoblasts, and other cells. Three different classes of receptors have been identified in mammals so far. TGFβ appears to have a regulatory role in the context of wound healing [1]. It can be either inhibitory or stimulatory, depending on concentration, the presence of other factors, and the receptor distribution on the cell membrane of the effector cells. At low concentrations, TGFβ exhibits chemotactic effects on granulocytes, T-lymphocytes, macrophages, and fibroblasts. At higher concentrations, however, the extracellular matrix (ECM) synthesis and the integrin expression in fibroblasts are augmented. In the remodeling phase of wound healing, TGFβ has a direct stimulatory effect on fibroblasts to synthesize extracellular matrix proteins. Of the different isoforms, TGFβ3 seems to have a more regulatory role during tissue repair. In experimental wounds, treatment with TGFβ3 not only accelerated wound healing but also had anti-scarring effects [14]. TGFβ activity is not restricted to skin defects. In an experimental model in rats, cryoinduced gastric ulcers healed more rapidly when TGFβ3 was either given systemically or applied as a perifocal infiltration [2] (Fig. 2). The cellular events in wound healing are not only regulated by growth factor activity. Collagen synthesis and remodeling plays an important role in all stages of wound healing. Collagen is a major component of the ECM. The ECM is composed of various polysaccharides and glycoproteins. The matrix itself affects the development, migration and proliferation, and metabolism of the cell types involved in wound healing. The ECM undergoes dynamic changes mainly induced by endogenous or exogenous collagenase activity. Imbalance in synthesis and degradation of collagen may result in deficient or excessive wound healing [3, 15].

Wound Healing and the Formation of Fibrous Adhesions

The conversion of fibrin deposits to fibrous adhesions after peritoneal injury may reflect the key event in the formation of peritoneal adhesions. At various stages (coagulation, growth factor action, proteolysis) the response to perito-

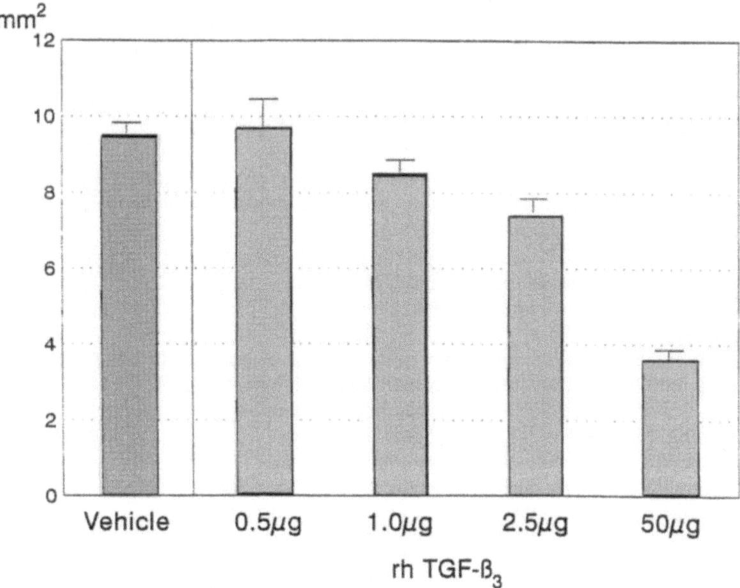

Fig. 2. Results of treatment of experimental gastric ulcers in rats. Ulcer size (mm^2: mean ± SEM) 7 days after local administration of vehicle alone (control) TGF-β3 (0.5, 1.0, 2.5, 50 μg) [2]

neal injury follows the rules of tissue repair. Fibroblasts and other tissue repair cells involved in adhesion formation are modulated by macrophages and growth factors [5]. Pharmaceutical strategies against adhesion formation seem to be possible in the future but may lead to undesired side effects.

References

1. Beck S, DeGuzman L, Lee WP, Xu Y, Siegel MW, Amento EP (1993) One systemic administration of transforming growth factor-β1 reverses age- or glucocorticoid-impaired wound healing. J Clin Invest 92: 2841–2849
2. Coerper S, Siegloch E, Köveker G, Starlinger M, Becker HD (1995) Stimulation der Heilung kryoinduzierter Magenulzera durch lokal injiziertes, rekombinantes TGF β3 im Tiermodell. Langenbecks Arch Chir 340–345
3. Falanga V (1992) Growth factors and chronic wounds: the need to understand the microenvironment. J Dermatol 19: 667–672
4. Folkman J (1992) Is there a field of wound pharmacology? Ann Surg 215: 1–2
5. Fukasawa M, Campeau JD, Yanagihara DL, Rodges KE, Di Zerega GS (1989) Mitogenic and protein synthetic activity of tissue repair cells: control by the postsurgical macrophage. J Invest Surg 2: 169–180
6. Knighton DR, Ciresi K, Fiegel VD (1990) Stimulation of repair of chronic nonhealing, cutaneous ulcers using platelet-derived wound healing formula. Surg Gynecol Obstet 170: 56–60
7. Lynch SE, Colvin RB, Antoniades HN (1989) Growth factors in wound healing. Single and synergistic effects on partial thickness porcine skin wounds. J Clin Invest 4: 640–646

8. Mustoe TA, Pierce GF, Morishima C, Deuel TF (1991) Growth factor-induced acceleration of tissue repair through direct and inductive activities in a rabbit dermal ulcer model. J Clin Invest 87: 694–703
9. Pierce GF, Mustoe TA, Lingelbach J, Masakowski R, Griffin GL, Senior RM, Deuel TF (1989) Platelet-derived growth factor and transforming growth factor-beta enhance tissue repair activities by unique mechanisms. J Cell Biol 109: 429–440
10. Pierce GF, Mustoe TA, Altrock BW (1991) Role of platelet-derived growth factor in wound healing. J Cell Biochem 45: 319–326
11. Pierce GF, Tarpley JE, Yangihara D (1992) Platelet-derived growth factor (BB homodimer), transforming growth factor-β1, and basic fibroblast growth factor in dermal wound healing. Am J Pathol 140: 1375–1388
12. Robson MC, Philips LG, Thomason A (1992) Platelet-derived growth factor BB for the treatment of chronic pressure ulcers. Lancet 339: 23–25
13. Ross R, Raines EW, Bowen-Pope DF (1986) The biology of platelet-derived growth factor. Cell 46: 155–159
14. Shah M, Foreman DM, Ferguson MW (1992) Control of scarring in adult wounds by neutralizing antibody to transforming growth factor β. Lancet 339: 213–214
15. Sporn MD, Roberts AB (1993) A major advance in the use of growth factors to enhance wound healing. J Clin Invest 92: 2565–2566
16. Steed DL (1995) Clinical evaluation of recombinant human platelet-derived growth factor for the treatment of lower extremity diabetic ulcers. J Vasc Surg 21: 71–81

1.4 Pathophysiology and Classification of Adhesions

E.P.M. Lorenz, H.V. Zühlke, R. Lange, and V. Savvas

Introduction

Intra-abdominal adhesions, as a result of damage to the peritoneum, continue to be a central and current problem in abdominal surgery. Adhesions also cause severe problems in other surgical specialties, for example in gynecological infertility surgery or in internal intraperitoneal chemotherapy and peritoneal dialysis. By far the majority of adhesions remain symptom-free or even promote intra-abdominal healing processes. However, 12% of adhesions cause recurring, chronic abdominal complaints and over 3% lead to serious symptoms requiring repeat laparatomies. The most severe complication, adhesion-related ileus, accounts for a considerable proportion of emergency operations.

Thus the surgeon is faced with a dilemma. On the one hand, adhesions are desirable in the normal course of healing, but on the other hand they lead to complications that should be avoided.

In addition to the anatomy of the peritoneum, knowledge of pathophysiology and peritoneal wound healing is necessary in order to intercede in the development of adhesions. Furthermore, it is necessary to have a generally accepted classification regarding the severity and organization of adhesions that includes a catalogue of criteria for measurability, comparability, and the exact description of findings.

Anatomy

Microscopically, the peritoneum consists of one layer of interlocking, flat, polygonal cells (surface and mesothelial cells), the surface of which is damp and reflective, thus forming the typically shiny aspect of the peritoneum. Underneath, there is a layer of connective tissue, in which fibroblasts, histiocytes, and lymphocytes as well as mastoid air and plasma cells can be detected. The subserous coat, as the gliding or displacement layer, is made up of blood and lymph vessels, nerves, and fat cells [10, 11].

Particularly in the area of the diaphragmatic peritoneum, there are so-called stomata, via which the exchange of corpuscular particles can take place.

Pathophysiological Aspects of Peritoneal Wound Healing

In contrast to the phase-like wound healing of external body surfaces, wound healing of the visceral and parietal peritoneum follows its own rules. Large serous defects are not covered in a stepwise manner starting at the wound edge, but quickly and synchronously over the entire surface by mesothelial cells. These cells come from the underlying connective tissue. The peritoneum is thus capable of reserosing even larger defects in a short period of time. The underlying tissue, however, lags behind this surface restitution, and scars remain after healing [5, 9].

It is now regarded as verified that, in addition to mechanical damage of the serosa, antibodies, necroses, residual blood, bacteria, and toxins as well as physical and chemical noxae lead to tissue damage. Following damage to very sensitive mesothelial cells, there is a flow of mediators, such as serotonin, bradykinin, histamine, and prostaglandin, which leads to an increase in vessel permeability and results in the extravasation of serosanguine liquid in the abdominal cavity. Through the concomitantly extravasated fibrogen, fibrin develops via the influence of released tissue thrombokinase, which goes on to form a loose three-dimensional network. This finally causes the adhesion of the adjacent serosal surfaces [1, 4].

In the course of normal healing, fibrin is broken down into fibrin degradation products by triggering the fibrinolytic system. Plasminogen is activated by endogenous activators as well as by the cytokinase of the mesothelial cells themselves. This step is the prerequisite for rapid reserosing and thus for adhesion-free healing.

Central to the pathophysiology of adhesions is, therefore, the dynamic balance between fibrin formation and fibrinolysis. Experimental studies showed that the spontaneous fibrinolytic activity of the peritoneum is reduced by trauma and above all by ischemia [4, 5, 9]. A decrease in plasminogen activator activity (PAA) was detected. As a result, fibrinous adhesions are not lysed, and a tighter fibrin network forms, which is the natural pathway for the proliferation of fibroblasts. Ergastoplasm-rich fibroblasts not only yield the raw material, mucopolysaccaride, but they also form collagen and tropocollagen.

In the temporal course of adhesion formation, fibrin can already be detected after 10 min. Maximal exudation occurs after 24 h, and resorption takes place within 5 days. The fibrin network is already so tight within the first 3 that separation is only possible in the case of defective formation of the mesothelium [8].

Further organization is introduced with the migration of fibroblasts within the first 3 days. Fibroblasts initially form precollagen and then collagen fibers; finally, the elastic fibers appear. Permanent adhesions i.e., ones that are no longer lysable, develop via differentiated collagen synthesis, proliferation of capillaries, and increased connective tissue organization before the surface is reserosed [1, 4, 8]. The complete formation of adhesions is finished after 10 days. The transformation to scar tissue occurs after 4–6 weeks at the earliest, and a possible regression can be documented within 2 months (Fig. 1).

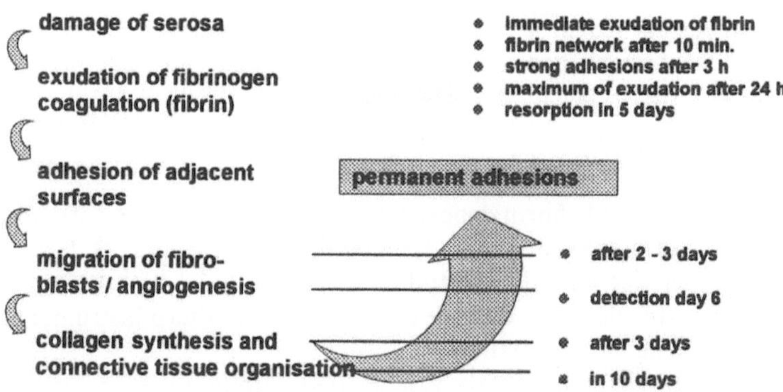

Fig. 1. Histiogenesis of adhesions

Classification of Adhesion

For clinical purposes, it is necessary to evaluate adhesions as objectively as possible according to the degree of severity and organization. In order to fulfill these requirements, classifications have been established on a pathological/anatomical basis [7, 11]. However, up to now these have been more or less subjective, particularly since each author uses his or her own classification [2].

In the older literature, classifications of intra-abdominal adhesions can be found based on etiology, clinical importance, topography, therapy, macroscopic morphology, histology, and histogenesis [3, 7, 11]. Classifications based on clinical importance followed. These were grouped into physiological, pathological, constructive or destructive adhesions. In the period that followed, classifications were reported according to topography and another with regard to therapeutic consequences.

The more criteria are applied, the less subjective and thus the more easily comparable classifications become. From the large number of classifications established according to this principle, two representative models were selected. Siegler and Luciano classified adhesions with four degrees of severity: from grade 0 with no adhesions to grade III with thick, extensive, vascularized adhesions including not directly adjacent organs [7, 11]. The classification of adhesions according to Knightly includes grades 0–IV, whereby grade IV consists of numerous extensive, thick adhesions with involvement of the mesenterium, intestine, and omentum as well as visceroparietal adhesions [6].

Method and Results

Within the framework of animal studies for adhesion prophylaxis, it seemed necessary to establish a new classification. Starting with preparations gained at different times in animal experiments and human preparations taken during routine operations, macroscopic documentation, histological processing, and evaluation of the preparations was carried out. The comparison of macroscopic and histological results led to a classification with four degrees of severity. Taking the previously established schemes as a starting point, we combined the most informative criteria, such as lysability, vascularization, and adhesion strength.

According to macroscopic criteria, the following classification can be made:

- *Grade I* adhesions include fibrin deposits, fine thread-like adhesion strands, or slight organ adhesions that can be lysed with blunt instruments.
- *Grade II* also includes adhesion strands that can be lysed with blunt instruments, but partly also ones that are only lysable with sharp instruments, with incipient fragile vascularization.
- *Grade III* adhesions include clearly vascularized, strong adhesion strands which are only lysable with sharp instruments (Fig. 2).
- *Grade IV* adhesions are firm, extensive organ adhesions, which are only lysable with sharp instruments and for which surgical treatment for organ damage is almost unavoidable.

In the histological evaluation, the following criteria were considered and included: fibrin, cell, and fiber content of the connective tissue, capillary or blood vessel formation, the detection of smooth muscle fiber, and antibody granulomas. Similar to the macroscopic evaluation, the following classification appeared to be practical according to the histomorphological criteria:

- *Grade I* adhesions have some fibrin and only very loose cell-containing connective tissue with fragile reticulin fibers.

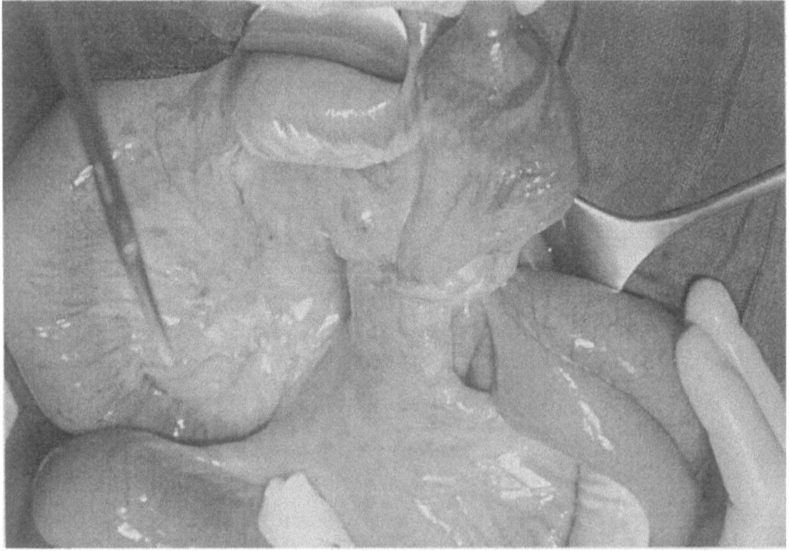

Fig. 2. Grade III adhesions in a human. Clearly vascularized strong adhesion strands, which are only lysable with sharp instruments

- In *grade II* adhesions, there is loose connective tissue containing cells and capillaries. Collagen fibers are already detectable.
- In *grade III* adhesions, the structure of the connective tissue is thicker; there is a reduction in the number of cells; there is an increased number of blood vessels, and occasionally elastic and smooth muscle fibers are found.
- *Grade IV* adhesions show older scar or callous tissue; the adjacent serosal surfaces are firmly grown together; smooth muscle fibers are occasionally found (Fig. 3).

Conclusion

The classification that we established does not take topography into consideration, since it is not important for the severity of adhesions. Acquired adhesions do not exhibit any regularity with regard to site [13]. If the classification grade is included in a topographical scheme – as Willital suggests for adhesion evaluation – then an adhesion index can be calculated, offering valuable assistance above all in the assessment and statistical calculation of animal studies [12].

The new classification presented here with the inclusion of macroscopic and microscopic criteria shows that uniform evaluation and description of adhesions can be carried out, enabling a comparable description in relaparotomies and easing advisory activities.

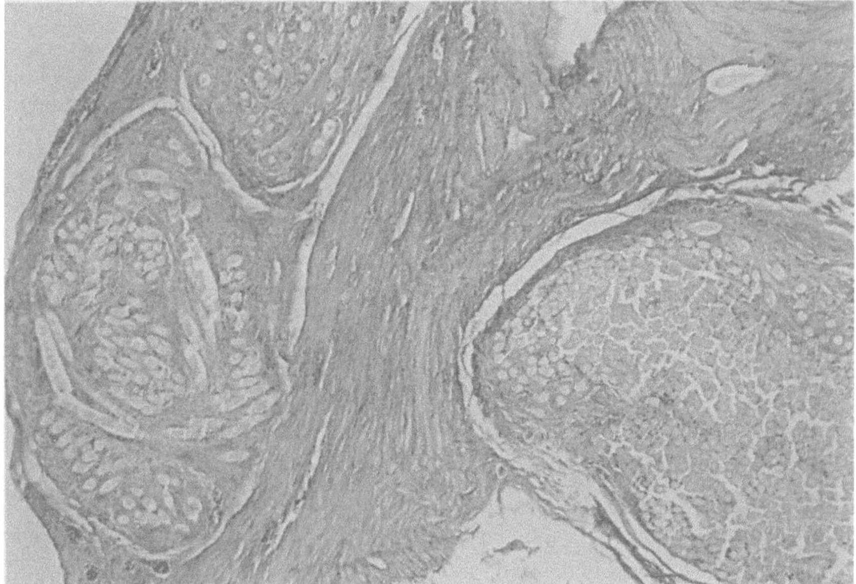

Fig. 3. Grade IV shows older scar or callous tissue; the adjacent serosal surfaces are firmly grown together; smooth muscle fibers are occasionally found

Summary

Central importance in the pathophysiology of adhesions is the shift dynamic balance between fibrinolysis and fibrin formation to fibrin formation. Permanent adhesions of very different morphology develop via fibroblast invasion of the fibrin network and fibrous organization. Classification into four degrees of severity is performed according to histological and morphological criteria. This is useful and feasible for objectifying and recording findings in repeat laparatomies, in expert ratings, and in animal experiments for adhesion research.

References

1. Bucman RF, Woods M, Sargent L, Gervin AS (1976) A unifying pathogenetic mechanism in the etiology of intraperitoneal adhesions. J Surg Res 20: 1–5
2. Clairmont P, Meyer M (1929) Bauchfellverwachsungen. Arch Klin Chir 157: 474–524
3. von Dembowski T (1888) Über die Ursachen der peritonealen Adhäsionen nach chirurgischen Eingriffen mit Rücksicht auf die Frage des Ileus nach Laparotomien. Langenbecks Arch Chir 37: 745–766
4. Ellis H, Harrison W, Hugh TB (1965) The healing of peritoneum under normal and pathological conditions. Br J Surg 52: 471–476
5. Ellis H (1978) Wound repair: reaction of the peritoneum to injury. Ann R Coll Surg Engl 60: 219–221
6. Knightly JJ, Agostino D, Cliffton EE (1962) The effect of fibrinolysin and heparin on the formation of peritoneal adhesions. Surgery 52: 250–257
7. Luciano AA, Hauser KS, Benda J (1983) Evaluation of commonly used adjuvants in the prevention of postoperative adhesions. Am J Obstet Gynecol 146: 88–92
8. Raftery AT (1981) Effect of peritoneal trauma on peritoneal fibrinolytic activity and intraperitoneal adhesion formation. Eur Surg Res 13: 397–401
9. Renvall SY (1980) Peritoneal metabolism and intra-abdominal adhesion formation during experimental peritonitis. Acta Chir Scand (Suppl) 508: 4–48
10. Schwemmle K (1990) Ursache von Verwachsungen im Abdomen. Langenbecks Arch Chir Suppl Kongressbd II: 1017–1021
11. Siegler AM, Kontopoulos V, Wang CF (1980) Prevention of postoperative adhesion in rabbits with ibuprofen, a non-steroidal anti-inflammatory agent. Fertil Steril 34: 46–49
12. Willital GH, Dietl KH, Meier H (1986) Ein neues Therapiekonzept zur postoperativen Adhäsionprophylaxe. Med Welt 37: 288–296
13. Zühlke HV, Lorenz EPM, Straub EM, Savvas V (1990) Pathophysiologie und Klassifikatione von Adhäsionen. Langenbecks Arch Chir Suppl Kongressbd II: 1009–1016

2 Animal Studies on Peritoneal Adhesions

2.1 Neoangiogenesis in Adhesion Formation and Peritoneal Healing

G. Bigatti, W. Boeckx, L. Gruft, N. Segers, and I. Brosens

Introduction

In 1971, Ellis [8] stated that "adhesions represent a vascular response by surrounding structures to the stimulus of ischemic tissue or foreign material within the peritoneal cavity."

He stressed the importance of ischemia and foreign body reaction as the primary cause of postsurgical adhesions and the role of neoangiogenesis in adhesion formation. Trauma and inflammation of the peritoneal membrane result in the release of kinin and histamine, increased permeability of blood vessels, and exudation of serosanguineous fluid in the peritoneal cavity with formation of fibrinous adhesions. These fibrinous adhesions are transient and lysed within 72 h if the fibrinolytic system is active, with perfect healing and no permanent adhesions. If the fibrinolytic system is depressed by the persistence of tissue ischemia, fibrinous adhesions become organized with ingrowth of blood vessels and fibroblast proliferation (Fig. 1).

The fibrinolytic activity of peritoneum resides in plasminogen activator activity (PAA), which is present in both mesothelial and submesothelial blood vessels and which activates plasmin to process fibrin with release of split products and reabsorption of fibrinous adhesions [2].

In 1973 Gervin [9] showed that massive adhesions occurred when the fibrinolytic activity was decreased by at least 50%.

Buckman [3] studied PAA of deperitonealized surfaces versus peritoneal grafts in rats (Fig. 2). A 2 × 2 cm area of parietal peritoneum was resected from the abdominal wall on both sides. On one side the peritoneal patch was immediately sutured back as a free peritoneal graft. On the other side, the peritoneal defect was left unsutured. PAA drastically decreased in the graft area compared to the unsutured defect. In addition, no adhesions were found in the unsutured area at 2 weeks, while all the peritoneal grafts showed dense adhesions (Table 1).

The overall incidence of adhesion formation following laparotomy is 93%, as reported by Menzies and Ellis [12] in a prospective analysis of 210 patients undergoing laparotomy who had previously had one or more abdominal operations.

The following complications can occur with intraperitoneal adhesions (Table 2):

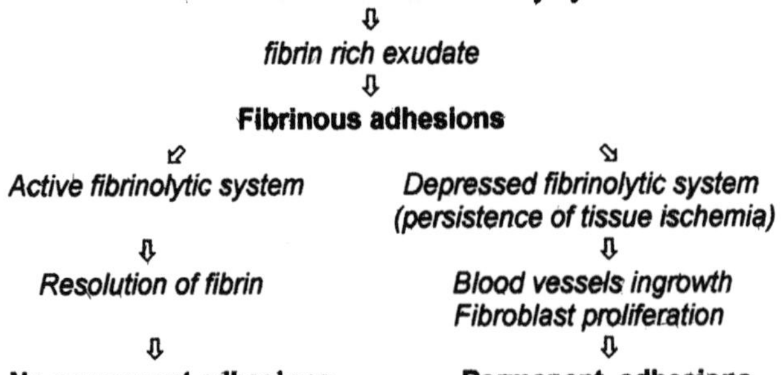

Fig. 1. Results of trauma and inflammation in peritoneal membrane. (From [2])

1. *Bowel obstruction.* Menzies and Ellis [12] reported intestinal obstruction in 1% of patients within 1 year of surgery (2708 laparotomies).
2. *Infertility.* Trimbos-Kemper [18] reported peritoneal adhesions in 55% of patients after tubal surgery at a laparoscopical control after 8 days (188 patients).
3. *Pelvic pain.* Rapkin [17] reported 12% of pelvic pain in 34 patients with adhesions undergoing laparotomy.

No treatment has yet proven to be uniformly effective in preventing post-operative adhesions [6]. At present the most promising treatments in the prevention of adhesion formation are the following:

- Interceed Tc7 (oxidized regenerated cellulose) (Johnson and Johnson Medical, Inc., Arlington, Texas USA) [10]
- Recombinant tissue-type plasminogen activator (rt-PA) [7]

Operative laparoscopy does not represent a solution to postsurgical adhesions. A recent multicenter study [14] reported an adhesion reformation rate of

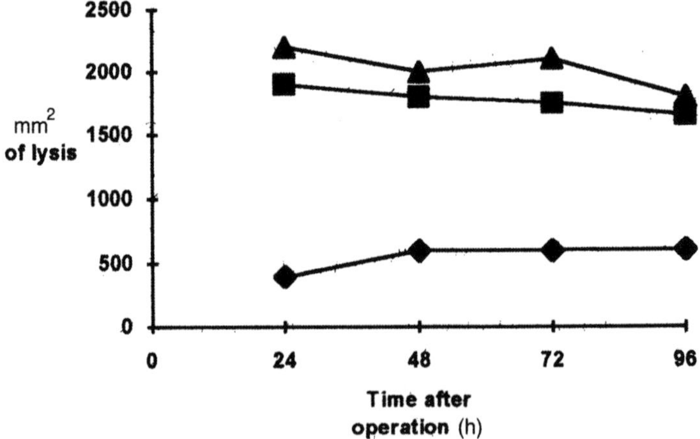

Fig. 2. Plasminogen activator activity (PAA) on deperitonealized surfaces (*squares*) versus peritoneal grafts (*diamonds*). *Triangles,* controls. (From [3])

Table 1. Incidence of formation of adhesions to grafted and deperitonealized surfaces [3]

	Grafted surface		Unsutured area	
	Adhesions (*n*)	Total (*n*)	Adhesions (*n*)	Total (*n*)
24 h	10	10	10	10
96 h	10	10	2	10
2 weeks	10	10	0	10

Table 2. Complications of postsurgical adhesions

Complication	Patients affected (%)	Total number of patients	Reference
Bowel obstruction	1	2708	[12]
Infertility	55	188	[18]
Pelvic pain	12	34	[17]

97% (66 of 68 patients) at second-look laparoscopy within 90 days of prior laparoscopic adhesiolysis. De novo adhesion formation occurred in eight of 68 women (12%), which was considerably less than the 51% reported by Diamond and DeCherney [5] after infertility abdominal surgery. The adhesion score showed a decrease of 52% from initial laparoscopical adhesiolysis (11.4) to second-look laparoscopy (5.5) [14].

These data confirm the importance of having a good experimental model to test the different techniques for the prevention of postoperative adhesions and to improve our knowledge on adhesion pathogenesis.

The aim of the present study was to create a standardized rat model to enable quantitative evaluation of adhesion growth and to establish the role of neoangiogenesis in adhesion formation and peritoneal healing.

Materials and Methods

Sixty Wistar rats weighing 250–300 g were used. The rats were anesthetized with an intramuscular injection of 0.3 ml Hypnorm (fluanisone and phentanylcitrate). The abdominal cavity was opened through a 4-cm midline incision using a clean, but not strictly aseptic operative technique. Using a steel spatula, we everted the abdominal wall, exposing the right side of the peritoneum. In this area, 1 cm lateral to the epigastric artery we fixed a square piece of Silastic (polymeric silicone) 0.5 cm × 0.5 cm × 0.2 mm with two separate angular stitches of nylon 9/0 (Fig. 3). All operations were performed using an operative microscope (Zeiss OPMI 6 or 7; Zeiss Belgium, Zaventem) fitted with a 200-mm focal length lens, 12 eyepieces, and 160-mm binocular tubes. This electrically foot-controlled zoom microscope provided a magnification of between × 8 and × 25. The silicon used was Silastic sheeting (nonreinforced 500-3; Dow Corning

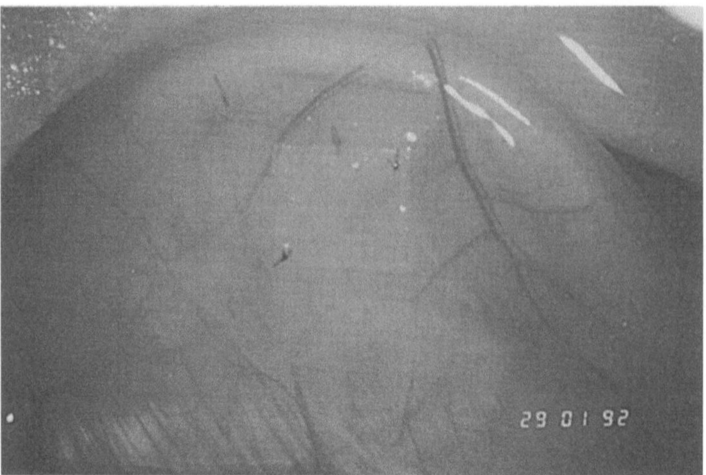

Fig. 3. Implantation of 0.5 × 0.5 cm², 0.2 mm thick silastic patch

Corporation Medical Products Midland, Michigan USA). The peritoneum was opened for approximately 10 min in each animal. The abdominal wall was sutured in a double layer, with separate stitches for the musculoperitoneal area and a continuous vicryl 3/0 stitch for the skin. The rats were randomized into six groups of ten animals each and reoperated on days 2, 4, 6, 8, 10, and 12, respectively. Inspection was performed through eversion of the abdominal wall exposing the peritoneal area where the piece of Silastic was fixed in order to observe the development of adhesions. Photographs were obtained at prefixed magnifications of ×10, ×15, ×20, and ×25 using a tungsten film of 170 ASA pushed at 320 ASA during the development. The camera used automatically performed three exposures one after the other for each single shot. For the first slide, the opening time of the shutter was automatically calculated by the camera according to the available light. The following two slides were over- and underexposed automatically to avoid any mistake. Instead of the direct light of the microscope, a special system of transillumination placed under the everted skin of the rat was used. This kind of illumination allowed clear slides without any shiny effect plus a good view of the vessels. On the side of each Silastic patch we placed a millimeter grid. This allowed measurements to the nearest one tenth of a millimeter. In addition, a 2×2-cm area of parietal peritoneum and underlying muscle around the Silastic (Silastic and adhesions included) was resected with complete removal of the tissue flap. Each specimen was fixed for scanning electron microscopy in order to evaluate the cellular tissue on the surface of the silastic.

The degree of adhesion was scored by our modified version of Diamond et al. 's classification [4] (Table 3). Omentoparietal adhesions to the piece of Silastic were scored according to their tenacity, type, and extent. The extent was measured by the percentage of Silastic surface covered by adhesions, which was made possible by the two-dimensional structure of our model. We

Table 3. Adhesion score system

Score	Tenacity	Adhesion type	Extent[a] (%)
0	None	None	0
1	Adhesion essentially fell apart	Dense avascular	< 25
2	Adhesion lysed with traction	Filmy avascular	< 50
3	Adhesion required sharp dissection	Dense vascular, small vessels (< 50 μm)	< 75
4	–	Dense vascular, large vessels (50–100 μm)	> 75

Modified from [4].

[a]Percentage of Silastic surface covered by adhesions.

studied the peritoneal neoangiogenesis (Fig. 4) by estimating the percentage of rats with measurable vascularization in order to better quantify the phenomenon. We chose rats that showed rows of parallel vessels with measurable length and diameter on the peritoneum around the Silastic. The two vascular parameters included vascular density (number of vessels per 5 mm) and distance between the edge and the center of Silastic (length of the vessels).

For each parameter we considered the arithmetic median. Concerning the length of vessels, we observed the distance from the edge to the center of Silastic and measured the longest vessel in each animal. We considered vessels with a diameter between 50 and 100 μm as large vessels and those with a diameter of less than 50 μm as small vessels.

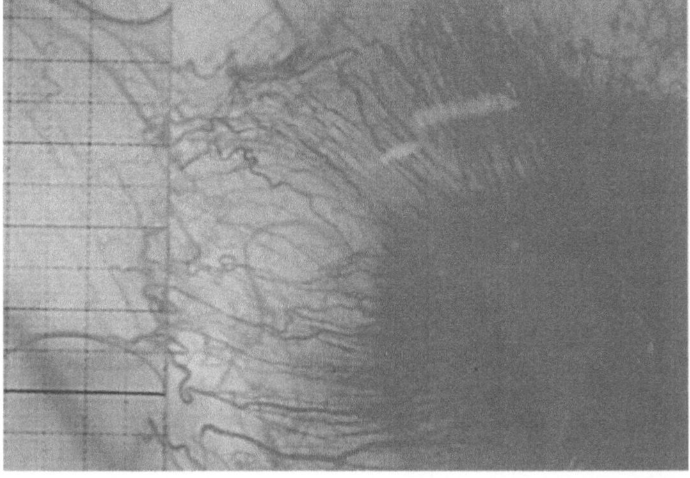

Fig. 4. Peritoneal neoangiogenesis; rows of parallel vessels extending towards the center of the silastic patch

Results

Extent of Adhesion

The extent was measured by the percentage of Silastic covered by adhesions, which was made possible by the two-dimensional structure of our model.

We noted a progressive increase in the extent of adhesions up to day 8, followed by a redistribution in the other ranges on days 10 and 12 (Fig. 5).

Type of Adhesion

On day 6, adhesions start to vascularize. In 60% of rats, adhesions are dense with small vessels, and only 40% show large vessels. On day 8 we found 100% of dense vascular adhesions with large vessels (Fig. 6).

Tenacity of Adhesions

On day 6, 80% of adhesions are lysed with traction and only 20% require sharp dissection, while on day 8 all adhesions require sharp dissection (Fig. 7).

Peritoneal Angiogenesis

Peritoneal angiogenesis began on day 4 in 20% of rats in the form of small spots around the implantation site. We observed a progressive increase up to day 12, at which point all animals showed peritoneal angiogenesis (Fig. 8).

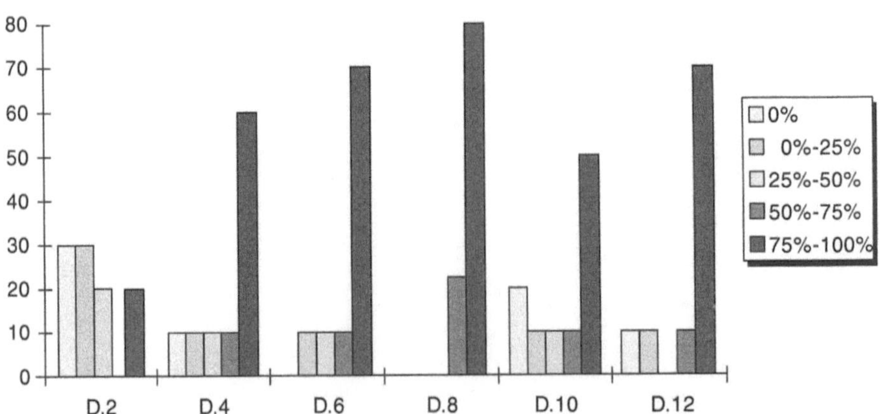

Fig. 5. Percentage of the Silastic surface covered by adhesions on days 2, 4, 6, 8, 10, and 12

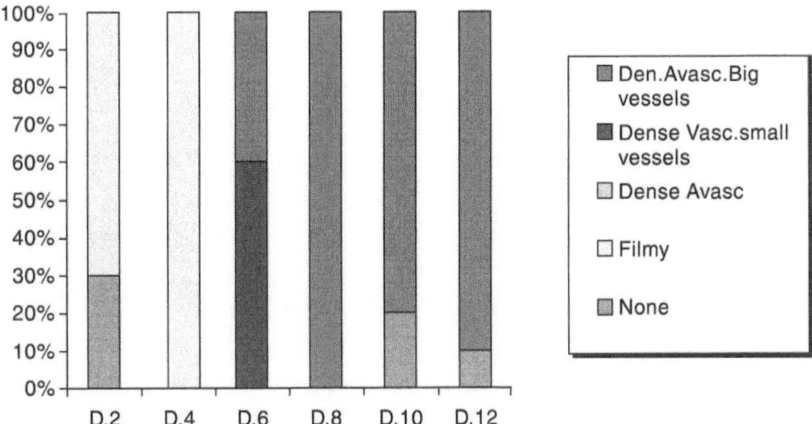

Fig. 6. Types of adhesions

Measurable Vascular Parameters

We were not able to evaluate vessel size until day 8. On day 8 we evaluated 33% of the rats, on day 10, 50%, and on day 12, 70%.

Vessel Length

The median vessel length was 0.7 mm on day 8, 1.6 mm on day 10, and 2.5 mm on day 12. It is important to note that on day 12 vessels reached the center of the Silastic patch.

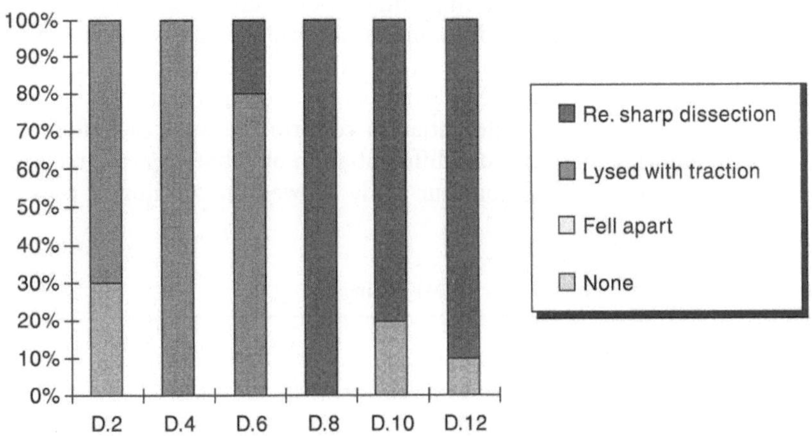

Fig. 7. Tenacity of adhesions

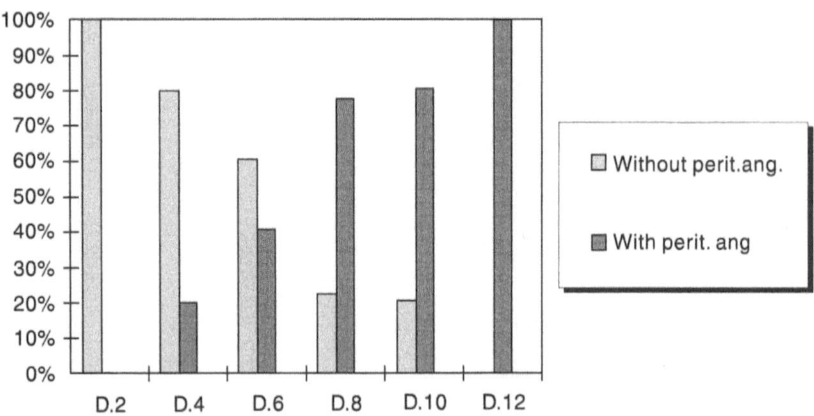

Fig. 8. Percentage of animals with and without peritoneal angiogenesis

Scanning Electron Microscopy

According to the findings of Raftery [15, 16] and Milligan and Raftery [13], scanning electron microscopy showed proliferation of mesothelial precursors on the Silastic patch from day 4 to day 8 (Table 4, Figs. 9–11). On day 8, these mesothelial precursors show microvilli on their surface equal to normal peritoneum. This confirms the ability of normal peritoneum to insulate the traumatized area.

Discussion

The aim of the present study was to clarify the natural history of neoangiogenesis in adhesion formation. The phenomenon has been standardized to allow a quantitative study of two parallel mechanisms that take part in the repair of trauma induced by the implantation of a silicon sheet on the peritoneum. While omentoparietal adhesions vascularize the Silastic surface, a new peritoneal tissue with its vascular network grows and covers the traumatized area. The findings concerning the Silastic surface of tissue repair cells on day 8 showing a clear mesothelial differentiation confirm the work of Raftery [15] and Ellis [8] showing a metaplastic differentiation of subperitoneal precursors into mesothelial cells. In addition, our study showed that peritoneal cells can

Table 4. Scanning electron microscopy (SEM) findings

Day	Findings
4	Tissue repair cells start to proliferate on the Silastic patch
6	Increase in cellular bindings
8	Complete mesothelial differentiation with microvilli on the surface

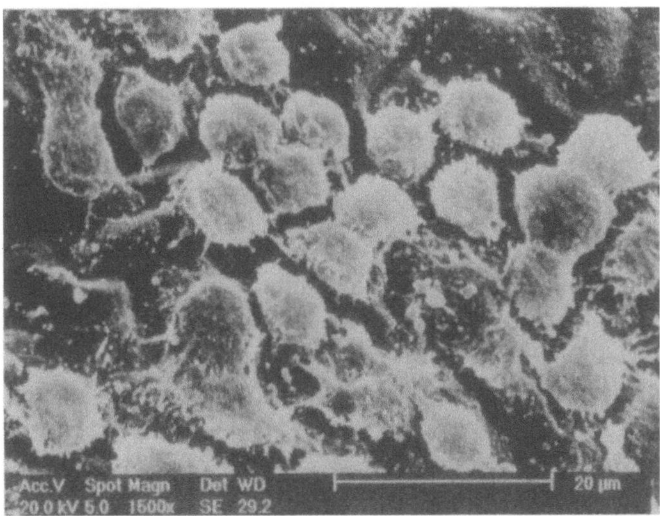

Fig. 9. Scanning electron micrograph taken on postoperative day 4. (Also see Table 4.) Mesothelial precursor cells over the silastic patch. Rare intercellular bindings

also originate from the edges of a wound, as found in studies by Johnson and Whitting [11] and Bridges and Whitting [1], and not only from the center. On day 8, perfectly differentiated mesothelial cells with clearly visible microvilli cover the Silastic surface. The growth on their surface of microvilli equal to the ones on normal peritoneum confirms our findings. The progression of re-

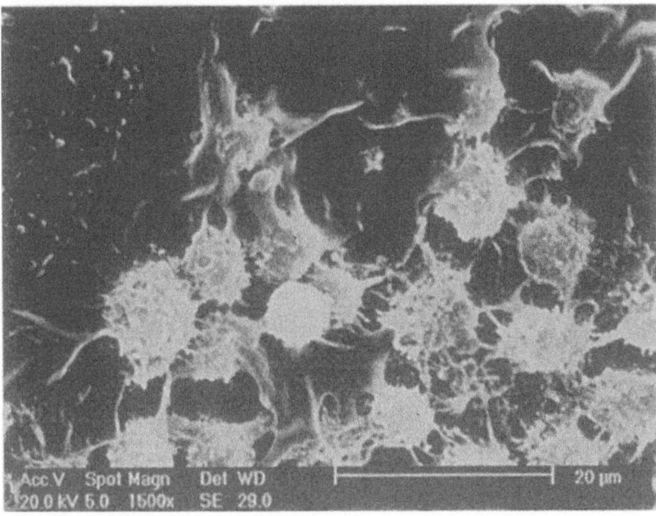

Fig. 10. Scanning electron micrograph taken on postoperative day 6. (Also see Table 4.) Increase of mesothelial precursor cells binding on silastic patch surface

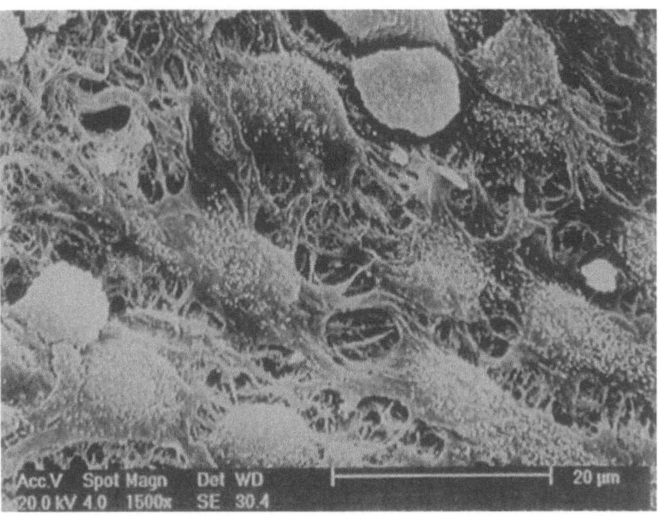

Fig. 11. Scanning electron micrograph taken on postoperative day 8. (Also see Table 4.) Microvilli on metaplastic differentiated mesothelial cells are clearly visible on the silastic patch surface

epithelization of the Silastic surface is seen from days 4 to 8 by the gradual increase of intercellular bindings. This confirms the peritoneal ability to insulate the foreign body by covering it with new mesothelial tissue. The use of a Silastic sheet offers a two-dimensional model that avoids neoangiogenesis under the patch and allows the growth of mesothelial cells only from the surrounding areas. It is not possible to check reperitonealization under the silicon patch. Concerning adhesion vascularization, we observed that between days 8 and 12 there is a rearrangement with a reduction in adhesions. At the same time, we reported the highest rate of adhesion vascularization and peritoneal neoangiogenesis. A theoretically valid treatment in preventing adhesion formation should increase peritoneal neoangiogenesis and repair of peritoneal lesions, but at the same time should decrease adhesion vascularization. The rearrangement observed is only temporary and needs further investigation. In our model, adhesion formation seems to be linked to the relationship between the speed of reperitonealization and omental ability to create vascular adhesions. The present model offers the possibility of testing, in a relatively short time, the effect of any treatment or device on the formation of postoperative adhesions and their resolution.

The major parameters for each series of animals are timed; they represent an easy tool for referral in prophylactic treatment to avoid adhesions and allow the standardization of a phenomenon currently described in the literature in a subjective way. Several experimental models report a traumatic approach to the genital tract far away from the site of normal surgical procedures. In this model, an inert material such as silicon of minimal size and thickness was used. The nylon 9/0 suture stitches were used following microsurgical principles. All these procedures were intended to minimize trauma according to the conservative surgical principle concerning the prevention of postsurgical adhesions. This study describes a detailed control group and represents the basis for further comparative investigations in order to find a concrete solution to this severe surgical complication.

Summary

This study presents an animal model for the observation of adhesion formation, from a vascular point of view. In 60 Wistar rats a 4cm-midline incision was performed and a 0.5 × 0.5 cm square piece of silastic 0.2 mm thick was fixed on the right side of the peritoneum with two separate angular stitches of nylon 9/0. The rats were randomized in six groups of ten animals which were reoperated respectively on days 2, 4, 6, 8, 10, and 12. Biopsies for scanning electron microscopy were obtained by resecting a 2 × 2 cm of parietal peritoneum around and covering the silastic patch. Foreign body reaction induced by the silastic and ischemia caused by stitching are the stimuli utilised for adhesion formation. The results showed a gradual progression in type and tenacity of adhesion formation. Between day 8 and day 12 we noted, together with a decrease and a redistribution in the extent of adhesions, the maximal degree of peritoneal reactive angiogenesis. In the early stages, vascularization is part of the organisation of adhesion while their extent is limited. Two parallel mechanisms take part in trauma healing. While omento-parietal adhesions are vascularized, a new peritoneal tissue with its vascular network develops and covers the silastic surface and the traumatized area. This theory is supported by the presence of mesothelial precursors differentiating into mesothelial cells on day 8. Theoretically, a valid treatment in preventing adhesions formation should increase the peritoneal neoangiogenesis and the repair of peritoneal lesions but at the same time prevent the vascularization of adhesions. The present model offers the possibility to test in a relatively short time the effect of any treatment or device for the prevention of postoperative adhesions.

References

1. Bridges JB, Whitting HW (1964) Parietal peritoneal healing in the rat. J Path Bact 87: 123
2. Buckman RF (1976) A unifying pathogenetic mechanism in the etiology of intraperitoneal adhesions. J Surg Res 20: 1–5
3. Buckman RF (1976) A physiologic basis for the adhesions free healing of deperitonealized surfaces. J Surg Res 21: 67–76
4. Diamond MP, Linsky CB, DiZerega GS (1987) A model for sidewall adhesions in the rabbit: reduction by an absorbable barrier. Microsurg 8: 197–200
5. Diamond MP, DeCherney AH (1987) Pathogenesis of adhesion formation/reformation. Application to reproductive pelvic surgery. Microsurgery 8: 103–107
6. DiZerega GS (1992) The peritoneum: postsurgical repair and adhesion formation. Rock JA, Murphy AA, Johns HW Jr (eds) Female Reproductive Surgery. William and Wilkins, Baltimore, pp 2–18

7. Doody K, Dunn RC, Buttram VC Jr (1989) Recombinant tissue plasminogen activator reduces adhesion formation in a rabbit uterus horn model. Fertil Steril 51(3): 509–512
8. Ellis H (1971) The cause and prevention of postoperative intraperitoneal adhesions. Surg Gyn Obstet 133(9): 497–511
9. Gervin AS (1973) Serosal hypofibrinolysis. A cause of post operative adhesions. Am J Surg 125: 80–88
10. INTERCEED (TC7) Adhesion Barrier Study Group (1989) Prevention of postsurgical adhesions by INTERCEED (TC7), an absorbable adhesion barrier: a prospective, randomised multicenter clinical study. Fertil Steril 51(6): 933–938
11. Johnson FR, Whitting HW (1962) Repair of parietal peritoneum. Br J Surg 49: 653
12. Menzies D, Ellis H (1990) Intestinal obstruction from adhesion – how big is the problem? Ann R Coll Surg Engl 72: 60–63
13. Milligan DW, Raftery AT (1974) Observations on the pathogenesis peritoneal adhesion: a light and electron microscopical study. Br J Surg 61: 274–280
14. Operative laparoscopy study group (1991) Postoperative adhesion development after operative laparoscopy: evaluation at early second-look procedures. Fertil Steril 55(4): 700–704
15. Raftery AT (1973) Regeneration of parietal and visceral peritoneum: a light microscopical study. Br J Surg 60(4): 293–299
16. Raftery AT (1981) Effect of peritoneal trauma on peritoneal fibrinolytic activity on intraperitoneal adhesion formation. An experimental study in the rat. Eur Surg Res 13: 397–401
17. Rapkin AJ (1986) Adhesions and pelvic pain: a retrospective study. Obstet Gynecol 68(1): 13–15
18. Trimbos-Kemper CM (1985) Adhesion formation after tubal surgery: results of the eighth-day laparoscopy in 188 patients. Fertil Steril 43(4): 395–400

2.2 A Three-Dimensional Cell Culture Method for Studying Peritoneal Adhesions

F. Bittinger, C.L. Klein, C. Skarke, C. Brochhausen, M. Otto, H. Köhler, and C.J. Kirkpatrick

Introduction

The peritoneum is a serous membrane of mesodermal origin which consists of mesothelial cells in a continuous layer which rests upon loose mesenchymal tissue, a basal lamina and basement membrane composed of a collagen lattice. The subperitoneal connective tissue contains collagen, fibroblasts, vascular and lymphatic vessels. This serous cavity is involved in several pathological processes, e.g. peritoneal adhesions. In this context, the interaction between different kinds of cells and extracellular matrix (ECM) components play an important role.

Muscatello [31] examined peritoneal inflammation and described serosal damage as the first step in peritoneal injury, followed by migration and accumulation of inflammatory cells, both under and above the mesothelial cell layer. Intraperitoneal adhesions are a result of this inflammation and often lead to intestinal obstruction [13]. Mesothelial and endothelial cells are actively involved in these inflammatory processes, although their exact roles in pathogenesis are still unclear.

Mesothelial cells cover the peritoneal surface and produce large amounts of phosphatidylcholine (PC) [12], which is important in maintaining gliding between cell surfaces. Moreover, mesothelial cells have been reported to be a non-thrombogenic surface [32] and to demonstrate fibrinolytic properties, as described by Merlo [28] and van Hinsberg [46]. Endothelial cells play an important role in the regulation of migrating granulocytes by expressing cell adhesion molecules (CAM) and in neovascularisation in inflamed areas.

The cellular mechanisms involved in the pathogenesis of peritoneal adhesions can be investigated either in vivo (animal experiments) or in vitro (cell culture). It is well known that cell culture offers the possibility of reproducing in vivo phenomena in vitro and of analysing cells, independent of systemic influences, which are constantly present in animal homeostasis. Nevertheless, several experimental studies have been carried out with animals [7, 9, 35].

Cell culture provides two possibilities, the two-dimensional and three-dimensional culture system. In a two-dimensional model, cells are cultivated on the bottom of a culture flask, whereas in the three-dimensional model the extracellular matrix first has to be prepared and then the cells have to be placed, depending on their origin, either in or on the resulting ECM. A gel culture appears to be an optimal in vitro system to analyse cell–cell and cell–matrix interactions. Collagen, a major component of ECM, plays an important role in the differentiation of cells and permits the in vitro reconstruction of tissues [30, 42, 44, 45].

In our study, a new three-dimensional model of the peritoneum will be presented which involves co-culture of human mesothelial and endothelial cells. In this model, it is possible to investigate cell–cell and cell–matrix interactions by using conventional histological and immunohistochemical methods. Furthermore, pre-formed fibrin, as well as other cell populations (e.g. inflammatory cells), can be employed to simulate specific pathological processes.

Material and Methods

Cell Culture

Mesothelial cells were obtained from human omental tissue (HOMES) by a modification of methods previously described by Nicholson et al. [32] and Stylianou et al. [41]. After incubation with 0.05% trypsin (type III, salt-free; Sigma, Germany) for 5 min, the cell pellet thus obtained was centrifuged and finally seeded in 75-cm^2 tissue culture flasks (GIBCO, Germany) with Ham's F-12/Iscove's medium (HIM; Gibco, Germany 50:50 v/v). Cells were maintained at 37 °C in an atmosphere of 5% CO_2.

Endothelial cells were obtained as follows:

Human umbilical endothelial cells (HUVEC) were isolated as previously described [23]. Umbilical veins were cannulated and incubated at 37 °C for 30 min with 0.25% collagenase I (Worthington). The cells were then separated by centrifugation at 600 g for 15 min. The cell pellet was resuspended in medium (HIM) and cultivated in 25-cm^2 tissue culture flasks (GIBCO, Germany).

Human microvascular endothelial cells (HOMEC) were obtained from omental tissue (10 g), which was previously used for the isolation of mesothelial cells using the technique described by Jackson et al. [22] and Bittinger et al. [4]. After incubation with collagenase I (30 min at 37 °C), the cell suspension contains microvascular endothelial cells and contaminant cells. In order to separate the endothelial cells, 0.5 mg *Ulex-europaeus* I-coated magnetic immunobeads (Immunotech, France) were used and added to 1 ml of a cell suspension in phosphate-buffered solution (PBS) + 20% fetal calf serum (FCS), resuspended and gently mixed. After incubation for 15 min at room temperature, the positive fraction of bead-coated target cells was separated with the help of a magnet concentrator. The cells obtained were cultivated in 25-cm^2 tissue culture flasks. The beads on the cell surface were eliminated by treating them with 0.1 M L-fucose (Sigma, Germany) for 10 min at 4 °C.

Three-Dimensional Cell Culture

Three different three-dimensional culture models were developed (Fig. 1), based on previous studies by Elsdale et al. [14], Enami et al. [15] and Bittinger et al. [5].

Mesothelial cells were cultivated on the pre-formed type I collagen gel and endothelial cells within the gel. Furthermore, a co-culture with mesothelial and endothelial cells was formed.

After reconstruction of type I collagen gel, as described by Sugihara et al. [42], the following procedures were used to achieve the cell culture models:

1. Mesothelial cells (5×10^4 cells/well) were layered out on the collagen matrix (0.5 ml) and covered with medium (HIM) containing 20% FCS.
2. Endothelial cells (HUVEC, HOMEC) were carefully embedded in 0.5 ml type I collagen gel and covered with medium.
3. To establish the co-culture model, mesothelial cells were seeded on the top of the matrix in which endothelial cells had been cultivated for 3–4 days, to allow vessel-like structures in the matrix to develop.

In order to characterise the functionality of the cell cultures, gels were additionally incubated with tumour necrosis factor (TNF)-α (300 U/ml; Sigma, Germany) for 5 h at 37 °C in order to study the expression of CAM by methods based on previous studies by Klein et al. [25, 26]. Furthermore, pre-formed

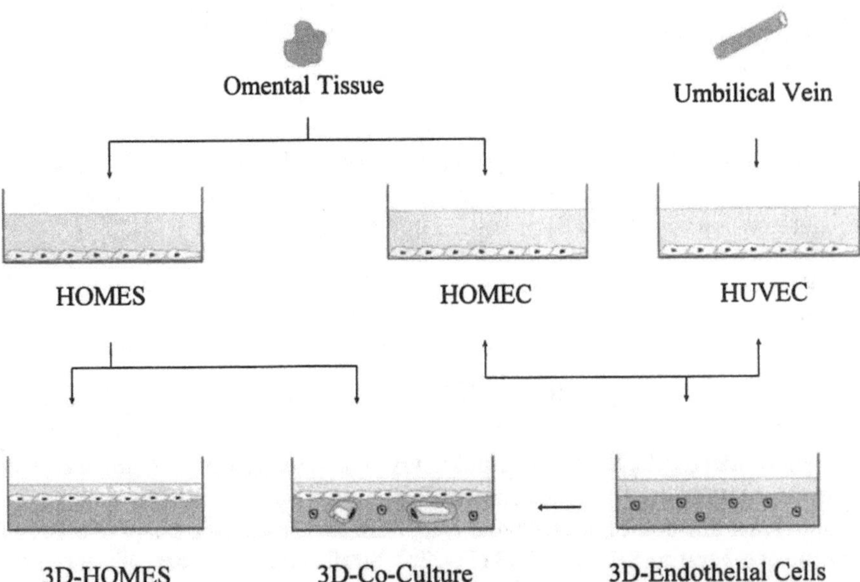

Fig. 1. Three-dimensional (*3D*) cell culture models. Human mesothelial (*HOMES*) and microvascular endothelial cells (*HOMEC*) from omentum and human endothelial cells from umbilical vein (*HUVEC*) were isolated and placed either *on* (HOMES) or *in* (HOMEC/HUVEC) type I collagen gel matrix. The co-culture model (in vitro peritoneum) was completed by seeding mesothelial cells on top of the gel matrix after the beginning of angiogenesis

blood clots were laid on the surface of the first model (see list above) and examined after 96 h.

Characterisation of Cell Cultures

Human mesothelial cells and endothelial cells were characterised in the two-dimensional cell culture by light microscopy and immunocytochemistry. For this purpose, cells were seeded in fibronectin-coated LAB-TEK culture chambers (Nunc, Germany) at a concentration of 25 000 cells per cm^2.

Using the indirect immunoperoxidase method, the expression of cytokeratin 8 (Becton Dickinson, MA), cytokeratin 18 (Progen, Germany), cytokeratin 7 (Progen, Germany), cytokeratin 19 (Boehringer, Mannheim), vimentin (Progen, Germany), factor VIII-related antigen (Dako, UK), *Ulex europaeus* agglutinin I (Sigma, Germany), anti-intercellular CAM (anti-ICAM), anti-vascular CAM (anti-VCAM), anti-E selectin and anti-platelet/endothelial CAM (anti-PECAM) (all CAM antibodies from British Biotechnology, UK) was analysed.

The three-dimensional collagen gel cultures were analysed by different methods:

1. Phase contrast microscopy was used to study cell growth.
2. For histological examination, the samples were fixed in 10% formalin, embedded in paraffin and stained with haematoxylin and eosin (H&E).
3. For immunocytochemical studies, paraffin-embedded samples were stained using the indirect immunoperoxidase method. Paraformaldehyde-fixed (4%) frozen sections of TNF-α-stimulated samples were used to demonstrate CAM by the alkaline phosphatase–anti-alkaline phosphatase (APAAP) method.
4. For ultrastructural studies, the collagen gel samples were fixed with 2.5% glutaraldehyde and processed by standard methods. The ultrastructural analyses were accomplished with the help of a Phillips 410 transmission electron microscope (TEM).

Results

Characterisation of Two-Dimensional Cell Cultures

The mesothelial cells are flat and polygonal with prominent nucleoli, and after confluence they have a "cobblestone" pattern (Fig. 2a). Using a panel of monoclonal antibodies, mesothelial cells were identified by a positive reaction for the cytokeratins 8/18 and 7/19 (Fig. 2b). Similar reactions were observed for vimentin in the same manner. Furthermore, a strong constitutive expression of ICAM-1 was demonstrated. VCAM-1 was only expressed after stimulation with TNF-α. E selectin was not detected. Electron microscopical studies showed numerous microvilli on the cell surface as well as intracytoplasmic tonofilaments.

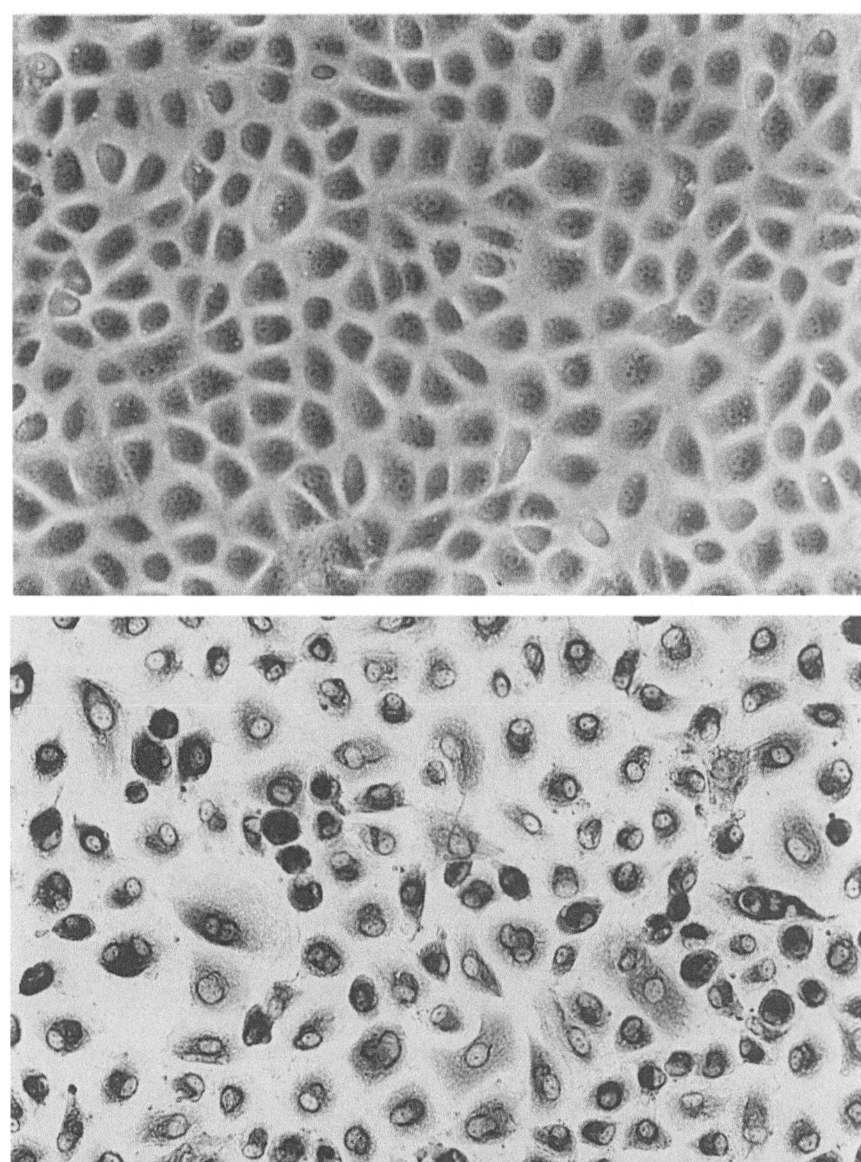

Fig. 2a,b. Human mesothelial cells (HOMES) show a polygonal shape and are strongly positive for cytokeratin. **a** Phase contrast microscope. × 200. **b** Cytokeratin 8. × 200

The endothelial cells from human umbilical veins (HUVEC) are polygonal and grow to form a regular, contact-inhibited monolayer of closely adherent cells ("cobblestone" pattern) (Fig. 3a). In contrast, microvascular endothelial cells (HOMEC) display a distinct morphology and after 12 h have a spindle-

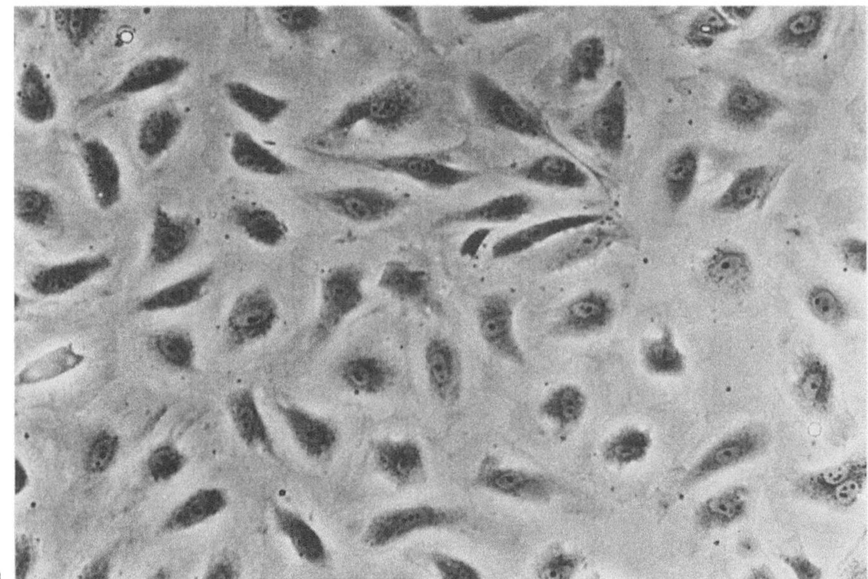

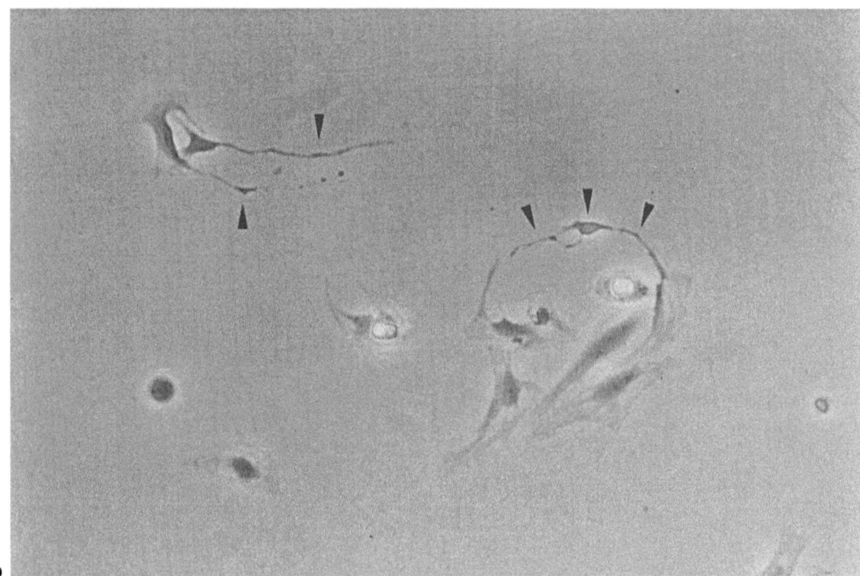

Fig. 3. a Primary monolayer culture of human umbilical endothelial cells (HUVEC) after confluence, with a typical "cobblestone" pattern. **b** Microvascular endothelial cells (HOMEC) with large cytoplasmic processes (*arrowheads*). Phase contrast microscopy. × 200

shaped form (Fig. 3b). However, a fibroblast morphology was not observed. After treatment with ʟ-fucose, no magnetic beads were found on the cell surface.

Immunocytochemical studies revealed a positive reaction for factor-VIII-related antigen and *Ulex europaeus* agglutinin I, as described by Stephenson et al. [40]. Like mesothelial cells endothelial cells show a strong expression of ICAM-1 and PECAM-1 in the absence of cytokine stimulation. Ultrastructural analyses demonstrated micropinocytotic vesicles at the cell surface. Furthermore, intracytoplasmic Weibel-Palade bodies confirmed the endothelial origin of the examined cells. HUVEC and HOMEC revealed no ultrastructural differences.

Characterisation of Three-Dimensional Cell Cultures

Mesothelial cells placed on a pre-formed type I collagen gel are completely adherent to the matrix after 1 h. After 4 days, HOMES build a close monolayer without penetration into the gel. Similar to conventional cell culture methods, cells show a polygonal form.

After embedding in type I collagen, endothelial cells have a round shape with large cytoplasmic processes. Within 24–48 h, small intracytoplasmic vesicles were evident as the initial stage of lumen formation. In the following 3–4 days, the cells proliferated and organised themselves into tube-like formations, each consisting of a few cells. After 5 days, cytoplasmic processes penetrated the gel and bound to other pre-formed neovessels, and at day 8, tube-like formation was replaced by the organisation of a complex network of vessel-like structures (Fig. 4a). These structures showed endothelial cells, which positively reacted with factor VIII-related antigen (Fig. 4b), *Ulex europaeus* I and vimentin. However, actin filaments were not observed. The microvascular endothelial cells became elongated and built only capillary-like formations. The newly formed vessels showed endothelial cells with in vivo-like characteristics.

On histological examination of three-dimensional cultures, the mesothelial cells were found to have a flat monolayer on the matrix (Fig. 5a). They showed positive staining for cytokeratin 8/18 (Fig. 5b) and 7/19, as well as for vimentin, whereas actin was not detected. These results were already demonstrated at the beginning of the three-dimensional experiments and were also observable during the entire time of culture. Furthermore, immunostaining for CAM on frozen sections revealed expression of ICAM-1 and PECAM-1 both in mesothelial and endothelial cells independent of stimulation (data not shown). VCAM-1 and E selectin were only expressed under TNF-α stimulation after 4 h. VCAM-1 was expressed in both cell types, whereas E selectin was only demonstrated in the endothelial cells (Fig. 6).

Human mesothelial cells exposed to a blood clot reacted by migrating into the gel as well as into the clot (Fig. 7).

Ultrastructural studies revealed mesothelial cells with several tight junctions as well as a matrix rich in collagen fibres beneath the mesothelial cell layer. Within the matrix, numerous vessel-like structures covered by endothelial cells were observed. In addition, numerous Weibel-Palade bodies, mitochondria, rough endoplasmic reticulum, Golgi complexes and tight junctions were found. A basal lamina was shown on the cell surface in contact with the collagen gel after 7 days in culture (Fig. 8).

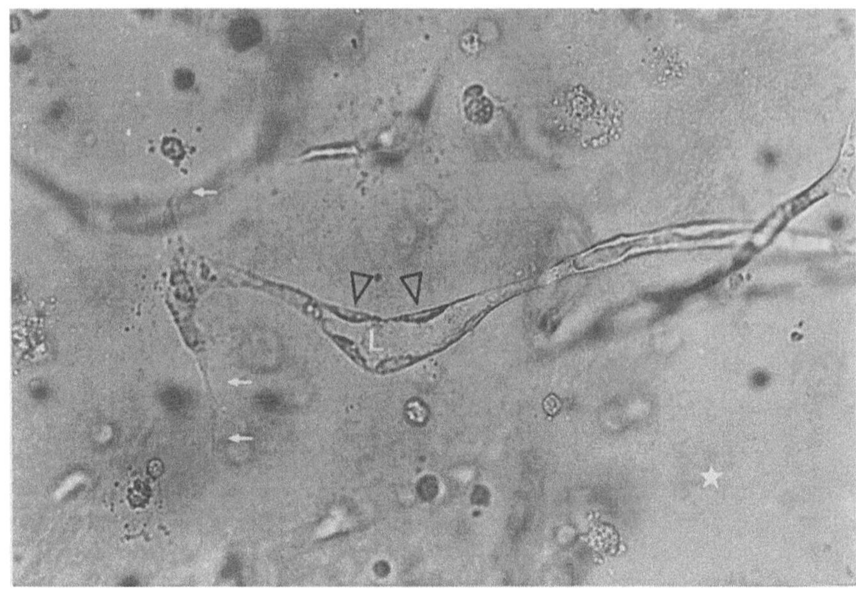

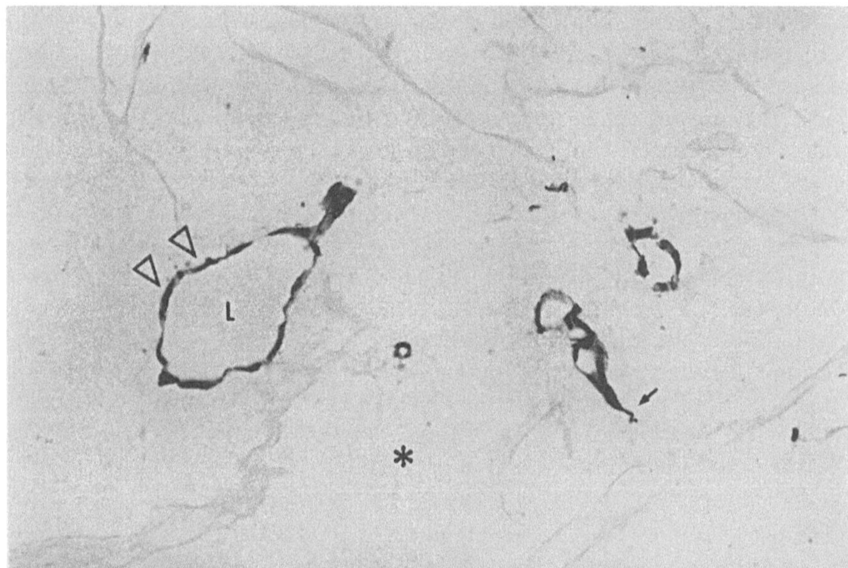

Fig. 4a,b. Reconstructed vessel-like structures in three-dimensional collagen gel (*asterisk*), with newly developed lumina (*L*) completely lined with endothelial cells (*arrowheads*). **a** Phase contrast micrograph shows the sprouting of cytoplasmic processes (*arrows*), × 200. **b** Light micrograph of paraffin sections stained with factor VIII-related antigen. × 200

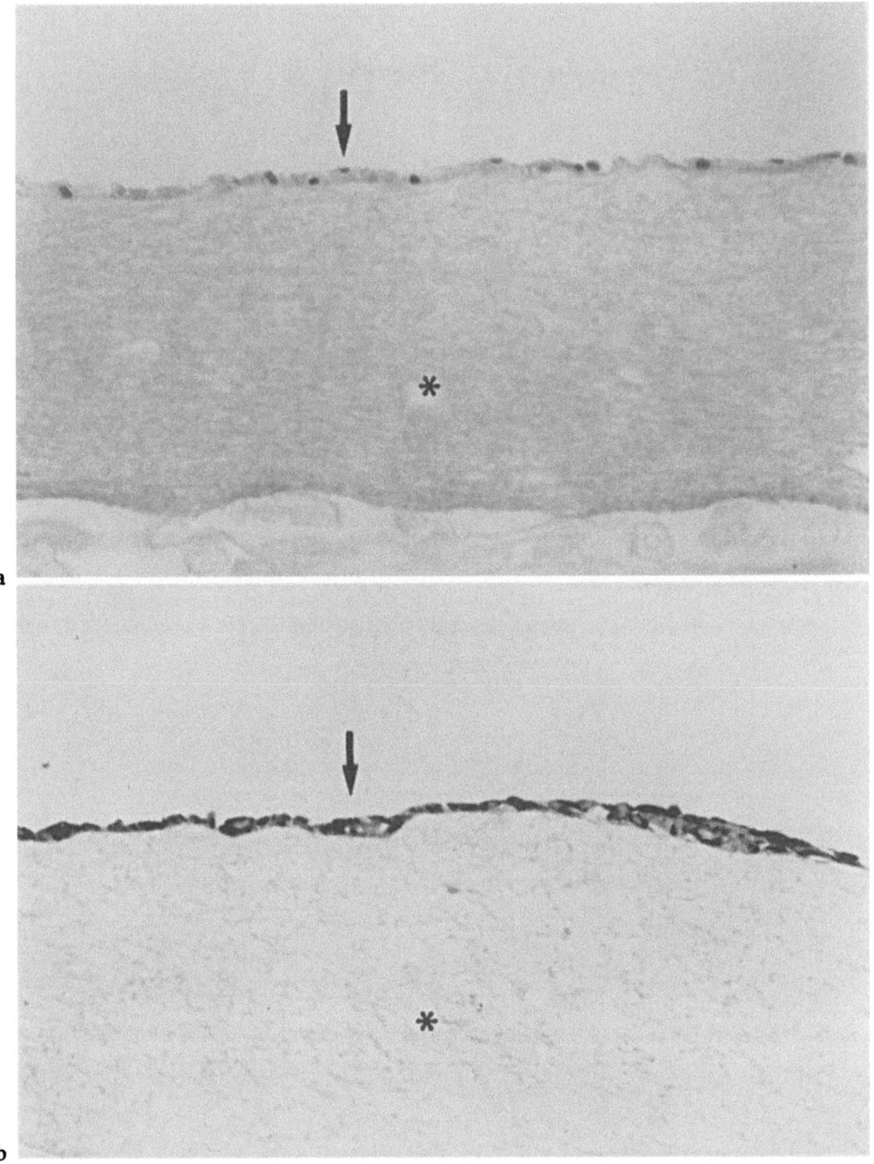

Fig. 5a,b. Light micrograph of paraffin sections shows mesothelial cells (*arrow*) covering the surface of the gel matrix (*asterisk*). **a** H&E. **b** Cytokeratin 8. × 200

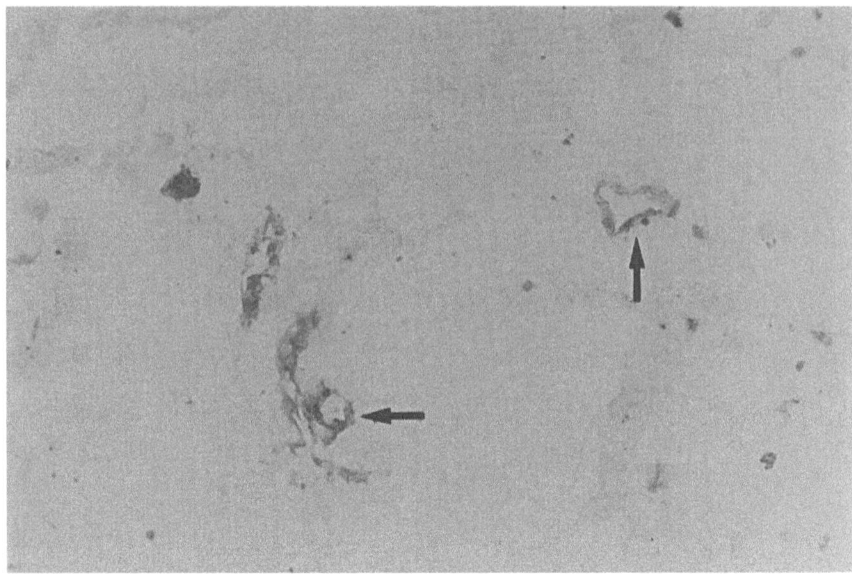

Fig. 6. Frozen section of three-dimensional in vitro model with neovessels (*arrows*) showing the expression of E selectin by the alkaline phosphatase–anti-alkaline phosphatase (APAAP) method. × 200

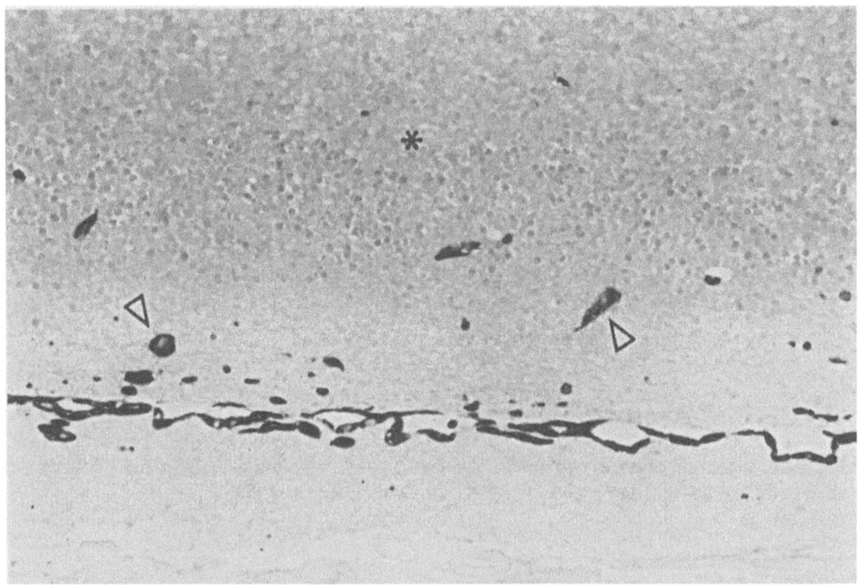

Fig. 7. Three-dimensional model with a lining of mesothelial cells stained by cytokeratin 8 show, after exposure to a blood clot (*asterisk*), a migration of cells (*arrowheads*) into the clot. × 200

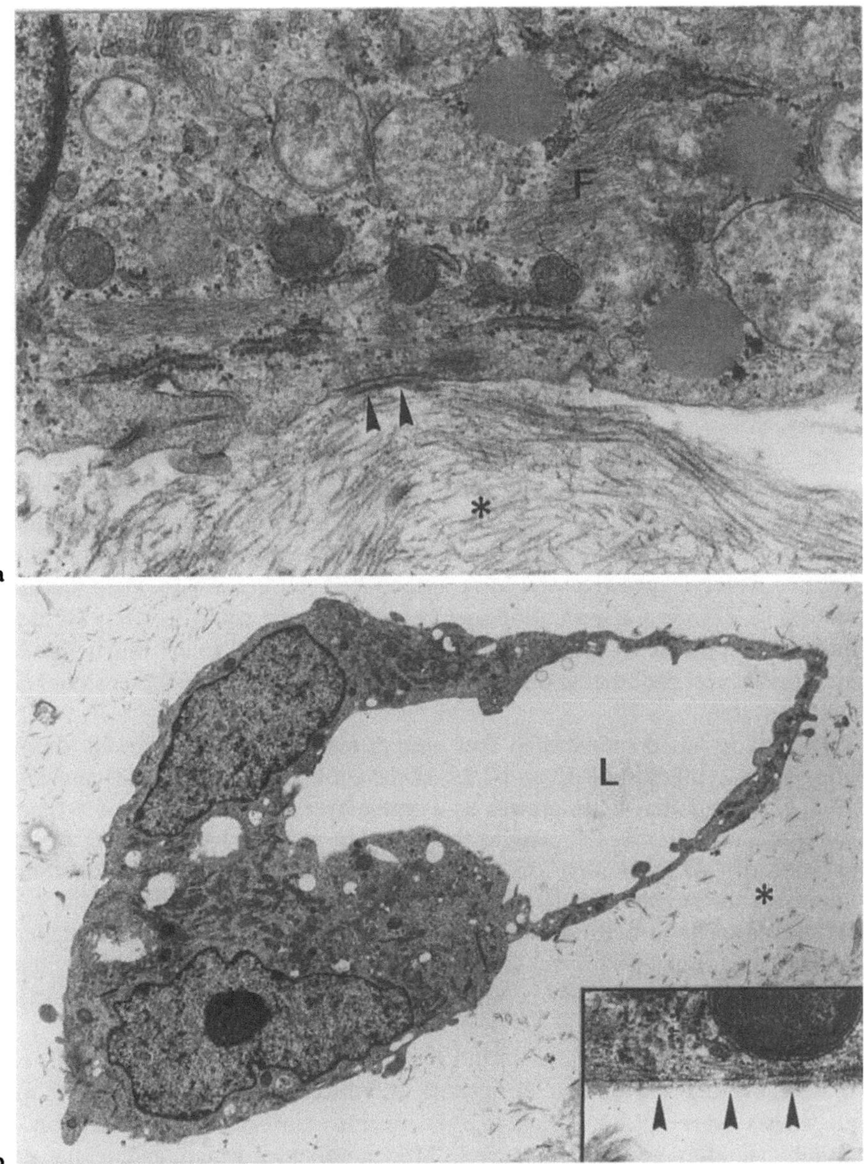

Fig. 8a,b. Ultrastructural analysis (transmission electron micrographs, TEM). **a** Mesothelial cells on type I collagen (*asterisk*) with bundles of tonofilaments (F). × 36 000. **b** Endothelial cells with lumina (*L*) surrounded by type I collagen (*asterisk*, × 5500) with a new basal lamina (*arrowheads* in *inset*) beneath the cell membrane in contact with the collagen gel. × 48 000

Discussion

Peritoneal inflammation and adhesion are grave complications after ischaemia, mechanical trauma, sepsis and surgery. The pathogenesis [3, 8, 33, 36, 47] and the role of mesothelial cells have been extensively investigated [10, 34, 46], although most steps are still incompletely understood. Endothelial cells, a fundamental part of the wound-healing process, play an important role in the development of peritoneal adhesions and therefore should be included in relevant experimental models.

The difficulties in understanding the cellular mechanisms resulting in adhesion formation have been added to by the fact that several of the models used up to now (especially animal experiments) do not provide comparable circumstances for investigation. Therefore, new models are necessary in which all the conditions are exactly known, so that experiments can be reduced to the essentials.

In contrast to animal experiments, cell culture offers the possibility of investigating the biology of cells in defined conditions and provides several options for developing different culture models, e.g. three-dimensional culture models. In this context and based on the role of collagen in morphogenesis, several investigators have established numerous in vitro culture models [2, 37]. As a major component of ECM, type I collagen offers an ideal matrix component to reconstruct the peritoneum in vitro in which human mesothelial and endothelial cells could be cultivated in a three-dimensional co-culture system.

Our study has demonstrated that human mesothelial cells showed the expression of cytokeratin 8/18 and 7/19, as described by Wu et al. [48] and Moll et al. [29], and that their growth as a monolayer on the surface of a type I collagen gel matrix was similar to the situation in vivo. Furthermore, the expression of CAM was identical to in vitro experiments [6]. Ultrastructurally, numerous microvilli were demonstrated on the cell surface of mesothelial cells [11, 41, 43]. The formation of a new basal lamina beneath the mesothelial cell layer similar to the peritoneal serosa [10, 19] and the migration into the blood clot confirm that in vivo-like conditions were achieved and should therefore be a matter of experimental research in future.

Endothelial cells cultivated within the gel showed a rearrangement of neovessels forming a wide-spread network in which the different stages of angiogenesis were visible [18, 24, 39]. In this context, the cytoskeleton is modulated after interaction with ECM components, which enable the endothelial cells to spread into the matrix.

This rearrangement into anastomosed neovessels has already been described by Folkman [16, 17], Ausprunk et al. [1], Maciag et al. [27], Sholley et al. [38], Ingber et al. [20] and Ishiwata et al. [21].

The three-dimensional co-culture model offers the possibility of analysing the mechanisms (cell–cell and cell–matrix interactions) involved in peritoneal inflammation and in the development of peritoneal adhesion under in vivo-like conditions. Such a model is not only valuable in investigating the pathogenesis of peritoneal adhesion, but, in addition, the present study gives us the opportunity to develop different tissue-like matrices to analyse other specific pathological processes. In conclusion, not only inflammatory processes, but also regulatory mechanisms in tumour metastasis (peritoneal carcinosis) could be subjects of further investigations.

Summary

Peritoneal adhesions are a common problem in abdominal and gynecological surgery. The pathogenesis of these processes remains unclarified in spite of intensive research. The aim of this study is to establish a new in vitro model for investigating the cellular mechanisms involved in the development of peritoneal adhesions. Such a model should include all components which play an important role in vivo, such as extracellular matrix and endothelial and mesothelial cells. We present a study on cultured omentum-derived mesothelial and microvascular endothelial cells on and in a three-dimensional collagen matrix, where both cell types maintain their characteristic morphology, forming an in vitro-like peritoneum. Cell–cell and cell–matrix interactions, which are involved in peritoneal adhesions, could be investigated in detail, including their kinetics. The present model provides a wide field for analysing the complex problems in adhesion formation. Furthermore, different cell types (e.g. inflammatory cells) can be employed to simulate acute peritonitis.

Acknowledgements. The authors express their gratitude to the State Ministry of Science of Rheinland-Pfalz for generous financial support. We also thank Miss M. Löbig and Miss L. Krecker for their technical assistance. Miss M. Müller for help in the electron microscopical analysis of this project and Mr P. Pulkowski for his excellent photographic assistance.

References

1. Ausprunk DH, Folkman J (1977) Migration and proliferation of endothelial cells in preformed and newly formed blood vessels during tumor angiogenesis. Microvasc Res 14: 175–202
2. Bennett DG (1980) Morphogenesis of branching tubulus in cultures of cloned mammary epithelial cells. Nature 285: 657–659
3. Benzer H, Blumel G, Piza F (1963) Über Zusammenhänge zwischen Fibrinolyse und intraperitonealen Adhäsionen. Klin Wochenschr 75: 881
4. Bittinger F, Salih V, Kirkpatrick CJ (1992) In Vitro-Modell zur Untersuchung der Angiogenese. Verh Dtsch Ges Pathol 76: 352 (abstr)
5. Bittinger F, Mühlbayer S, Kirkpatrick CJ (1993) Dreidimensionales Modell für die in vitro-Untersuchung der zellulären Dynamik des Mesotheliums bei Verwachsungen. Verh Dtsch Ges Pathol 77: 388 (abstr)
6. Bittinger F, Köhler H, Klein CL, Kirkpatrick CJ (1995) Expression of adhesion molecules ICAM-1, VCAM-1 and E-selectin on human mesothelial cells in vitro and in vivo. Pathol Res Pract 191: 208 (abstr)
7. Boys F (1942) The prophylaxis of peritoneal adhesions: a review of the literature. Surgery 11: 118–168
8. Buckman RF, Woods M, Sargent L, Gervin AS (1976) A unifying mechanism in the etiology of intraperitoneal adhesions. J Surg Res 20: 1–5

9. Connolly JE, Smith JW (1960) The prevention and treatment of intestinal adhesions. Int Abstr Surg 110: 417–431
10. Davila RM, Crouch EC (1993) Role of mesothelial and submesothelial stromal cells in matrix remodeling following pleural injury. Am J Pathol 142(2): 547–555
11. Dobbie JW (1989) Morphology of the peritoneum in CAPD. Blood 7: 74–85
12. Dobbie JW (1990) New concepts in molecular biology and ultrastructural pathology of the peritoneum: their significance for peritoneal dialysis. Am J Kidney Dis 15(2): 97–109
13. Ellis H (1971) The cause and prevention of postoperative intraperitoneal adhesions. Surg Gynecol Obstet 133: 497–511
14. Elsdale T, Bard J (1972) Collagen substrate for studies on cell behavior. J Cell Biol 54: 626–637
15. Enami J, Enami S, Kawamura K, Kohmoto K, Hata M, Koezuka M, Koga M (1987) Growth of normal and neoplastic mammary epithelial cells of the mouse by mammary fibroblast-conditioned medium factor. In: Enami J, Ham RG (eds) Growth and differentiation of mammary epithelial cells in culture. Japan Scientific Societies Press, Tokyo, p 125
16. Folkman J (1972) Anti-angiogenesis: new concept for therapy of solid tumors. Ann Surg 175: 409–416
17. Folkman J (1985) Tumor angiogenesis. Adv Cancer Res 43: 175–202
18. Folkman J, Haudenschild C (1980) Angiogenesis in vitro. Nature 288: 551–556
19. Gay S, Viljanto J, Raekkallio J, Penttinen R (1978) Collagen types in early phases of wound healing in children. Acta Chir Scand 144: 205
20. Ingber DE, Folkman J (1989) Mechanochemical switching between growth and differentiation during fibroblast growth factor-stimulated angiogenesis in vitro: role of extracellular matrix. J Cell Biol 109: 317–330
21. Ishiwata I, Ishiwata C, Soma M, Naik DR, Hashimoto H, Sudo T, Ishikawa H (1990) Effect of tumour angiogenesis factor on proliferation of endothelial cell and tube formation. Virchows Archiv A Pathol Anat 417: 473–476
22. Jackson CJ, Garbett PK, Nissen B, Schrieber L (1990) Binding of human endothelium to Ulex europaeus I-coated dynabeads. Application to the isolation of microvascular endothelium. J Cell Sci 96: 257–262
23. Jaffe EA, Nachman RL, Becker CG, Minick CR (1973) Culture of human endothelial cells derived from umbilical veins. J Clin Invest 52: 2745–2756
24. Klagsbrun M, D'Amore PA (1991) Regulators of angiogenesis. Annu Rev Physiol 53: 217–239
25. Klein CL, Bittinger F, Skarke C, Wagner M, Köhler H, Walgenbach S, Kirkpatrick CJ (1995) Effects of cytokines on the expression of cell adhesion molecules by cultured human omental mesothelial cells. Pathobiology 63: 204–212
26. Klein CL, Köhler H, Bittinger F, Wagner M, Hermanns I, Grant K, Lewis JC, Kirkpatrick CJ (1994) Comparative studies on vascular endothelium in vitro. I. Cytokine effects on the expression of adhesional molecules by human umbilical vein and femoral artery endothelial cells. Pathobiology 62: 199–208
27. Maciag T, Kadish J, Wilkins L, Stemerman MB, Weinstein R (1982) Organizational behavior of human umbilical vein endothelial cells. J Cell Biol 94: 511–520
28. Merlo G, Fousoni G, Barbero C, Castagna B (1980) Fibrinolytic activity of the human peritoneum. Eur Surg Res 12: 433–438
29. Moll R (1993) Cytokeratine als Differenzierungsmarker: Expressionsprofile von Epithelien und epithelialen Tumoren. Progr Pathol 142: 112–117
30. Murray JC, Stingle G, Kleinman HK, Martin GR, Katz SI (1987) Epidermal cells adhere preferentially to type IV (basement membrane) collagen. J Cell Biol 80: 197–202
31. Muscatello G (1895) Ueber den Bau und das Aufsaugungsvermögen des Peritonäum. Virchows Archiv 142: 327–358
32. Nicholson LJ, Clarke JMF, Pittilo RM, Machin SJ, Woolf N (1984) The mesothelial cell as a non-thrombogenic surface. Thromb Haemost 52: 102–104
33. Raftery AT (1981) Effect of peritoneal trauma on peritoneal fibrinolytic activity and intraperitoneal adhesion formation. Eur Surg Res 13: 397–401
34. Renvall S, Lehto M, Penttinen R (1987) Development of peritoneal fibrosis occurs under the mesothelial cell layer. J Surg Res 43: 407–412

35. Richardson KH (1911) Studies on peritoneal adhesions with a contribution to the treatment of denuded bowel surfaces. Am Surg 54: 758–797
36. Ryan GB, Grobety BS, Majno G (1971) Postoperative peritoneal adhesions. Am J Pathol 65: 117–148
37. Schor AM, Schor SL, Kumar S (1979) Importance of a collagen substratum for stimulation of capillary endothelial cell proliferation for tumor angiogenesis factor. Int J Cancer 24(2): 225–234
38. Sholley MM, Ferguson GP, Seibel HR, Montour JL, Wilson JD (1984) Mechanisms of neovascularization: vascular sprouting can occur without proliferation of endothelial cells. Lab Invest 51: 624–634
39. Speidel CC (1933) Studies of living nerves: activities of ameboid growth cones, sheath cells, and myelin segments, as revealed by prolonged observation of individual nerve fibers in frog tadpoles. Am J Anat 52: 1–79
40. Stephenson TJ, Griffiths DW, Mills PM (1986) Comparison of Ulex europaeus I lectin binding and factor VIII-related antigen as markers of vascular endothelium in follicular carcinoma of the thyroid. Histopathology 10(3): 251–260
41. Stylianou E, Jenner LA, Davies M, Coles GA, Williams JD (1990) Isolation, culture and characterization of human peritoneal mesothelial cells. Kidney Int 37: 1563–1570
42. Sugihara H, Toda S, Miyabara C, Yonemitsu N (1993) Reconstruction of alveolus-like structure from alveolar type II epithelial cells in three-dimensional collagen gel matrix culture. Am J Pathol 142: 783–792
43. Thomas N (1987) Embryology and structure of the mesothelium. In: Jones JSP (ed) Pathology of the mesothelium. Springer, Berlin Heidelberg New York, pp 1–13
44. Toda S, Sugihara H (1990) Reconstruction of thyroid follicles from isolated porcine follicle cells in three-dimensional collagen gel culture. Endocrinology 126: 2027–2034
45. Toda S, Yonemitsu N, Hikichi Y, Sugihara H (1992) Differentiation of human thyroid follicle cells from normal subjects and Basedow's disease in three-dimensional collagen gel culture. Pathol Res Pract 188: 874–882
46. van Hinsbergh VWM, Kooistra T, Scheffer MA, van Bockel JH, van Murjen GNP (1990) Characterization and fibrinolytic properties of human omental tissue mesothelial cells. Comparison with endothelial cells. Blood 75: 1490–1497
47. Weibel MA, Majno G (1973) Peritoneal adhesions and their relation to abdominal surgery. Am J Surg 126: 345–353
48. Wu YJ, Parker LM, Binder NE, Beckett MA, Sinard JH, Griffiths CT, Rheinwald JG (1982) The mesothelial keratins: a new family of cytoskeletal proteins identified in cultured mesothelial cells and nonkertinizing epithelia. Cell 31: 693–703

2.3 Zinc Induces Heat Shock Protein-70 and Metallothionein Expression in the Small Bowel and Protects Against Ischemia

B. Klosterhalfen, C. Töns, H.M. Klein, L. Tietze, C. Mittermayer, M. Anurov, B.S. Titkova, and A. Öttinger

Introduction

Mesenteric ischemia as an acute disease has a fatal outcome in about 60% of all patients [1]. Small intestinal ischemic necrosis occurs predominantly in elderly individuals with cardiovascular disease, artherosclerosis, and coagulative disorders [1, 2]. Intestinal damage occurs within minutes of total circulatory arrest, with the mucosa most sensitive to injury, followed by edema, hemorrhage, and sloughing. Within 1 h, the upper two thirds of the villi are denuded. If the blood supply is cut off for more than 2 h, the mucosa becomes progressively destroyed with subsequent development of transmural necrosis [3–5].

At the level of a single cell, nature has evolved a system that allows the cell and virtually all organ systems, from bacteria to mammals, to tolerate stresses that might be otherwise lethal. The defense mechanism is commonly referred to as the stress response and can be initiated by a wide variety of different agents, including ischemia, several types of metabolic stress, and hyperthermia [6–9]. The general pattern of the stress response in all organisms is the rapid and almost exclusive synthesis of a small number of intracellular proteins, the so-called stress proteins, including heat shock proteins (HSP) and metallothionein (MT).

HSP and MT have proven in many in vivo and in vitro studies to have beneficial effects in ischemic heart, skeletal muscle, and brain disease [10–13], septic shock [14–16], and radiation disease [17].

From all we know about stress protein expression in various organs due to different stress factors, it can be postulated that these proteins are also induced in intestinal ischemia. Furthermore, stress protein induction promises to be the basis of an effective therapeutic approach in intestinal ischemia of various etiologies and the development of protective effects in major gut surgery.

The present study was designed to prove whether preinduction of HSP-70 and MT with zinc protects the small bowel of rats against ischemia.

Materials and Methods

Animal Model

Male Wistar rats weighing 250 g were subjected to ischemia of the small bowel by isolation of a defined small-bowel segment. The test group ($n=12$) received zinc bis-(DL-hydrogen aspartate) (UNIZINK, Köhler Pharma, Germany) at a dose of 50 mg/kg (i.e., 10 mg zinc/kg) intraperitoneally 24 h before ligation; the control group ($n=12$) received the same amount of saline solution. Four animals each in the test and the control group were killed 24 h after zinc or saline administration, but without ligation of the small bowel, in order to determine the stress response to zinc before ischemia. Tissue samples of the small bowel were collected before and 2, 4, and 6 h after ligation. The specimens were finally investigated by conventional histology with hematoxylin and eosin (H&E) stains and immunohistochemistry against HSP-70 and MT by the indirect immunoperoxidase reaction. The histological alterations of the tissue specimens were assessed according to a modified version of the classification by Park [18] (Table 1).

All operations on the control and test animals were done under i.p. anesthesia with xylazine (Rompun; 8mg/kg) and Ketamine (Ketanest; 80 mg/kg) simultaneously.

Table 1. Modified classification of Park [18] used in this study to divide the extent of ischemic tissue necrosis into defined stages

Injury type	Grade	Histologic features
No injury	0	Normal mucosal villi
Superficial mucosal injury	1	Development of subepithelial Gruenhagen's space, usually at the apex of the villus; often with capillary congestion or extension of the subepithelial space with moderate lifting of epithelial layer from the lamina propria
	2	Massive epithelial lifting and desintegration of the epithelial layer; denuded villi with lamina propria and dilated capillaries exposed; increased cellularity of lamina propria
	3	Digestion and disintegration of lamina propria; hemorrhage and ulceration
Deep mucosal injury	4	Injury of the crypt layer with incomplete or complete necrosis
	5	Complete transmucosal necrosis including the muscularis mucosae
Mural injury	6	Incomplete transmural necrosis
	7	Complete transmural necrosis
	8	Complete transmural necrosis with intramural gas formation

Antibodies

Antibodies used included monoclonal mouse anti-MT E9, M639, 1:200 (DAKO, Hamburg, Germany) and polyclonal rabbit anti-HSP-70 A500, 1:200 (DAKO, Hamburg, Germany). Anti-HSP-70 reacts strongly with the two major HSP-70 proteins (HSP-72 and HSP-73). Anti-MT is directed against the products of two separate groups of genes in the human genome, MT-1 and MT-2. The products are a group of low molecular weight proteins (approximately 6 kDa) containing a single chain of 61 amino acids which is folded doubly within two domains, A and B.

Light Microscopy and Immunohistochemistry

Tissue samples were fixed in 10% formalin and embedded in paraffin, and sections were stained with H&E and periodic acid–Schiff (PAS) plus diastase and Alcian blue for mucin. Immunohistochemistry was performed on the paraffin-embedded material using the avidin–biotin complex method, with diaminobenzidine as a chromogen. The same staining method was used in all test and control animals, and each stain was performed twice on separate days. The immunohistological staining intensity in viable gut parts was scored as nonreactive (–), low (+), moderate (++), and intense (+++).

Statistics

Statistical analysis was carried out using Statistical Package for Social Sciences (SPSS) software. The two-tailed Fisher exact test was used to compare the staining intensity for the various reactions. Student's *t* test was used to examine the results of the histological determination of ischemic small-bowel injury, and p values less than 0.01 were considered to be significant.

Results

Immunohistochemistry of the test animals (n=4) receiving zinc showed a significant induction of HSP-70 and MT in the small bowel. HSP-70 was expressed in the mucosa, in particular in the tips of the villi (Fig. 1A). In addition, the gut wall structures, including the smooth muscle, the vessel walls, and endothelial and mesothelial cells, showed a significantly increased staining pattern against the HSP-70 antibody. In contrast, MT was mainly expressed in the basal mucosa (Fig. 1B), whereas gut wall structures showed only weak MT expression. The control animals showed no or only focal HSP-70 or MT antibody reaction by immunohistochemistry (Table 2).

Histology of small-bowel tissue specimens showed no significant morphological alterations at 0 h in either the test or the control group. At 2 h, the control group already showed complete transmucosal necrosis, whereas the

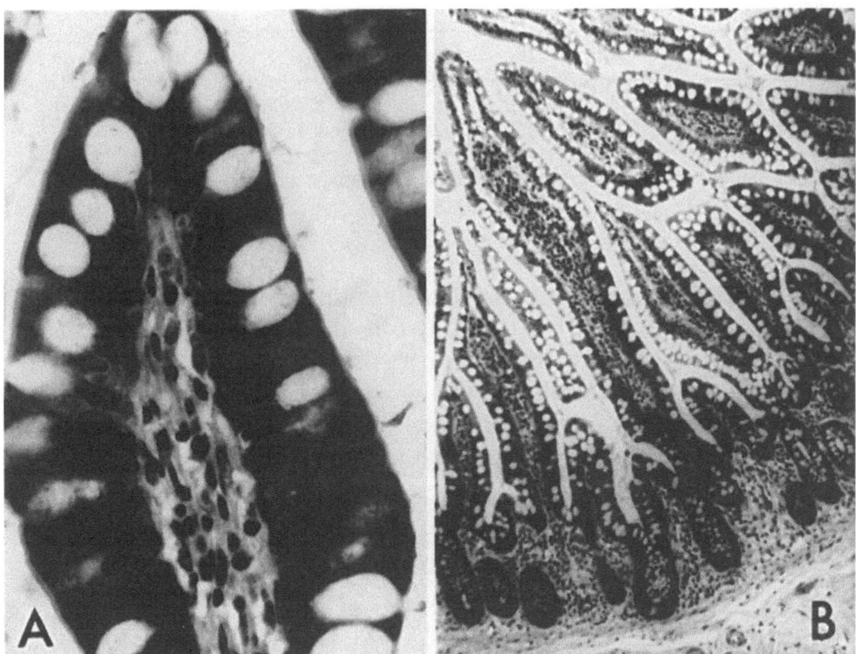

Fig. 1A,B. Induction of **A** heat shock protein (HSP)-70 and **B** metallothionein (MT) in the small bowel of the test group after 24 h by zinc bis-(DL-hydrogen aspartate); HSP-70 is mainly expressed in the tips of the villi, and MT mainly in the crypt layer. x 40

test group showed superficial mucosal lesions (4.8 ± 1.46 versus 1.71 ± 0.62; $p < 0.01$) (Table 3). At 4 h, histology of the controls revealed incomplete transmural necrosis, while histology of the test group showed complete disturbance of the epithelial cell layer with denuded villi and digestion and des-

Table 2. Summary of the immunohistological staining results after induction of heat shock protein (HSP)-70 and metallothionein (MT) with zinc bis-(DL-hydrogen aspartate)

	Control Group		Test Group	
	MT	HSP70	MT	HSP70
Tips of villi	–	–	+	+++[*]
Basal mucosa	+	–	+++[*]	+/++
Smooth muscle	–	+	+	+++[*]
Vessel walls	–	+	+	+++[*]
Endothelial cells	–	(+)	+	++[*]
Mesothelial cells	–	–	+	++[*]

–, No reaction; +, low reaction; ++, moderate reaction; +++, intense reaction.
[*]$p < 0.01$.

Table 3. Time course of ischemic small-bowel necrosis after 0, 2, 4 and 6 h in the control and test group

	0 h	2h	4 h	6 h
Control group	0	4.8 ± 1.46	6.34 ± 2.63	7.13 ± 2.05
Test group	0	1.71 ± 0.62[*]	3.49 ± 1.37[*]	6.78 ± 2.8

Values given are given in average grades of tissue damage ± S.D.
[*]$p < 0.01$.

integration of the lamina propria, as well as injury of the crypt layer (6.34 ± 2.63 versus 3.49 ± 1.37; $p < 0.01$). At 6 h, the histological picture in both groups showed incomplete or complete transmural necrosis (7.13 ± 2.05 versus 6.78 ± 2.8; $p > 0.01$). While the test group revealed significantly decreased ischemic tissue injury in the small bowel within the first 4 h, no difference was observed after 6 h between control and test group animals.

Discussion

As previously shown in many studies [19–21], the first detectable sign of gut ischemia is increased permeability. With long-term ischemia, the permeability is further increased, with subsequent mucosal epithelial cell injury that is morphologically detectable. Intestinal mucosal injury should be considered as a continuum of injury ranging from increased permeability to definite tissue destruction in the small bowel and the large intestines. The extent and duration of ischemia appears to directly correlate with the depth of tissue injury [19]. Altogether, the reaction pattern in the small bowel and the large intestine is similar, although the small bowel showed an increased vulnerability to ischemia compared to the large intestine.

The intact gut mucosa serves as a barrier between the nonsterile lumen and the sterile peritoneal cavity. Bacteria sometimes penetrate this barrier, a process referred to as translocation [22]. Recent publications have increasingly focused on the role of the gastrointestinal tract as a reservoir of pathogens that can enter the circulation by translocation, initiating septic processes and eventually leading to multiple organ failure [23]. While systemic circulatory disturbances generally lead to ischemic lesions limited to the tips of the villi, complete circulatory arrest within the mesenteric arteries induces rapid and severe tissue damage and translocation of pathogens. In patients with mesenteric artery occlusion, the dysfunction and destruction of the mucosal gut barrier become manifest as septic and organ failure complications in the majority of these patients.

The immunological system of the gut, functioning as an effective barrier against intraluminal pathogens, is supported by different mechanisms. The Peyer's patches of the intestinal wall, together with the lymphocytes, macrophages, and local immunoglobulin A (IgA) production combined with IgA present in bile, provides a special defense system [24]. The Kupffer cells and endothelial cells of the liver serve as a cellular back-up system before entrance into the systemic circulation. Bacterial particles entering the circulation can also be cleared and detoxified to some extent in the serum. Serum proteins, predominantly lipopolysaccharide-binding proteins, bactericidal or permeability-increasing protein, and high-density lipoprotein, play an important role in this system. An additional immunological defense system of the gut might be the expression of intracellular stress protein with an increased stress resistance of the gut, in particular in mucosal epithelial gut cells.

The present study proves that induction of HSP-70 and MT by zinc is an effective strategy to protect the small bowel against ischemia with total circulatory arrest for about 4 h. After 6 h arrest, even the HSP-70- and MT-protected test animals developed incomplete transmural necrosis of the isolated segment.

In agreement with this study, in 1991 Yoshikawa et al. [25] reported that a novel synthetic zinc–carnosine chelate compound provided a protective effect against aggravation of gastric mucosal injury by ischemia-reperfusion in rats.

The mechanism of stress protein induction by zinc remains unclear. Pretreatment with zinc with a subsequent increase of MT expression can be interpreted by the increased flow of zinc into the subcellular fractions [26]. A recent study showed that MT gene expression is markedly induced by zinc at day 18 of fetal life in the rat intestine to a level that remains constant throughout postnatal life [27]. Furthermore, MT has a central role in heavy metal absorption in the intestinal tract [28] with increased MT levels after increased intestinal heavy metal uptake.

The interrelation between zinc and HSP-70 expression is still unclear. Recent studies, however, show that zinc induces cytokines in human peripheral blood mononuclear cells [29] and that it regulates cytokine induction by superantigens and lipopolysaccharide in polymorphonuclear cells and whole blood cultures [30]. Cytokines likely stimulate HSP-70 production, but this is not yet completely understood, whereas the induction of MT by cytokines in rat tissues was recently shown by Sato et al. [31]. On the other hand, recent studies proved that the expression of HSP-70 concomitantly inhibits the production of these cytokines in human monocytes and mouse macrophages activated by lipopolysaccharide [32].

In conclusion, our study shows that induction of HSP-70 and MT by zinc is an appropriate method to reduce ischemic small-bowel tissue damage in rats. The underlying mechanisms are still poorly understood and urgently need further investigation. Understanding the molecular mechanisms that lead to increased HSP-70 expression and decreased cytokine biosynthesis may help us to establish new strategies to prevent ischemic intestinal lesions in future.

Summary

To investigate whether preinduction of HSP-70 and MT with zinc protects the small bowel of rats against ischemia, ischemia was induced in 16 male Wistar rats weighing 250 g by isolating a defined small bowel segment. The test group (n=12) was injected with zinc-bis-(DL-hydrogen aspartate) (UNIZINK, Köhler Pharma, FRG) at a dose of 50 mg/kg (i.e., 10 mg zinc/kg) intraperitoneally 24 h before ligation. The control group (n=12) received the same amount of saline solution. Four animals each from both the test and the control group were killed 24 h after zinc or saline application, but without ligation of the small bowel to determine the stress response to zinc before ischemia.

Tissue samples of the small bowel were collected before and 2, 4 and 6 h after ligation and investigated histologically, immunohistochemically and by Western blotting. The test group showed a significantly increased intracellular expression of HSP-70 and MT after zinc injection. Histology after ischemia showed significantly decreased tissue necrosis in the test group compared with the controls.

In conclusion, induction of HSP-70 and MT by zinc is an effective strategy to protect the small bowel against ischemia in rats.

References

1. Moore WM, Hollier LH (1991) Mesenteric artery occlusive disease. Cardiol Clin 9: 535–541
2. Böttger T, Alpern S, Schäfer W, Weber W, Junginger T (1990) Value of preoperative diagnostics in acute mesenteric vascular occlusion – a prospective study. Lang Arch Chir 375: 278–282
3. Wagner R, Gabbert H, Hohn P (1979) The mechanism of epithelial shedding after ischemic damage to the small intestinal mucosa. Virch Arch (Cell Pathol) 30: 25–31
4. Wagner R, Gabbert H, Hohn P (1979) Ischemia and post-ischemic regeneration of small intestinal mucosa. Virch Arch (Cell Pathol) 31: 259–276
5. Ming SC, McNiff J (1976) Acute ischemic changes in intestinal muscularis. Am J Pathol 82: 315–326
6. Lindquist S, Craig EA (1988) The heat-shock proteins. Annu Rev Genet 22: 631–677
7. Nover L (ed) (1984) Heat shock response of eukaryotic cells. Springer, Berlin Heidelberg New York, pp 7–10
8. Riabowol KT, Mizzen LA, Welch WJ (1988) Heat shock is lethal to fibroblasts micro-injected with antibodies against HSP 70. Science 242: 433–436
9. Schlesinger MJ (1990) Heat shock proteins. J Biol Chem 265: 12111–12114
10. Hutter MM, Sievers RE, Barbosa V, Wolfe CL (1994) Heat-shock protein induction in rat hearts. A direct correlation between the amount of heat shock protein induced and the degree of myocardial protection. Circulation 89(1): 355–360
11. Garramone RR, Winters RM, Das DK, Deckers PJ (1994) Reduction of skeletal muscle injury through stress conditioning using the heat-shock response. Plast Reconstr Surg 93(6): 1242–1247
12. Andres J, Sharma HS, Knoll R, Stahl J, Sassen LM, Verdouw PD, Schaper W (1993) Expression of heat shock proteins in the normal and stunned porcine myocardium. Cardiovasc Res 27(8): 1421–1429
13. Marber MS, Latchman DS, Walker JM, Yellon DM (1993) Cardiac stress protein elevation 24 hours after brief ischemia or heat stress is associated with resistance to myocardial infarction. Circulation 88(3): 1264–1272
14. Ribeiro SP, Villar J, Downey G, Edelson JD, Slutsky AS (1994) Sodium arsenite induces heat shock protein-72 kilodalton expression in the lungs and protects rats against sepsis. Crit Care Med 22: 922–929
15. Villar J, Ribeiro SP, Mullen BM, Kuliszewski M, Post M, Slutsky AS (1994) Induction of heat shock response reduces mortality rate and organ damage in a sepsis-induced acute lung injury model. Crit Care Med 22: 914–921

16. Abe S, Matsumi M, Tsukioki M, Mizukawa S, Takahashi T, Iijimu Y, Itano Y, Kosaka F (1987) Metallothionein and zinc metabolism in endotoxin shock rats. EXS 52: 587–594
17. Matsubara J (1987) Alteration of radiosensitivity in metallothionein induced mice and a possible role of Zn-Cu-thionein in GSH-peroxidase system. EXS 52: 603–612
18. Park PO, Haglund U, Bulkley GB, Fält K (1990) The sequence of development of intestinal tissue injury following strangulation ischemia and reperfusion. Surgery 107: 574–580
19. Haglund U, Bulkley GB, Granger DN (1987) On the pathophysiology of intestinal ischemic injury. Acta Chir Scand 153: 321–324
20. Haglund U (1994) Gut ischaemia. Gut [Suppl] 1: S73–S76
21. Chiu CJ, McArdle AH, Brown R, Scott HJ, Gurd FN (1970) Intestinal mucosal lesion in low-flow states. Arch Surg 101: 478–483
22. Van Leeuwen PAM, Boermeester MA, Houdijk APJ, Ferwerda CHC, Cuesta MA, Meyer S, Wesdorp RIC (1994) Clinical significance of translocation. Gut [Suppl]: S28–S34
23. Van Deventer SJH, Ten Cate JW, Tytgat GNJ (1988) Intestinal endotoxemia. Gastroenterology 94: 824–831
24. Dobbins WO (1982) Gut immunopathology: a gastroenterologist view with emphasis on pathophysiology. Am J Phys 242: 91–98
25. Yoshikawa T, Naito Y, Tanigawa T, Yoneta T, Yasuda M, Ueda S, Oyamada H, Kondo M (1991) Effect of zinc-carnosine chelate compound (Z-103), a novel antioxidant, on acute gastric mucosal injury induced by ischemia-reperfusion in rats. Free Radic Res Commun 14(4): 289–296
26. Cosson RP (1994) Heavy metal intracellular balance and relationship with metallothionein induction in the gills of carp. After contamination by Ag, Cd, and Hg following pretreatment with Zn or not. Biol Trace Elem Res 46(3): 229–245
27. Mengheri E, Murgia C, Vignolini F, Nobili F, Gaetani S (1993) Metallothionein gene is expressed in developing rat intestine and is induced by zinc but not by corticosteroids. J Nutr 123(5): 817–822
28. Cousins RJ (1985) Absorption, transport, and hepatic metabolism of copper and zinc: special reference to metallothionein and ceruloplasmin. Physiol Rev 65(2): 238–309
29. Driessen C, Hirv K, Rink L, Kirchner H (1994) Induction of cytokines by zinc ions in human peripheral blood mononuclear cells and seperated monocytes. Lymphokine Cytokine Res 13(1): 15–20
30. Driessen C, Hirv K, Kirchner H, Rink L (1995) Zinc regulates cytokine induction by superantigens and lipopolysaccharide. Immunology 84(2): 272–277
31. Sato M, Sasaki M, Hojo H (1994) Differential induction of metallothionein synthesis by interleukin-6 and tumor necrosis factor-alpha in rat tissues. Int J Immunopharmacol 16(2): 187–195
32. Hall TJ (1994) Role of HSP70 in cytokine production. Experientia 50(11–12): 1048–1053

2.4 Anti-interleukin-10: Effect on Postoperative Intraperitoneal Adhesion Formation in a Murine Model

F.J. Montz, P.M. Cristoforoni, C. Holschneider, M. Punyasavatsut, and E. Abed

Introduction

Despite the expenditure of millions of dollars in the development of agents intended to limit their occurrence, intraperitoneal adhesions remain a major source of surgery-related morbidity and mortality as well as a financial burden on Western health care systems [1, 2]. The inadequacies of presently available antiadhesion modalities probably arise from the inability or failure to employ evidence based on rational drug and device development, as much of what occurs at a molecular biologic level following the occurrence of a peritoneal injury is unknown. Drugs and devices such as barriers have often been selected based on their theoretical potential for success, and not on a thorough understanding of the cellular or molecular changes that lead to adhesion formation and what happens when these predictable changes are modified. Though the serial cellular events that transpire following a peritoneal injury have been defined [3], the exact role of cytokines in peritoneal repair and adhesion formation has only been partially elucidated. Preliminary data exist demonstrating that numerous cytokines such as interleukin (IL)-1 [4, 5], IL-2, transforming growth factor (TGF)-β, and platelet-derived growth factor (PDGF)-β [6] are potentiators of postoperative adhesion formation, while IL-10 (cytokine synthesis-inhibiting factor, CSIF) significantly inhibits such adhesion formation [7]. We proposed to confirm our prior findings regarding the adhesion prevention properties of IL-10. Secondly, we were interested in determining whether there was a pronounced increase in IL-10 production following peritoneal injury. Lastly, we were interested in evaluating what effect an anti-IL-10 monoclonal antibody (mAb) would have on the development of postsurgical adhesion formation in a well-standardized animal model. This latter investigation would be undertaken in an attempt to determine whether endogenous IL-10 production that may not be appreciated by enzyme-linked immunosorbent assay (ELISA) determination of IL-10 concentrations in lavage fluids is a significant component in the cytokine response to peritoneal injury.

Materials and Methods

After obtaining approval from the UCLA Animal Research Committee, a total of 220 6-week-old female Swiss Webster mice (Simonsen Laboratories, Inc.,

Gilroy, CA) were used for our series of investigations. The animals were housed at the UCLA Vivarium. All animal procedures were performed in accordance with the standards described in the National Institute of Health (NIH) Guide for the Care and Use of Laboratory Animals, in compliance with the Federal Animal Welfare Act. Prior to surgery, the animals were allowed access to water and chow ad lib. Anesthesia was induced with inhaled halothane. Adequate anesthesia was maintained as necessary with halothane via a cotton ball. A sharp midline incision was made extending 2 cm from the symphysis to the upper abdomen. Intraperitoneal exploration was performed and any adhesions present quantified. Subsequently, a standardized left lower abdominal wall injury was induced using sharp abrasion so as to induce microhemorrhage and peritoneal disruption over an area of 2 cm^2. The anterior abdominal wall was closed using a running 3 0 Maxon suture (American Cyanamid Company, Danbury, CT) for the peritoneum/fascia/muscle in an en bloc technique, and the skin was closed using a running 3 0 silk suture. After recovery from anesthesia, animals were allowed immediate and unlimited access to water and chow.

The first 150 animals were used for an investigation of the in vivo role of IL-1α in postoperative adhesion formation, the results of which are reported elsewhere [8]. As part of this investigation, animals were randomized into 14 groups of ten animals each. These groups were serially killed at 8, 16, 24, 32, 40, 48, 56, 64, and 72 h and 4, 5, 6, 7, and 14 days postoperatively. A 15th group of ten animals served as nonoperative controls. At the time the animals were killed, the peritoneal cavity of each mouse was lavaged with 2 ml endotoxin-free phosphate-buffered saline (PBS) using 100% endotoxin-free plastics, needles, and glass. Samples were first centrifuged at 4 °C at 1200 g for 10 min, and then the supernatant was filter sterilized with a 0.22-micropore sterilizer. Filter-sterilized supernatants were stored at –20 °C in 0.5-ml aliquots.

For the investigations of the effects of anti-IL-10 mAb on adhesion formation, 70 animals were randomized into seven separate groups. Group I underwent induction of anesthesia, but had no surgical procedure performed (sham surgery). These animals received 1 ml endotoxin-free PBS administered transabdominally into the peritoneal cavity using an aseptic technique at time 0 and then 24, 48, and 72 h thereafter. Group II also did not undergo surgery and received 30 ng recombinant IL-10 (Peprotec, Rocky Hill, NJ; 98% purity, biological activity at 0.2–20.0 ng/ml) in 1 ml PBS intraperitoneally in the time schedule described above. Group III served as anti-IL-10 controls and received 30 ng rat anti-mouse IL-10 mAb (Pharmingen, San Diego, CA) in 1 ml PBS intraperitoneally on the same time schedule. Group IV underwent surgery only and received no postoperative injections. Group V underwent surgery and then received intra-abdominal vehicle alone in a manner similar to group I, with the first dose administered immediately after closure of the anterior abdominal wall via the percutaneous route. Group VI underwent surgery and IL-10 treatment like group II, while group VII was treated postoperatively using the same mAb and schedule as group III with, in both groups, the first administration being immediately after closure of the anterior abdominal wall. On postoperative day 7, the animals were killed using carbon dioxide euthanasia;

Table 1. Adhesion scoring

	Adhesion score
Extent	
None	0
Confined to traumatized area	1
Confined to nontraumatized area	2
In traumatized and nontraumatized areas	3
Type	
Filmy	1 × extent
Opaque, nonvascular	2 × extent
Opaque, vascular	3 × extent
Dense	4 × extent

Modified from [5].

they were examined and adhesions were quantified employing a modification of the method by Hershlag and associates [5]. This technique quantifies adhesions by extent and type to obtain a composite adhesion score for a given animal (Table 1).

Peritoneal lavage fluids collected at 0, 8, 16, and 32 h and at 3, 7, and 14 days were assayed using Endogen murine IL-10 ELISA (EM-IL10; Endogen Inc., Boston, MA), a commercially available ELISA kit. EM-IL10 is standardized to detect a minimum level of 0.14 units/ml of biologically active murine IL-10. EM-IL10 results in U/ml were converted to pg/ml using a conversion coefficient of 262 supplied by the manufacturer. EM-IL10 is specific for the measurement of natural and recombinant murine IL-10. It is reported to not crossreact with murine IL-2, IL-3, IL-4, granulocyte-macrophage colony-stimulating factor (GM-CSF), or tumor necrosis factor (TNF)-α.

Statistical analysis was performed using the SAS statistical package (SAS Institute, Inc., Cary, NC). Student's *t* test was employed to evaluate the differences between the means in group data, as was one-way ANOVA for the differences between all groups respectively. To correct for multiple comparisons, Bonferroni adjustment was carried out. The data were log-transformed prior to statistical analysis to account for heterogeneous variance.

Results

EM-IL10 was able to detect IL-10 in all lavage fluids assayed. These concentrations, regardless of time of collection, were consistently less than 0.2 ng/ml (Fig. 1). IL-10 biological activity is reported to be within the range of 0.2–20 ng/ml [9]. Therefore, there was no increase in intraperitoneal concentrations of IL-10 that would be considered biologically significant.

Regarding the group of animals in which we investigated the effects of anti-IL-10, there were no instances where intraperitoneal adhesions were evident at the time of the initial laparotomy. No abnormalities of healing of the anterior abdominal wall incision (e.g., wound disruption, infection) were noted in any

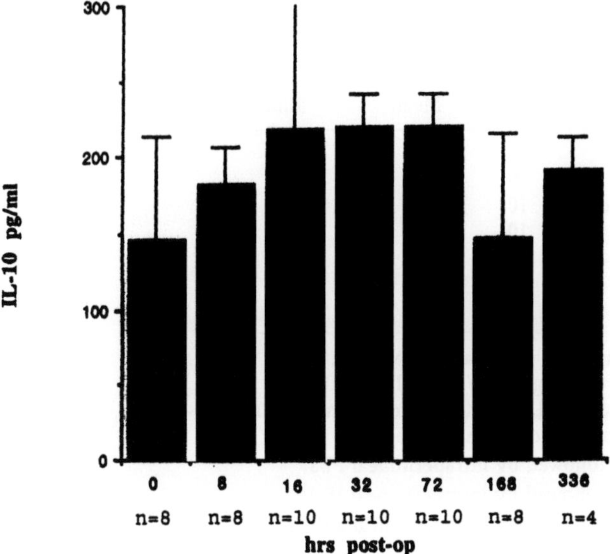

Fig. 1. Mean interleukin (IL)-10 concentrations in peritoneal lavages obtained at time of autopsy

of the animal groups that had undergone surgery, regardless of which of the study regimens they were assigned to. Four animals (one each in groups I and II that only underwent sham surgery and one each in groups VI and VII that underwent intraperitoneal surgery) died in the immediate perioperative period, presumably from anesthetic complications. Therefore, the total number of animals from whom data are available is 66.

There were no adhesions observed at posteuthanasia autopsy in mice that had not undergone surgery but had only been injected with PBS. Adhesions were rare in those animals receiving IL-10 or anti-IL-10 mAb without concomitant surgery. Remarkably, at the time of exploration, postoperative adhesions were universally found in animals which were either injected with PBS only (group V) or PBS with anti-IL-10 mAb (group VII) or which received no postoperative intraperitoneal injections (group IV).

There were no significant differences as regards postoperative adhesion scores between the three operative groups that did not receive IL-10 (group IV, 8.4 ± 5.3; group V, 8.1 ± 3.0; group VII, 10.5 ± 4.1; $p > 0.05$). In contrast, adhesions were noted to a lesser extent and degree in the majority of the IL-10-treated animals (group VI) (Table 2). Postoperative adhesion scores were significantly lower in the mice that were treated with IL-10 than in those that underwent surgery alone or surgery followed by intraperitoneal PBS administration or in similar animals that received anti-IL-10 mAb ($p < 0.005$).

Table 2. Adhesion scores

Group	Treatment	Mice	Adhesion scores	
		(n)	Mean	Range
I	PBS, control	9	0 ± 0	0–0
II	IL-10, control	9	0.1 ± 0.1	0–1
III	Anti-IL-10, control	10	0.3 ± 0.2	0–2
IV	Surgery, control	10	8.4 ± 5.3	1–16
V	Surgery + PBS[a]	10	8.1 ± 3.0	2–12
VI	Surgery + IL-10[b]	9	4.8 ± 2.2	2–9
VII	Surgery + anti-IL-10[c]	9	10.5 ± 4.1	4–16

Group V vs. VI, $p < 0.5$ (analysis of variance, ANOVA); group V vs. VII, not significant ($p = 0.1$); group VI vs. VII, $p < 0.001$.
PBS, phosphate-buffered saline; IL-10, interleukin-10; anti-IL-10, goat anti-mouse interleukin-10 monoclonal antibody.
[a]Surgically induced injury followed by intraperitoneal PBS.
[b]Surgically induced injury followed by intraperitoneal IL-10.
[c]Surgically induced injury followed by intraperitoneal anti-IL-10 monoclonal antibody.

Discussion

Cytokines are ubiquitous mediators of the immune response, affecting T cell, B cell, and macrophage function [10]. These molecules comprise a heterologous group of glycosylated proteins, all of which are of low molecular weight, but which share only small percentages of amino acid sequence concordance. Cytokines are extremely potent, demonstrating their effects locally and in a transient manner, with such effects occurring after binding to cell surface receptors. Cytokines are commonly grouped into families based on structural similarities. These major families are the hematopoietins, TNF, chemokines, interferons (INF), and IL.

There appear to be specific patterns of cytokines response to an immunologic challenge [11]. A type I response which involves type I T helper cells (Th-1) has an associated production of IL-2, INF-γ, TNF-α and -β, GM-CSF, and IL-3. These cytokines potentiate cell-mediated immune and inflammatory responses.

In contrast, a type II response involving type 2 T helper cells (Th-2) appears to revolve around the production of IL-4, IL-5, IL-6, and IL-10. The type II response has an associated increase in humoral (i.e., B cell-based) immune function with a relative suppression of cell-mediated and inflammatory responses.

The exact roles that cytokines play in the body's complex response to peritoneal injury is currently being defined. Though our understanding of the quantitative and temporal order of the cytokine response to a peritoneal injury is still somewhat primitive, it appears that IL-1α [4, 5] IL-2, PDGF, and TGF-β [6] all act potentiate adhesion formation. Recently it has been demonstrated that fibrous adhesive tissues actually have higher concentrations of TGF-β_1,

TGF-β_2, and TGF-β_3 than does intact peritoneum [12]. In contrast, IL-10, or CSIF as it has been labeled, curtails adhesion formation [7] while serving an autocrine function in the general inflammatory response [13]. It is IL-10's ability to suppress the proadhesion cytokines produced by Th-1 cells that is responsible for its adhesion and inflammation-preventing activities [14–20]. Based on the cumulative data, it appears that the extent to which postoperative adhesion formation occurs is probably a result of enhanced deposition of fibrin, decreased endogenous fibrinolytic activity, and the degree of cytokine-mediated stimulation of fibroblast proliferation and collagen production [7, 21, 22].

Whether IL-10 plays any role in counteracting the excess production of proadhesion cytokines in the untreated peritoneal milieu is unknown. As we have demonstrated, changes in peritoneal lavage concentrations of IL-10 following a standard adhesion-inducing injury are biologically insignificant.

Thus we administered high titers of anti-IL-10 mAb to block any small amounts of endogenous IL-10 that might be secreted in an autocrine/paracrine fashion. This blocking was manifested by a potentiation of postoperative intraperitoneal adhesion formation. As we failed to see adhesion potentiation in the anti-IL-10 mAb-treated animals, our data suggest that IL-10 probably does not play a significant role in the autocrine/paracrine regulation of proadhesion cytokines and subsequent adhesion formation.

This lack of a role for IL-10 is somewhat surprising. Though Th-2 helper T cell clones (the most potent endogenous source of IL-10) do not predominate at the site of peritoneal injury during repair, blood monocytes, which later differentiate into macrophages, are commonly found at the healing defect [23]. These later cells have been demonstrated to produce IL-10. It may be that the level of production is biologically insignificant and fails to induce a CSIF-like effect.

As this study has confirmed the adhesion-inhibiting effect of exogenous IL-10 while demonstrating that it is highly likely that surgical peritoneal injury fails to induce an increased level of intraperitoneal IL-10, we are investigating what steps could be taken to potentiate the production of endogenous IL-10 following a peritoneal injury in an attempt to improve natively occurring, biologic antiadhesion therapy.

Summary

The objective of this study was to determine the ability of an anti-IL-10 mAb to modify postoperative intraperitoneal adhesion formation. Six-week-old Swiss Webster mice were randomized to groups undergoing surgery or no surgery. The surgery group underwent a standardized intraperitoneal adhesion-inducing operative procedure. Animals were then further randomized to receive no further intervention or intraperitoneal injection of 1 ml PBS, IL-10 (30 ng) in 1 ml PBS, or rat anti-mouse IL-10 mAb (30 ng) in 1 ml PBS. All intraperitoneal injections were given immediately after surgery and then every 24 h for a total of four injections. Animals were killed 7 days after surgery and adhesion formation assessed.

Animals treated with PBS vehicle, IL-10, or anti-IL-10 but not undergoing surgical intervention had no or only minimal intraperitoneal adhesions. Animals undergoing surgery who were treated with IL-10 had significantly lower postoperative adhesion scores than did control animals who postoperatively received PBS only or anti-IL-10 mAb (4.6 ± 2.2 vs. 8.1 ± 3.0 and 10.5 ± 4.1, respectively; $p < 0.005$). Anti-IL-10 mAb did not significantly increase adhesion scores when compared to surgery alone or surgery together with vehicle treatment.

IL-10 is effective at limiting postoperative intraperitoneal adhesion formation. When administered in pharmacologic doses, an anti-IL-10 mAb does not appear to significantly block any endogenously produced IL-10 to a degree that facilitates postoperative adhesion formation. Therefore, it is probable that biologically significant IL-10 production is not part of the normal physiologic response to peritoneal injury.

References

1. Ray NF, Larsen JW Jr, Stillman RJ (1993) Economic impact of hospitalizations for lower abdominal adhesiolysis in the United States in 1988. Surg Gynecol Obstet 176: 271–276
2. Stangel JJ, Nisbet JD II, Settles H (1984) Formation and prevention of postoperative abdominal adhesions. J Reprod Med 29: 143–156
3. Milligan DW, Raftery AT (1974) Observations on the pathogenesis of peritoneal adhesions: a light and electron microscopical study. Br J Surg 61: 274–280
4. McBride WH, Mason K, Withers HR, Davis C (1989) Effect of interleukin 1, inflammation, and surgery on the incidence of adhesion formation and death after abdominal irradiation in mice. Cancer Res 49: 169–173
5. Hershlag A, Otterness IG, Bliven ML, Diamond MP, Polan ML (1991) The effect of interleukin 1 on adhesion formation in the rat. Am J Obstet Gynecol 165: 771–774
6. Kovacs EJ, Brock B, Silber IE, Neuman JE (1993) Production of fibrogenic cytokines by Interleukin 2 treated peripheral blood leukocytes: expression of TGF-β amd PDGF B chain genes. Obstet Gynecol 82: 29–36
7. Montz FJ, Holschneider CH, Bozuk M, Gotlieb WH, Martinez-Maza O (1994) Interleukin-10: ability to minimize postoperative intraperitoneal adhesion formation in a murine model. Fertil Steril 61: 1136–1140
8. Carlton AD, Holschneider CH, Gotlieb WH, Montz FJ. Interleukin-1α: in vivo role in murine peritoneal healing and postoperative adhesion formation (in preparation)
9. Zlotnik A, Moore KW (1991) Interleukin-10. Cytokine 3: 366–371
10. Roitt I (1994) Essential immunology, 8th edn. Blackwell, London pp 173–181
11. Romagnani S (1992) Type 1 helper and type 2 helper cells: functions, regulations, and role in protection and disease. Int J Clin Lab Res 21(2): 152–158
12. Chegini N, Gold LI, Williams RS, Masterson BJ (1994) Localization of transforming growth factor beta isoforms TGF-$\beta 1$, TGF-$\beta 2$, and TGF-$\beta 3$ in surgically induced pelvic adhesions in the rat. Obstet Gynecol 83: 449–454
13. Feng L, Tang WW, Chang TC, Wilson CB (1993) Molecular cloning of rat cytokine synthesis inhibiting factor (IL-10) cDNA and expression in spleen and macrophages. Biochem Biophys Res Commun 192: 452–458
14. Fiorentino DF, Bond MW, Mossman TR (1989) Two types of mouse T helper cell IV. Th2 clones secrete a factor that inhibits cytokine production by Th1 clones. J Exp Med 170: 2081–2095
15. Taga K, Tosato G (1992) IL-10 inhibits human T cell proliferation and IL-2 production. J Immunol 148: 1143–1148

16. Mosmann TR, Moore KW (1991) The role of IL-10 in crossregulation of TH1 and TH2 responses. Immunol Today 12: A49–A53
17. Fiorentino DF, Zlotnik A, Mosmann TR, Howard M, O'Garra A (1991) IL-10 Inhibits cytokine production by activated macrophages. J Immunol 147: 3815–3822
18. Gérard C, Bruyns C, Marchant A et al. (1993) IL-10 reduces the release of TNF and prevents lethality in experimental endotoxemia. J Exp Med 177: 547–550
19. Rousset F, Garcia E, Defrance T et al. (1992) Interleukin 10 is a potent growth and differentiation factor for activated human B-lymphocytes. Proc Natl Acad Sci USA 89: 1890–1893
20. Howard M, O'Garra A (1992) Biological properties of interleukin 10. Immunol Today 13: 198–200
21. Montz FJ, Fowler JM, Wolff AJ, Lacey SM, Mohler M (1991) The ability of recombinant tissue plasminogen activator to inhibit post radical pelvic surgery adhesions in the dog model. Am J Obstet Gynecol 165: 1539–1542
22. Montz FJ, Monk BJ, Lacey SM, Fowler JM (1993) Ketorolac tromethamine, a nonsteroidal anti-inflammatory drug: ability to inhibit post-radical pelvic surgery adhesions in a porcine model. Gynecol Oncol 48: 76–79
23. DiZerega GS (1990) The peritoneum and its response to surgical injury. In: DiZerega GS, Diamond MP, Malinak R, Linsky CB (eds) Postoperative adhesion development. Wiley-Liss, New York, pp 1–11

2.5 A New Technique for Surgical Treatment of Large Abdominal Wall Defects: An Experimental Study

A. Iuppa, M. Migliore, D. Santagati, G. Petralia, C. Sapienza, A. Sciuto, and G. Romeo

Introduction

In recent years, there have been significant advances in the surgical treatment of large abdominal wall defects using prosthetic materials. Meanwhile, several studies have indicated that 30% of patients who underwent repair for abdominal wall defects without the use of a prosthetic material will have a recurrence [1, 2].

A new prosthesis, made of expanded polytertrafluoroethylene (PTFE) or Gore-tex (soft tissue patch), has been introduced. It presents several advantages over previous meshes in that it has greater strength (more than twice the most commonly used meshes), easier handling and conformability, low infectability, a minimal foreign body reaction, and a low rate of adhesion formation [3–6].

The aim of our experimental study was to test the use of a new, very thin Gore-tex prosthesis (surgical membrane), as a peritoneal substitute. We propose that this prosthesis, which is only 0.1 mm thick and already used as a pericardial substitute [7, 8], may be positioned between the bowel and the prosthetic patch to avoid adhesion formation and the risk of obstructive complications [9, 10]. This property is related to the low porosity of the surgical membrane. It has a microfibrillary structure with fibrils shorter than 1μm, thereby avoiding cellular invasion from the surrounding tissues.

Materials and Methods

The study was performed on 24 adult male rats weighing 300–400 g each. The rats were divided into two groups (A and B) of 12 and anesthetized with fentanyl and droperidol (0.7 ml/kg), administered intramuscularly. Their abdomens were sterilized with a 10% iodine solution. All rats had 4 cm long midline skin incisions made through the linea alba. The subcutaneous tissues were dissected from the abdominal wall muscles and a defect of about 1 cm^2 was created in the anterior abdominal wall.

In the first group (A), the defects were replaced by a soft tissue patch (3 cm^2) positioned intraperitoneally in contact with the viscera and fixed with interrupted 3-0 polypropylene sutures to the abdominal wall margins.

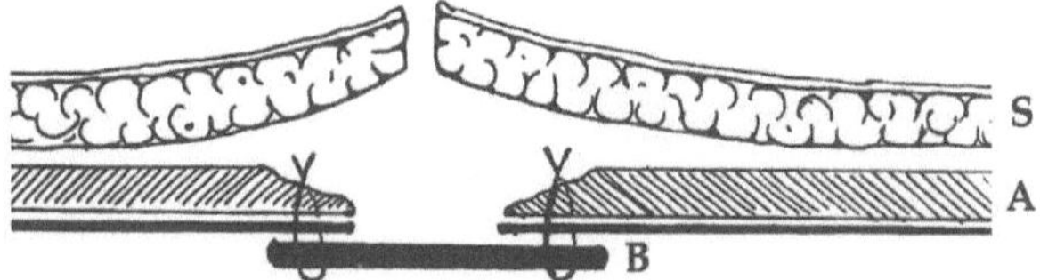

Fig. 1. In group A, the soft tissue patch (*B*) is placed directly onto the abdominal viscera. *S*, subcutaneous tissue; *A*, abdominal fascia

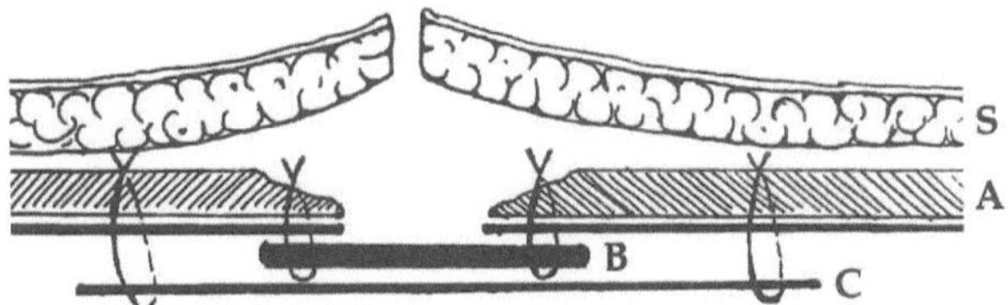

Fig. 2. In group B, the surgical membrane (*C*) is placed between the bowels and the soft tissue patch (*B*). *S*, subcutaneous tissue; *A*, abdominal fascia

In the second group (B) two prosthetic material patches were used. The first patch (4 cm^2) was the surgical membrane. Used as peritoneal substitute, it was placed intraperitoneally in contact with the viscera and fixed to the internal surface of the abdominal wall, 1.5 cm from the edge of the defect, using interrupted 3-0 polypropylene sutures. Thus, group A had the soft tissue patch intraperitoneally (Fig. 1), while group B had a surgical membrane between the bowels and the soft tissue patch (Fig. 2).

All rats had their muscle sheaths closed over the prosthesis with 4-0 running polypropylene sutures. The skin was sutured with 2-0 continuous silk sutures and sterilized again with 10% iodine solution.

All rats were killed 60 days after surgery. The skin was dissected from the abdominal wall muscle to display the adhesion on the peritoneal surface. Evaluation of the adhesions was assessed in this way: 0, no adhesion; 1, minimal adhesions requiring gentle blunt dissection; 2, moderate adhesions requiring aggressive blunt dissection; 3, dense adhesions requiring sharp dissection.

We also evaluated the incidence of sepsis, the histological changes of the patches and the space between the two prostheses (group B only). The results were compared using a χ^2 test for determining statistical significance.

Results

No rats died before the end of the experiment, and none of the rats became infected.

In group A, we found that all rats had grade 1 and 2 adhesions between the inferior surface of the prosthesis and the abdominal viscera. These adhesions required aggressive blunt dissection (grade 2) with the omentum, bowel and in three cases (25%) with the liver (Fig. 3).

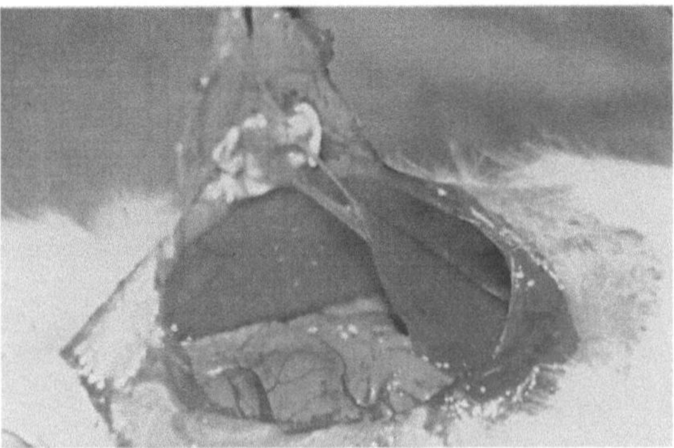

Fig. 3. Group A, 60 days after surgery: dense adhesions between the soft tissue patch and the abdominal viscera

In group B, there were no adhesions between the surgical membrane and the abdominal viscera ($p < 0.001$) (Fig. 4); in two rats (16.6%), grade 1 adhesions were found between the omentum and the polypropylene surgical knots. In one rat (8.3%), the surgical membrane had been folded due to a technical mistake, resulting in an area of grade 2 adhesion.

In group A, the foreign body reaction completely encompassed the soft tissue patch and entered the individual fibers of the mesh, both on the inferior and superior surfaces. The granulation tissue was rich in new capillaries (Fig. 5). Group B showed no reactive tissue attachment to the surgical membrane; its inferior surface was covered by hyperplastic mesothelial cells resembling a neoperitoneum (Fig. 6).

We did not find any serum or infected abscesses between the prostheses in group B; the two prostheses remained free and completely separated.

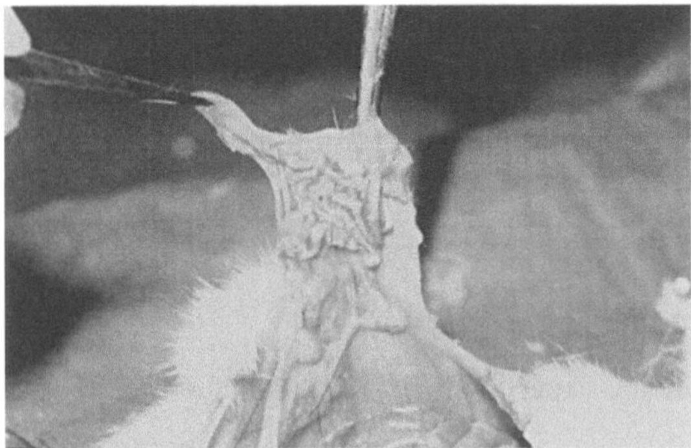

Fig. 4. Group B, 60 days after surgery: total absence of adhesions between the surgical membrane and the abdominal viscera

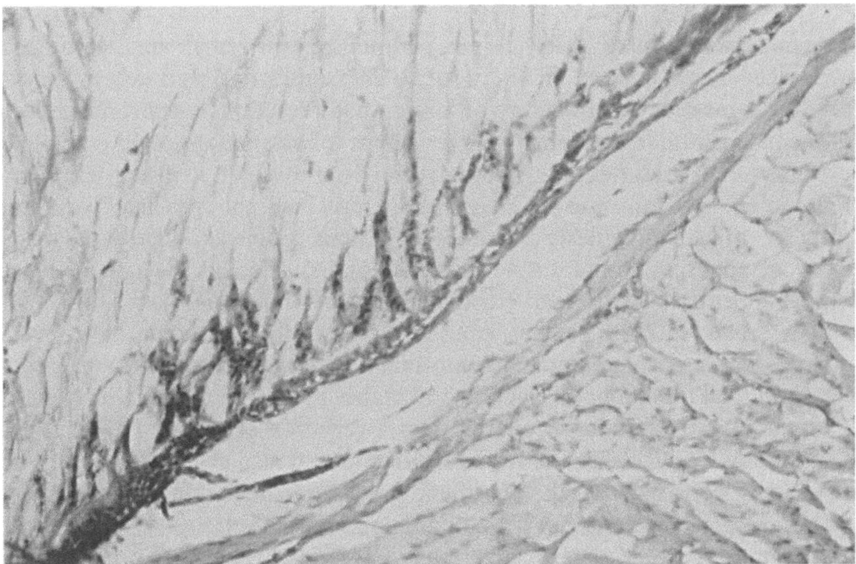

Fig. 5. Group A histological findings. The foreign body reaction completely encompassed the soft tissue patch, entering the individual fibers of the mesh, both on the inferior and superior surfaces

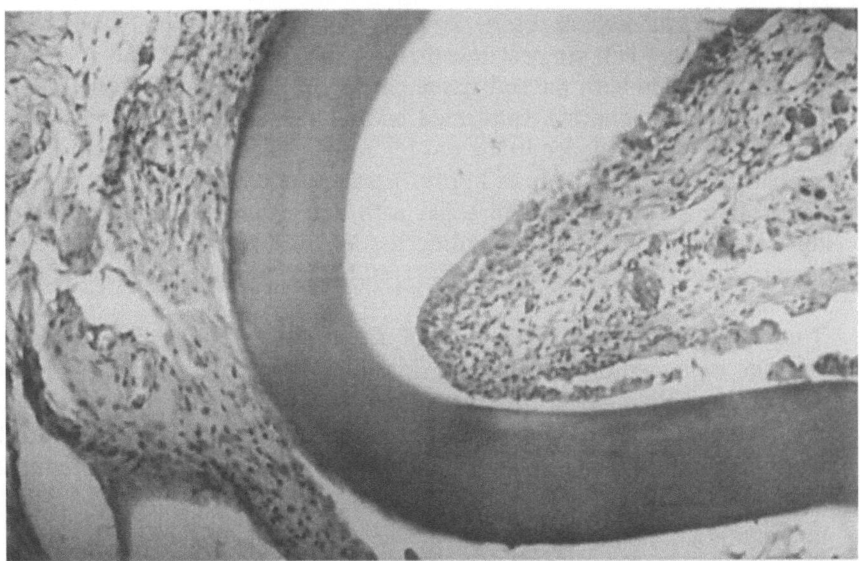

Fig. 6. Group B histological findings. No reactive tissue attachment to the surgical membrane; its inferior surface was covered by a hyperplastic mesothelial cell, resembling a neoperitoneum

Discussion

The most widely used materials for abdominal wall repair are Dacron and Mersylene mesh (Ethicon Inc.) [3, 11–13]. These are strong and easy to handle, produce a massive inflammatory or foreign body reaction, support fibroblastic tissue incorporation, and offer little resistance to infection. Another commonly used material is Marlex mesh or polypropylene mesh (C.R. Bard, Inc.). It is more resistant to infection but is rigid and poorly malleable. The intraperitoneal placement of the prosthesis creates other serious problems, such as the possibility of adhesion formation with the abdominal viscera, the risk of bowel occlusion, enteric fistulas and erosion into intraabdominal organs [14–17].

The expanded PTFE patches, compared to the other materials, have several advantages: easier handling and conformability, lower rate of adhesion formation, minimal foreign body reaction and higher resistance to infection [18–20].

Some investigators have reported that a very thin expanded PTFE surgical membrane is valuable as a pericardial substitute. It also produces significantly fewer adhesions between the prosthetic patch and the abdominal viscera following surgical treatment of large abdominal wall defects.

The results of our experimental study have clearly shown that the surgical membrane functions very well as a peritoneal substitute, avoiding any adhesion formation with the abdominal viscera. The χ^2 test for statistical significance comparing groups A and B showed a $p < 0.001$.

The adhesion formation observed in three animals of group B was not due to the surgical membrane; in two cases adhesions were related to the polypropylene sutures. Thus, we suggest using PTFE sutures to fix the prosthesis to the abdominal wall.

The expanded PTFE surgical membrane proved to be safe and inert, remaining apart from both the soft tissue patch and the abdominal viscera.

Our histological findings confirmed several earlier studies [19, 21]. The expanded PTFE surgical membrane was microscopically unchanged. There was no evidence of a foreign body or fibrous tissue reaction, probably because the microfibrillary structure of the material, with fibrils shorter than 1 μm, avoids cellular invasion from the surrounding tissues. It is remarkable that the inferior surface of the prosthesis was covered by hyperplastic mesothelial cells resembling a neoperitoneum.

The results of our study support the use of the expanded PTFE surgical membrane as a peritoneal substitute in abdominal wall repair [22, 23]. It should be clinically used in patients with a very large abdominal wall defect, when the peritoneum cannot be closed under the prosthesis or the great omentum cannot be placed between the prosthetic patch and the abdominal viscera.

References

1. Langer S, Christiansen J (1985) Long-term results after incisional hernia repair. Acta Chir Scand 151: 217–219

2. Larson GM, Harrower HW (1978) Plastic mesh repair of incisional hernia. Am J Surg 135: 559–563
3. Romeo G, Catania G, Basile F et al. (1988) L'impiego delle protesi nella chirurgia delle ernie e dei laparoceli. Proceedings Italian Society of Surgery, Rome, pp 221–236
4. Bauer JJ, Salky BS, Gelernt IM, Kreel I (1987) Repair of large abdominal wall defects with expanded polytetrafluoroethylene (PTFE). Ann Surg 206: 765–769
5. Harada Y, Imai Y, Kurosawa H, Hoshino S, Nakano K (1988) Long-term results of the clinical use of an expanded polytetrafluoroethylene surgical membrane as a pericardial substitute. J Thorac Cardiovasc Surg 96: 811–815
6. Heydorn WH, Daniel JS, Wade CE (1987) A new look at pericardial substitutes. J Thorac Cardiovasc Surg 94: 291–296
7. Notaras MJ (1974) Experience with mersylene mesh in abdominal wall repair. Proc Roy Soc Med 67: 1187–1190
8. Chevrel JP (1985) Surgery of the abdominal wall. Springer, Berlin Heidelberg New York
9. Arnaud JP, Eloy R, Adloff M, Greiner JF (1977) Critical evaluation of prosthetic materials in repair of abdominal wall hernias. Am J Surg 133: 338–345
10. Stone HH, Fabian TC, Turkelson MI, Jurkiewicz MJ (1981) Management of acute full-thickness losses of the abdominal wall. Ann Surg 193: 612–618
11. Schneider R, Herrington JL Jr, Granada AM (1979) Marlex mesh in repair of a diaphragmatic defect later eroding into the distal esophagus and stomach. Am J Surg. 45: 337–339
12. Kaufman Z, Engelberg M, Zager M (1981) Fecal fistula: a late complication of marlex mesh repair. Dis Colon Rectum 24: 543–544
13. Voyles CR, Richardson JD, Bland KI (1981) Emergency abdominal wall reconstruction with polypropylene mesh. Short-term benefits versus long-term complications. Ann Surg 194: 219–223
14. Law NW, Ellis H (1988) Adhesion formation and peritoneal healing on prosthetic materials. Clinical Materials 3: 95–101
15. Sher W, Pollack D, Paulldes CA, Matsumoto T (1980) Repair of abdominal wall defects – Goretex vs marlex grafts. Am Surg 46: 618–623
16. Brown GL, Richardson JD, Malangoni MA (1985) Comparison of prosthetic materials for abdominal wall reconstruction in the presence of contamination and infection. Ann Surg 201: 705–711
17. Revuelta M, Garcia-Rinaldi R, Val F, Crego R, Durar CMG (1985) Expanded polytetrafluoroethylene surgical membrane for pericardial closure. J Thorac Cardiovasc Surg 89: 451–455
18. Sakamoto T, Imai Y, Koyanagi H, Hayashi H, Hashimoto A (1987) Clinical application of a new material, "expanded polytetrafluoroethylene". Kyobu Geka 31: 23–29

2.6 Influence of Peritoneal Transplants in an Experimental Animal Model for the Study of Readhesion Formation

M. Korell

Introduction

The development of postoperative adhesions is a frequent occurrence after laparotomy and endoscopic surgery. It is well accepted that careful preparation for surgery and atraumatic surgical technique can prevent adhesions [3]. The effectiveness of several additive agents used for prophylaxis is not yet proven [4]. To study the influence of closing the serosal defects on the incidence of adhesions we carried out an animal study with the use of peritoneal transplants [5].

Materials and Methods

The abdominal walls of 58 female Wistar rats were opened by midline incision. In 33 animals, an area (1.5 cm^2) of psoas muscle on one side was deperitonealized and the wound bed was squeezed in a standardized manner with a clamp to induce necrosis. The rats were randomized into different groups to evaluate the effect of leaving the peritoneal defect uncovered (group I; $n=12$) or covering it with a peritoneal transplant taken from the opposite side (group II; $n=21$). The graft was fixed with four 8-0 nylon interrupted sutures (group IIa; $n=11$) or fibrin glue (group IIb; $n=10$). Two weeks after the initial surgery the animals were reopened and the presence or absence of adhesions was explored.

In group III ($n=25$), both horns of the uterus were scratched with a toothbrush in a standardized manner (Fig. 1). The traumatized areas were sutured together using two 8-0 nylon interrupted sutures (Fig. 2). During relaparotomy 14 days later the tight connection between both sides was cut using a microelectrode. The resulting defect (Fig. 3) was covered by a peritoneal transplant on one horn and left open on the control side. The transplant was taken from the peritoneum over the psoas muscle of the same animal and fixed with four 8-0 nylon interrupted sutures. All animals were relaparotomized after 14 days and the presence or absence of adhesions was evaluated. A p value of < 0.05 was established for statistical significance using Fisher's exact test for statistical analysis.

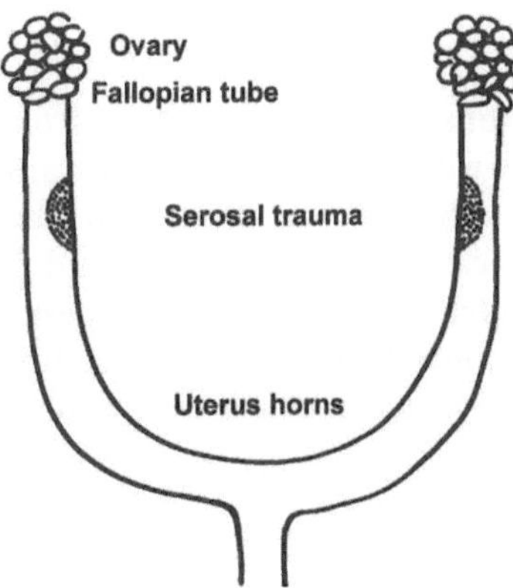

Fig. 1. Peritoneal injuries on both uterine horns by brushing

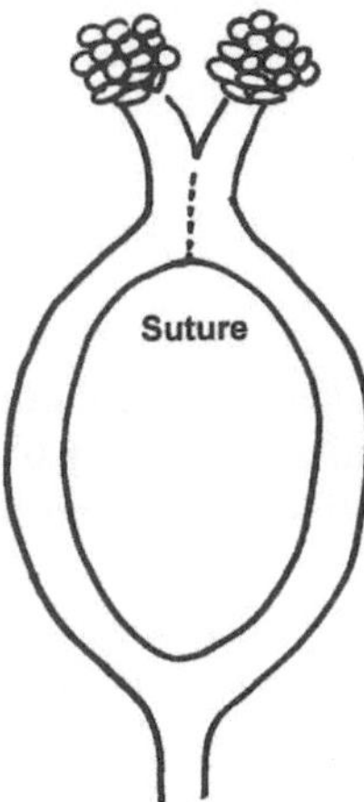

Fig. 2. Suturing together the traumatized areas by two interrupted 8-0 nylon sutures

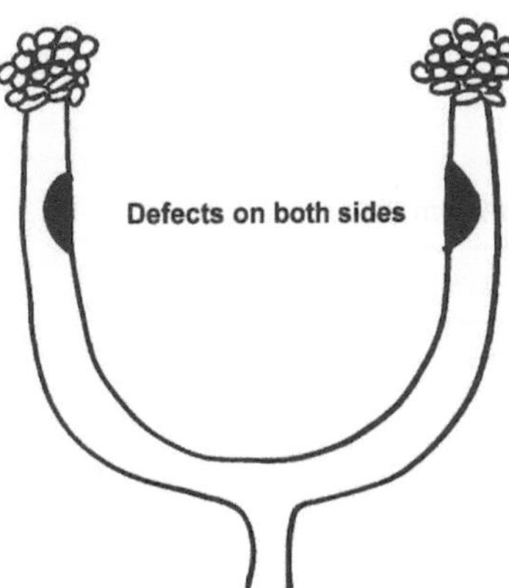

Fig. 3. Defects on both uterine horns during re-laparotomy to cut the tight connection between both uterine horns

Results

In group I, four of 12 animals developed adhesions at the defect area. In group II, adhesions were found in four of 11 animals with sutured peritoneal transplants (group IIa) and in five of 10 rats in which the graft was secured in place by fibrin glue (group IIb). No statistically significant differences were noted. In the uterine horn model, seven of 25 covered uterine horns showed adhesion formation compared with 21 of 25 uncovered control sides. This was statistically different ($p < 0.001$). Figure 4 gives the incidence of adhesions in the different groups.

Discussion

The problem of postoperative adhesions is of great importance. Various studies have been undertaken to evaluate the effects of multiple agents on adhesion formation but have failed to demonstrate a clear benefit [4]. In reconstructive tubal surgery the prevention of adhesions is of special interest. After salpingolysis the resulting defects on the visceral peritoneum often lead to re-formation of adhesions and lower postoperative pregnancy rates. This is the case in both, laparotomy (Table 1) and endoscopic surgery (Table 2). Here, the risk of readhesions reaches up to 96% [2].

We have developed an animal model to investigate the influence of peritoneal transplants on reformation of adhesions. In our modified uterine model in rats the induced injuries on visceral peritoneum are similar to defects observed in the clinic after salpingolysis. The induced connection of both horns of the rat uterus seems to be comparable to the adhesions between ovary and tube observed clinically. After salpingolysis the resulting peritoneal defects are similar to the injuries of both uterine horns. Furthermore, we used the pelvic sidewall model to study the different action of visceral and parietal peritoneum. No grading system was used to estimate the amount of adhesions. Only the absence or presence of adhesions was taken into account. Different grading systems have been developed and applied, but they are not comparable and may be subjectively influenced [1]. Some results of our study are remarkable. There was no significant difference among the groups regarding the parietal peritoneum. Using the pelvic sidewall model, the closure of the defect by

Table 1. Readhesions after microsurgical salpingolysis (from [2])

Reference	Time after surgery	n	Readhesions (%)
Diamond (1987)	1–12 weeks	106	86
DeCherney (1984)	4–6 weeks	20	75
Surrey (1982)	6–8 weeks	31	71
Pittaway (1985)	4–6 weeks	23	23
Trimbos-Kemper (1985)	8 days	188	55
Daniell (1983)	4–6 weeks	25	96

Table 2. Readhesion rate after endoscopic reconstructive surgery (from [2])

Reference	n	Readhesions	De novo
Diamond (1991)	68	67% Fallopian tubes 80% ovary	23%
Canis (1992)	42	82% adnexa	21%
Lundorff (1991)	31	60% Fallopian tube	17%

peritoneal transplant did not reduce the incidence of adhesion. In group I, four of 12 rats (33.3%) with peritoneal transplants developed adhesions compared with nine of 21 rats (42.9%) in group II (Fig. 4). It may very well be that the use of fibrin glue for fixing the graft (group IIb; 5 of 10) actually induces adhesion formation (group IIa; 4 of 11). Taking into account that the closure of parietal peritoneum has no significant effect, it may be justified to leave operative defects open in certain indications such as oncologic surgery.

The visceral peritoneum seems to act differently. In our uterine horn model, the incidence of adhesions was significantly higher after peritoneal injury ($p < 0.01$). Of 25 uterine horns with uncovered defects, 21 (84% vs 33.3% in group I) developed adhesions. Despite different surgical methods inducing the injuries in parietal vs visceral peritoneum, the difference seems to be relevant. This confirms the clinical experience that there is a high incidence of readhesions following salpingolysis (Tables 1, 2). The closure of the defect on the uterine horn leads to a significant reduction of adhesion formation. Only seven of 25 covered uterus sides (28%) showed adhesions ($p < 0.001$).

These results are very important for all reconstructive surgery. Because of the high incidence of adhesion formation, the amount of injuries on visceral peritoneum in ovary, fallopian tubes, uterus and bowel must be minimized by using atraumatic surgical techniques. In case of large defects, the traumatized area must be closed either by suture or peritoneal transplant. The preparation of the graft is not only time-consuming but leaves a peritoneal defect that may

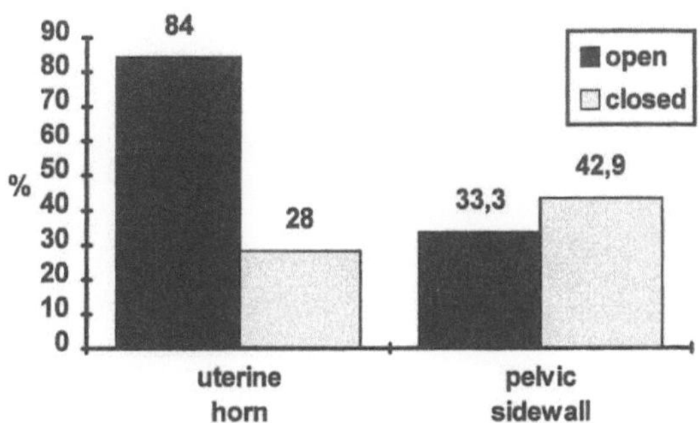

Fig. 4. Influence of peritoneal transplants on the adhesion rate (%) following defects on visceral (uterine horn) and parietal (pelvic sidewall) peritoneum in the rat

itself cause adhesions. Synthetic barrier methods e.g., Interceed TC7 (Johnson & Johnson Medical GmbH, Norderstedt, Germany) and Goretex surgical membrane (W.L. Gore & Associates , Flagstaff, AZ) can perhaps offer a solution in reducing adhesion formation.

Conclusion

Parietal and visceral peritoneum seem to act differently in adhesion formation. Injuries on visceral peritoneum should be avoided or closed. In contrast, parietal peritoneum defects are of less clinical significance. Our rat uterine horn model seems to provide results equivalent to those observed in the clinic for tubal reconstructive surgery. It is thus recommended that the effect of barrier methods in preventing readhesion formation be investigated.

References

1. American Fertility Society (1988) The AFS classifications of adnexal adhesions, distal tubal occlusion, tubal occlusion secondary to tubal ligation, tubal pregnancies, mullerian anomalies and intrauterine adhesions. Fertil Steril 49: 944
2. diZerega G, Rodgers KE (1992) The peritoneum. Springer, Berlin Heidelberg New York
3. Ellis H (1982) The causes and prevention of intestinal adhesions. Br J Surg 69: 241–243
4. Holtz G (1984) Prevention and management of peritoneal adhesions. Fertil Steril 41: 497
5. Korell M, Scheidel P, Hepp H (1994) Experimental animal model for readhesion formation study. J Invest Surg 7: 409–415

2.7 Postoperative Adhesions – Laparoscopy Versus Laparotomy

A. Tittel, E. Schippers, M. Anurov, K.-H. Treutner, A. Öttinger, and V. Schumpelick

Introduction

A total of 4%–10% of all laparotomized patients suffer from adhesion-related problems [6], and 2.5% develop a postoperative intestinal obstruction [9]. Intestinal obstruction is caused by postoperative adhesions in 65%–80% of all cases [6, 8]. These facts show how important it is to minimize adhesion after abdominal surgery. Although laparoscopic surgery is suspected to induce less adhesions, objective data concerning adhesions is still missing. The purpose of our study was to compare adhesions following identical laparoscopic and conventional operations in a dog model.

Methods

Fourteen mongrel dogs were divided into a laparoscopic and a conventional operation group. Their body weight ranged from 15 to 27 kg. All dogs underwent a Trapanal-Ketanest endotracheal anesthesia.

In the laparoscopy group, four trocars with a diameter of 5–11 mm were inserted after insufflation of CO_2. The trocars were placed supraumbilically, subcostally, and through the left and right flank. Starting from the terminal ileum, 50 cm of the small bowel was explored with two atraumatic forceps. The cecum was resected with linear stapler (endo-GIA) (Fig. 1). A small part of the omentum majus was ligated and resected, and 2 cm^2 of the lateral abdominal wall was deserosated by electrocoagulation.

In the laparotomy group, the abdomen was opened by an incision 7 cm in length, which was widened by a self-retaining tissue retractor. Starting from the terminal ileum, 50 cm of the small bowel was eventrated out of the abdominal cavity and manually explored. After 15 min, the bowel was put back into the abdominal cavity and the cecum was resected with a linear stapler (TA-30). As in the laparoscopic operation, 2 cm^2 of the right lateral abdominal wall was deserosated by electrocoagulation, and a small tip of the omentum majus was ligated and resected. Finally, the peritoneum was closed by a running suture and the abdominal wall by single sutures.

All dogs were reexplored after 8 days. Areas of adhesions were dissected and their extent was quantified using a digitizing tablet and a personal computer. Statistical analysis was done using Student's t test.

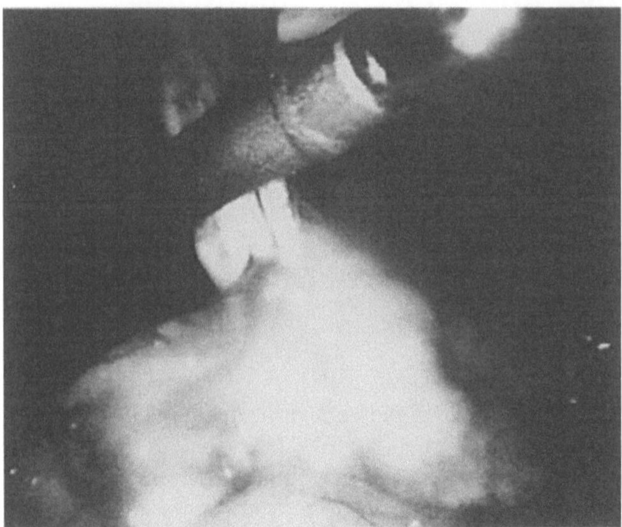

Fig. 1. Cecal resection with endo-GIA

Results

The time of operation did not differ significantly in the two groups (72 min for the laparoscopies versus 58 min for the conventional operations).

Adhesions occurred in both groups. Adhesions were localized at all sites of intra-abdominal manipulations and at peritoneal wounds (Table 1).

The overall extent of adhesions was significantly smaller after laparoscopy (630 mm^2) than after laparotomy (3300 mm^2). A highly significant difference in the area of trocar wounds and abdominal incision was found (155 mm^2 versus 1006 mm^2). We found adhesions to all laparotomies (Fig. 2), but only to 22% of the trocar wounds. Open manipulation of the gut resulted in significantly more enteric adhesions than laparoscopic manipulation (157 mm^2 versus 1840 mm^2). No significant difference in the extent of adhesions due to cecal resection and deserosation of the lateral abdominal wall was found.

Table 1. Extent of adhesions in both operation groups (data expressed as mean ± standard deviation; $p < 0.001$; * = n.s.)

	Laparoscopy (mm^2)		Laparotomy (mm^2)	
	Mean	SD	Mean	SD
Total	630	360	3300	1007
Trocar wounds or laparotomy	155	101	1006	381
Cecal resection	163	55	159	66*
Abdominal deserosation	180	94	195	102*
Enteroenteric adhesions	157	108	1840	606

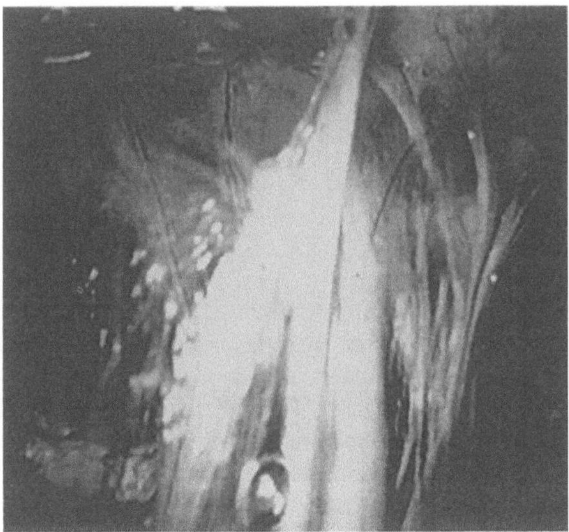

Fig. 2. Adhesion to laparotomy

Table 2. Morphological characteristics of adhesions in the two operation groups

	Laparoscopy (n)	Laparotomy (n)
Conglomerate of adhesions	1/7	3/7
Adhesive bands	–	2/7
Intestinal kinking	3/7	7/7
Number of adhesions to trocar or laparotomy wound	6/28	7/7

Not only the extent but also the form of adhesions differed in the two groups (Table 2). Conventional operations more often led to a conglomerate of adhesions (three versus one dog). Adhesive bands were found only in two laparotomized dogs. Enteroenteral adhesions with intestinal kinking were observed in all laparotomized but only in three laparoscopied dogs.

Discussion

Laparoscopic surgery is thought to be less traumatic than open surgery. Therefore, it should induce less adhesions. The data in the literature is still contradictory concerning the formation of postoperative adhesions after laparoscopic and conventional operations.

Filmar [1] was unable to find an advantage of the laparoscopic operative technique in the rat model, whereas Luciano [2] saw significantly less adhesions after laparoscopic operations in the rabbit model. In both studies, gynecological operations were simulated by iatrogenic injuries of a uterine horn.

Lundorf [3] studied the formation of adhesions after laparoscopically or laparotomically treated tubar gravidity in a prospective and randomized clinical trial. A total of 73 of his 105 patients underwent a second-look laparoscopy to explore the extent of the postoperative adhesions. Lundorf found significantly less adhesions in the laparoscopically treated group.

The basic principle of the formation of adhesions is the dynamic balance between fibrinogenesis and fibrinolysis, which is mostly influenced by the damage and regeneration of the peritoneum [4, 5, 10].

The lesser extent of postoperative adhesions after laparoscopic operations can be explained on the one hand by the smaller defect in the parietal peritoneum caused by the laparoscopic approach compared to a conventional abdominal incision. Furthermore, laparoscopic handling of the gut constitutes a less severe trauma for the visceral peritoneum than manual handling during open surgery. Desiccation of the gut – another cause of peritoneal damage – is reduced by laparoscopic surgery [7].

Similar manipulations at identical anatomical structures caused equal alterations in the peritoneum and therefore led to identical adhesions after laparoscopic and conventional operations.

The overall extent of postoperative adhesions is less after laparoscopic surgery than after identical conventional operations. This may reduce the risk of adhesion-related complications.

Summary

The purpose of the study was to compare adhesions following laparoscopic and conventional operations. In 14 dogs, a cecal resection and a deserosation of the abdominal wall (2 cm^2) were performed laparoscopically ($n=7$) or by laparotomy ($n=7$). After 8 days, all dogs were reexamined, and the adhesions were quantified by computer-aided measurements. Laparoscopic surgery was followed by significantly less adhesions ($p < 0.001$). After conventional operations, extensive adhesions to the abdominal incision and interenteric adhesions were found. Identical manipulations, such as cecal resection or deserosation of the lateral abdominal wall, led to the same frequency and extent of adhesions in the two groups.

References

1. Filmar S, Gomel V, McComb PF (1987) Operative laparoscopy versus open abdominal surgery: a comparative study on postoperative adhesion formation in the rat model. Fertil Steril 48: 486–489
2. Luciano AA, Maier DB, Koch EI, Nulsen JC, Whitman GF (1989) A Comparative study of postoperative adhesions following laser surgery by laparoscopy versus laparotomy in the rabbit model. Obstet Gynecol 74: 220–224

3. Lundorf P, Hahlin M, Kallfelt B, Thorburn J, Lindblom B (1991) Adhesion formation after laparoscopic surgery in tubal pregnancy: a randomized trial versus laparotomy. Fertil Steril 55: 911–915
4. Raferty AT (1981) Effect of peritoneal trauma on peritoneal fibrinolytic activity and intraperitoneal adhesion formation. Eur Surg Res 13: 397–401
5. Renvall SY (1980) Peritoneal metabolism and intra-abdominal adhesion formation. Acta Chir Scand [Suppl] 508: 4–48
6. Schwemmle K (1990) Ursachen von Verwachsungen im Abdomen. Landgenbecks Arch Chir Suppl II: 1017–1021
7. Tittel A, Schippers E, Grablowitz V, Pollivoda M, Anurov M, Öttinger A, Schumpelick V (1995) Intra-abdominal humidity and electromyographic activity of the gastrointestinal tract – laparoscopy versus laparotomy. Surg Endosc 9: 786–790
8. Treutner KH, Winkeltau G, Lerch MM, Stadel R, Schumpelick V (1989) Postoperative, intraabdominelle Adhäsionen – ein neues standardisiertes und objektives Tiermodell und Testung von Substanzen zur Adhäsionsprophylaxe. Langenbecks Arch Chir 374: 99–104
9. Willital GH, Dietl KH, Meier H (1986) Ein neues Therapiekonzept zur postoperativen Adhäsionsprophylaxe. Med Welt 37: 288–296
10. Zühlke HV, Lorenz EMP, Straub EM, Savas V (1990) Pathophysiologie und Klassifikation von Adhäsionen. Langenbecks Arch Chir Suppl II: 1009–1016

3 Aetiology and Pathogenesis of Adhesions

3.1 Studies on the Aetiology and Consequences of Intra-abdominal Adhesions

H. Ellis

Introduction

Adhesions are the commonest cause of intestinal obstruction in the western world. For example, McEntee and colleagues [13] investigated 288 patients with obstruction admitted to four neighbouring district general hospitals over a 12-month period studied prospectively. Adhesions accounted for 75 admissions (32%), malignant disease for 61 (26%) and strangulated hernias for a further 59 (25%). Adhesive obstruction is practically confined to the small intestine, and there are numerous large series reported which show that this cause accounts for some 60% of all small-bowel obstructions [19, 20].

Intra-abdominal adhesions may occasionally be congenital or inflammatory in origin, but the great majority result from previous surgery. We carried out a prospective analysis of 210 patients undergoing laparotomy who had previously had one or more abdominal operations [16]. Of these, 195 (93%) were found to have adhesions which we attributed to previous surgery. In addition, two had adhesions due to their current disease alone and one had adhesions that were considered to be congenital in origin. Seven of the 12 patients with no adhesions had undergone previous appendectomy, and three had undergone lower segment caesarean section. In contrast, of 115 patients undergoing first-time laparotomy, only 12 (10.4%) were found to have adhesions. Of these, 11 were considered to be inflammatory and one congenital.

Obviously, the majority of people who have undergone previous abdominal surgery (and almost invariably if that surgery has been major or repeated) will have abdominal adhesions, and yet only a small number will ever develop subsequent adhesive obstruction. Since this may occur many years after surgery (see below), the true proportion of patients at risk is not accurately known. Menzies and Ellis [16] carried out a prospective study of 2708 laparotomies followed up for an average of 14.5 months (range, 0–91 months) and found that 26 developed intestinal obstruction due to postoperative adhesions within 1 year of surgery (1%), and 14 (0.5%) did so within 1 month of the initial surgery. Of these 2708 laparotomies, 80 were performed for intestinal obstruction from adhesions. Of these 80, 38.7% occurred within 1 year of the initial surgery, 21.25% between 1 and 5 years, 6.25% between 5 and 10 years and no less than 21.25% more than 10 years after the initial operation. Ten patients (12.5%) could not recall the date of their initial operation. There is obviously, therefore, no time limit following operation after which we can say that a patient is no longer at risk of developing adhesive obstruction. Indeed, we have encountered a patient who developed intestinal obstruction from an adhesive band 38 years after his original surgery, which was performed at the age of 1 year for intusussception.

It should be noted that these cases of adhesive obstruction were ones that required surgery. Almost an equal number were admitted and treated conservatively. The majority of patients (75%) developing adhesive obstruction have had operations involving the peritoneal cavity below the transverse mesocolon; these include appendectomy, colectomy and gynaecological surgery. Adhesions almost invariably occur after upper abdominal procedures, but these adhesions involved diaphragm, liver, stomach, transverse colon and transverse mesocolon; it is lower abdominal procedures which are likely to implicate the small intestine and which may therefore proceed to small-bowel obstruction. It would seem that infants are at greater risk of adhesive obstruction than adults. In a study of 649 neonates undergoing laparotomy, 54 (8.3%) required subsequent surgery for adhesive obstruction, 75% of these within 6 months and 90% within 1 year of the initial operation [23].

One question that we cannot answer, and which is perhaps the most important question of all, of interest not only to surgeons but particularly to their patients, is the risk of recurrence of adhesive obstruction following lysis of the adhesion. Intelligent patients will certainly wish to know what their prognosis is likely to be for further episodes of obstruction following operative cure of such an obstructive episode. Obviously, no accurate figure can be given, because we have already noted that there is a life-time risk of an episode of adhesive obstruction following any abdominal surgery. A number of authors have given follow-up figures but, of course, none of these cover the life-span of the patient. Figures for recurrence of obstruction vary widely from 9% to as high as 32% [1].

Aetiology

From the earliest days of abdominal surgery, surgeons became familiar with the fibrinous adhesions that develop within a few hours of operative trauma. This fibrin can either reabsorb completely, leaving a completely clear peritoneal cavity, or become organised by the ingrowth of fibroblasts to form established fibrous adhesions. It soon became apparent that the important thing to determine is the factor that decides whether the adhesions are to be absorbed or to become organised into persistent and potentially dangerous fibrous strands [3]. Fibrous adhesions may result from three groups of conditions, which as a result of major abdominal surgery may often co-exist. These are the following:

1. The apposition of two deperitonealised surfaces. It is well recognised that isolated peritoneal defects heal without adhesion formation [3]. However, Lamont et al. [10] demonstrated in the rat model that, when an area of

   caecal serosa and an area of adjacent parietal peritoneum are denuded, adhesions occurred in 80% cases.

2. Ischaemic tissue is a potent stimulus to the development of fibrous adhesions. This ischaemia may result from some pathological process within the abdomen, such as a gangrenous appendix or gallbladder, or may result from ischaemia produced by sutures or the devascularisation along the line of an anastomosis. We have shown by injection studies that the adhesions that developed to areas of vascular damage comprise active vascular ingrowth of newly formed vessels. In many instances, these vascular grafts are undoubtedly life-saving, preserving the viability of an anastomosis, reinforcing the integrity of a traumatised segment of intestine or preventing an ischaemic appendix or gallbladder from perforating into the general peritoneal cavity. Indeed, we were able to show experimentally that prevention of adhesions from developing to a segment of intestine deprived of its blood supply was followed by gangrene of the segment, whereas if adhesions were allowed to develop the bowel segment up to a certain critical level remained viable [3].

3. The presence of foreign material (almost invariably introduced at operation by the surgeon) into the peritoneal cavity. This includes suture material, glove dusting powder, antibiotic powder and various synthetic materials.

A common pathway in fibrous adhesion production which links all these three mechanisms is a reduction in local plasminogen activator activity of the mesothelial cells of the peritoneum in the presence of trauma or ischaemia [15, 17].

Surgical Glove Powders

In this presentation I shall consider in detail just one aspect of the three aetiological modalities listed above, i.e., the production of granulomas and adhesions by surgical glove powders. This is because this topic has been a particular interest of mine over the past 25 years. A detailed bibliography will be found in two recent reviews [4, 5]. Rubber gloves were introduced into the operating theatre over 100 years ago, not only as part of the new antiseptic technique but also to protect the hands of both the surgeon and the nurse from the powerful antiseptic agents which were then in use. Originally, gloves were sterilised by boiling and then put on wet over the wet hands. With the introduction of dry sterilisation, it was necessary to use a dusting powder to facilitate the donning of the gloves. The first agents used were lycopodium (the spores of club moss) or talcum powder, which is mainly magnesium silicate.

It was only in the 1930s that examples of postoperative foreign body granulomas due to talc were reported in various sites after operation. By the early 1940s, the dangers of talc were well recognised and a search was made for substitutes. Lee and Lehman [12] reported the use as a glove lubricant of corn starch powder treated with epichlorhydrin mixed with 2% magnesium oxide as a desiccating agent. This was later marketed as Biosorb (Regent Hospital

Products, London, UK), and it is this material that remains in use today. It should be noted that, by 1952, one of these authors reported inflammatory reactions and adhesions in the peritoneal cavity of dogs produced by implantation of starch [11].

The initial hope that the new glove lubricant would prove inert in clinical practice was unfounded. In 1955, two cases of wound granuloma due to starch were reported [21], and in the following year McAdams [14] reported three patients with granulomatous intraperitoneal foreign body reaction due to starch powder. Cases have also been reported of pelvic starch granuloma in women who have undergone previous vaginal examinations and as a result of dusting powder on a condom.

Myers et al. [18] introduced the term "granulomatous peritonitis due to starch," describing three patients with this syndrome; over the following years, numerous reports of this condition were published from centres worldwide. This syndrome is now well recognised; 10 days to 4 weeks after laparotomy, the patient develops abdominal pain, distension, vomiting and a low-grade pyrexia. Examination reveals a distended and tender abdomen. The white cell count is often elevated. A plain radiograph of the abdomen demonstrates distended loops of intestine. A diagnosis of intestinal obstruction caused by postoperative adhesions or intra-abdominal infection or a combination of both is made. Because of this, the majority of these patients have undergone a second laparotomy, at which time the typical findings are of ascitic fluid (which may be yellow, green or serosanguineous) or a thickened nodular omentum, small miliary nodules scattered over the surface of the peritoneum and dense adhesions. If the surgeon is not familiar with this condition, miliary tuberculosis or even carcinomatosis may be diagnosed [6].

The diagnosis is made by examination of a biopsy of one of the nodules examined under polarised light using the frozen section technique, which will reveal the typical Maltese crosses of starch. Starch granules can be also seen if the ascitic fluid is examined under polarised light.

Although the majority of studies deal with the intra-peritoneal reactions to starch, a number of other syndromes have been noted. These include pleural effusion after thoracotomy, pericardial effusion and adhesions after cardiac surgery, meningism after craniotomy and retroperitoneal fibrosis.

We have shown [9] that peritoneal contamination with starch probably occurs with every laparotomy using conventional starch-powdered gloves, yet the clinical manifestations of reaction to this material are comparatively rare. There is evidence that the more florid reactions to starch may be as a result of starch sensitivity. It has been shown, for example, that patients after starch peritonitis showed a brisk skin reaction to intradermal injection of starch, whereas no reaction was observed in control subjects [7]. The same workers demonstrated that delayed hypersensitivity to starch could be induced in guinea pigs innoculated intradermally with starch and Freund's adjuvant. When these immunised animals were then challenged with an intraperitoneal injection of starch in saline, florid omental granulomas developed in eight of 36 animals. The rest of the group, together with 36 controls, showed only a low-grade microscopic inflammatory reaction [8]. The experimental studies on surgical dusting powders that we and many other investigators have carried out are somewhat artificial. The important question is what happens when powder contaminations occur at the same time as surgical trauma. After all, the usual state of affairs is that powder contamination takes place at the time of some operative procedure. Jagelman and Ellis [9] showed that an innoculum of 0.1 g starch was completely absorbed from the peritoneal cavity of the rat within 1 week on macroscopic inspection, but when such a dose was introduced in the presence of peritoneal injury, adhesions invariably developed. Also working in my laboratory, Walker [22] showed that the peritoneal reaction to blood and to bile was greatly enhanced by the addition of starch. Obviously, there are two ways to prevent the occurrence of starch powder contamination at operation. The first is to remove all traces of powder, and the second is to develop a powder-free surgical glove. We have shown that conventional washing of the donned gloves in saline solution is ineffective. Washing the gloves in two successive bowls of saline failed to remove all the starch and, indeed, resulting in clumping of the residual starch granules [9]. The most effective technique of removing starch comprises a 1-min cleansing with povidone iodine, followed by a rinse with sterile water. This technique, although effective, is time consuming, costly and must be repeated every time the gloves are changed by any member of the surgical team.

In 1982, a surgical glove was produced in which lubrication was effected by a process which bonded a film of hydrogel polymer to the surface of the glove. This is the material used in the manufacture of soft contact lenses and has been determined in numerous studies to be entirely non-reactive. It also has the advantage of protecting the health worker using the glove from developing latex-starch sensitivity. The widespread use of such gloves, marketed under the name Biogel (Regent Hospital Products, London UK), should almost eliminate the hazard of starch contamination in our operating theatres.

Summary

Adhesions are the commonest cause of small bowel obstruction in the Western world. The great majority of these follow previous abdominal surgery. About 1% of patients will obstruct within 1 year of abdominal surgery, but there is no time limit after which it can be said that the patient is free from this danger. The risk of recurrent obstruction after lysis of the adhesion is not accurately known, but published figures vary from 9% to 32%.

Fibrous adhesions result from (1) denudation of adjacent peritoneal surfaces, (2) from the presence of intra-abdominal ischaemic tissue, or (3) as a reaction to a variety of intra-peritoneal foreign materials introduced by the surgeon. One of these, glove powder, can be eliminated by using starch-free gloves.

References

1. Brightwell NL, McFee AS, Aust JB (1977) Bowel obstruction and the long tube stent. Arch Surg 112: 505–511
2. Ellis H (1962) The aetiology of post-operative abdominal adhesions. Br J Surg 50: 10–16
3. Ellis H (1982) The causes and preventions of intestinal adhesions. Br J Surg 69: 241–243
4. Ellis H (1990) The hazards of surgical glove dusting powders. Surg Gynecol Obstet 171: 521–527
5. Ellis H (1994) Review-pathological changes produced by surgical dusting powders. Ann R Coll Surg Engl 76: 5–8
6. Giercksky KE, Quist H, Giercksky TC, Warloe T, Nesland JM (1994) Multiple glove powder granulomas masquerading as peritoneal carcinomatosis. J Am Coll Surg 179: 299–304
7. Grant JBF, Davies JD, Espiner HJ, Eltringham WK (1982) Diagnosis of granulomatous starch peritonitis by delayed hypersensitivity skin reactions. Br J Surg 69: 197–199
8. Grant JBF, Davies JD, Jones JV (1976) Allergic starch peritonitis in the guinea pig. Br J Surg 63: 867–869
9. Jagelman D, Ellis H (1973) Starch and intraperitoneal adhesion formation. Br J Surg 60: 111–114
10. Lamont PM, Menzies D, Ellis H (1992) Intra-abdominal adhesion formation between two adjacent deperitonealized surfaces. Surg Res Commun 133: 127–130
11. Lee CM, Collins WT, Largen TL (1952) A reappraisal of absorbable glove powder. Surg Gynecol Obstet 95: 725–728
12. Lee CM, Lehman EP (1947) Experiments with non-irritating glove powder. Surg Gynecol Obstet 84: 689–695
13. McEntee G, Pender D, Mulvin D et al. (1987) Current spectrum of intestinal obstruction. Br J Surg 74: 976–980
14. McAdams GB (1956) Granulomata caused by absorbable starch glove powder. Surgery 39: 329–336
15. Menzies D, Ellis H (1989) Intra-abdominal adhesions and their prevention by topical tissue plasminogen activator. Proc R Soc Med 82: 534–535
16. Menzies D, Ellis H (1990) Intestinal obstruction from adhesions – how big is the problem? Ann R Coll Surg Engl 72: 60–63
17. Menzies D, Ellis H (1991) The role of plasminogen activator in adhesion prevention. Surg Gynecol Obstet 172: 362–366
18. Myers RN, Deaver JM, Browne CE (1960) Granulomatous peritonitis due to starch glove powder. Ann Surg 151: 106–112
19. Raf LE (1969) Causes of abdominal adhesions in cases of intestinal obstruction. Acta Chir Scand 135: 73–76
20. Stewardson RH, Bombeck T, Nyhus LM (1978) Critical operative management of small bowel obstruction. Ann Surg 187: 189–193
21. Sneierson H, Woo ZP (1955) Starch powder granuloma. A report of two cases. Ann Surg 142: 1045–1050
22. Walker EM (1978) Effects of blood, bile and starch in the peritoneal cavity. J Anat 126: 495–507
23. Wilkins BM, Spitz L (1986) Incidence of post-operative adhesion obstruction following neonatal laparotomy. Br J Surg 73: 762–764

3.2 Aetio-pathogenesis of Peritoneal Adhesions with Respect to Post-traumatic Fibrinolytic Activity

D. Menzies

Type and Incidence of Adhesions

Adhesions are either congenital or acquired. Congenital adhesions include the nameless adhesions across the lesser sac or Ladd's bands. Acquired adhesions arise from either an intra-abdominal infection or episode of inflammation such as cholecystitis or diverticulitis or they are post-traumatic. The commonest form of post-traumatic adhesions are those that develop after surgery. Approximately 85% of adhesions that cause intestinal obstruction are post-surgical, 10% are inflammatory and 5% are congenital [1].

Postoperative adhesions occur after 95% of all abdominal operations [2]. Their frequency and extent increases with the size of the operation performed [3]. These adhesions produce intestinal obstruction in 3% of all laparotomies, 0.5% occurring within 1 month of surgery and 1% within 1 year [2]. The remainder may obstruct at any time after surgery.

Theories of Adhesion Formation

According to the primitive theory of adhesion formation, adhesions were thought to be due to peritoneal injury healing by scar formation which developed adhesions between adjacent viscera (Fig. 1).

Later, specific stimuli were identified which were known to cause adhesion production. These included trauma, infection and ischaemia. These stimuli created an acute inflammatory intraperitoneal response, which resulted in a fibrin-rich inflammatory exudate. Fibrin was laid down and produced fibrinous adhesions. In the presence of an intact peritoneum, these fibrinous adhesions were inhibited and the fibrin dissolved. In the absence of a healthy peritoneum, the fibrinous adhesions persisted and became organised to develop fibrous adhesions.

This theory has been labelled the classical pathway for adhesion formation (Fig. 2).

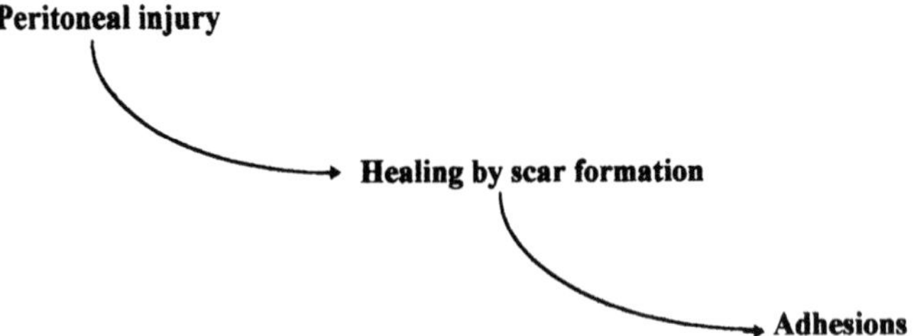

Fig. 1. Primitive theory of adhesion formation

Fibrinolytic Activity of the Peritoneum

In 1969, Myrhe-Jensen identified the peritoneum as having a fibrinolytic capability due to plasminogen activation [4]. This plasminogen activation was isolated as plasminogen activator activity (PAA). In 1976, Buckman found that PAA was reduced after peritoneal trauma or in the presence of ischaemic tissue [5, 6]. These findings were confirmed by Raftery in 1981 [7]. It was found that different types of insult to the peritoneum created differing degrees of depression of PAA, e.g. ischaemic trauma caused a greater depression of PAA than abrasive trauma [5]. These observations resulted in a modification of the classical pathway of adhesion formation to that shown in Fig. 3.

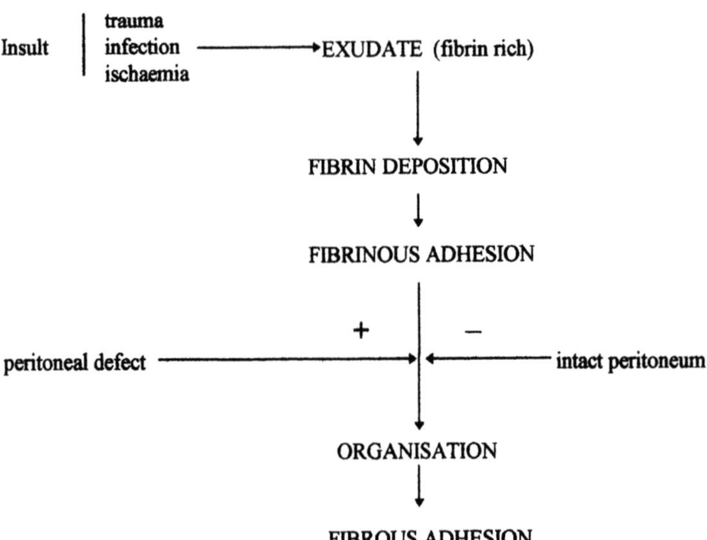

Fig. 2. Classical pathway of adhesion formation

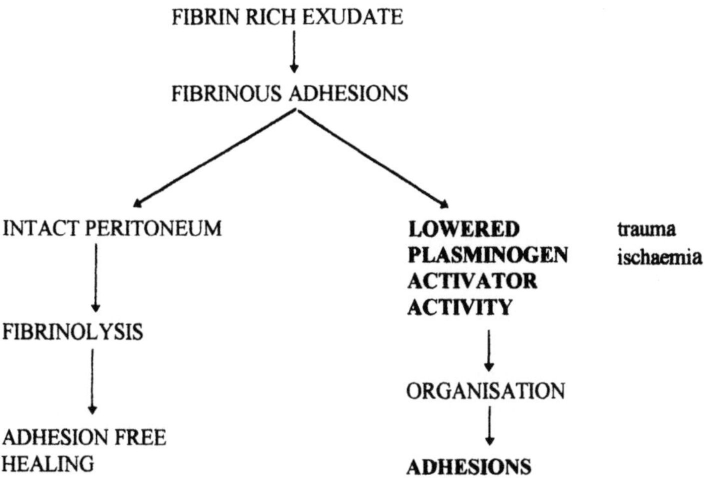

Fig. 3. Modification to classical pathway

Recombinant Tissue Plasminogen Activator and Studies on Adhesion Prevention

The identification of a reduction in PAA in adhesion formation led to several attempts to replace this deficit with fibrinolytic agents. The results of these studies met with varying success. The production of recombinant tissue plasminogen activator (rt-PA) from *Escherichia coli* cultures [8] and later from Chinese hamster ovaries (CHO) allowed its use in studies to prevent adhesion formation.

The effect of rt-PA upon primary adhesion formation and recurrent adhesion formation was studied in a rabbit model [9]. The peritoneum over a section of the caecum and an apposing portion of the parietal peritoneum was stripped to create adhesions. These were divided after 1 week to allow recurrent adhesions to form. The preventative properties of rt-PA were studied by application of rt-PA to the initial strips and to divided adhesions at 1 week, and rt-PA was compared to a placebo (hyaluronic acid) and a control group. The results showed that primary and recurrent adhesions were prevented from forming in more than 90% of cases [9]. Other workers have since confirmed these findings [10]. It was of concern that rt-PA may interfere with wound and colonic anastomotic healing, but studies on the strength of both of these features with the use of rt-PA failed to show any clinical or mechanical effect [9]. There is some evidence that a biochemical reduction in hydroxyproline in wounds treated with rt-PA does occur [11]. This implies that such a wound may be weaker, but this has yet to be proven.

During these experimental studies on colonic anastomotic healing, it was noted that adhesions still occurred to the anastomosis despite the application of a dose of rt-PA that prevented adhesion formation after simple peritoneal trauma. This raised the question of whether there was any additional stimulus to adhesion formation that was present with inflammation or ischaemia, but not with simple trauma.

Plasminogen Activator Activity and the Peritoneum – Suppression After Peritoneal Insult

The studies by Buckman in 1976 [5, 6] identified the inhibition of fibrinolysis on a fibrin plate by the presence of ischaemic tissue. This suggested that, rather than there being a simple absence of PPA in the presence of ischaemia, there was active inhibition of activity. This was not followed up until 1990, when Vipond et al. [11] identified the presence of plasminogen activator inhibitor-1 (PAI-1) in inflamed and ischaemic peritoneum. In 1993, Whawell et al. [12] found that PAI-2 was present in similar tissue samples, but that tissue plasminogen activator (t-PA) was also present in normal quantities. Evaluation of the presence of PAI-1 or PAI-2 after simple trauma has not been carried out, but measurements by Buckman [5] failed to indicate PAA inhibition after simple trauma. It would appear that after simple trauma PAA is reduced secondary to the reduction in the presence of t-PA. In the presence of inflammation or ischaemia there are normal levels of t-PA, but there is inhibition of PAA by PAI-1 and PAI-2. This suggests that there are two variations on the pathogenesis of adhesions; indeed, there may be two types of adhesions.

Are There Two Types of Adhesions?

In terms of pathogenesis, there appear to be two types of adhesions: those that are formed after simple trauma and those that develop after inflammation or ischaemia. This may be of clinical significance with respect to adhesion prevention. The majority of adhesions that form after surgery are not related to the site of surgery, but involve the wound or loops of the small bowel [2]. These adhesions between loops of bowel are the main cause of postoperative adhesive intestinal obstruction [2] and are probably produced due to local simple trauma reducing the level of t-PA at the time of surgery. Adhesions at the site of surgery may be beneficial, as they can support a precarious anastomosis, introduce a new blood supply to ischaemic tissue and wall off areas of sepsis to prevent spread. These adhesions are probably facilitated by suppression of PAA by PAI-1 and PAI-2. It may be possible to selectively inhibit the formation of adhesions that may produce intestinal obstruction and to permit the formation of adhesions that are beneficial.

Degree of Trauma and Extent of Adhesion Formation

It seems likely that less trauma means less adhesion formation. It has always been recommended that one aspect of general adhesion prevention is the careful handling of tissue [13]. The recent explosion of laparoscopic surgery has allowed further study of this phenomenon. It is professed by laparoscopists that laparoscopic surgery provides less traumatic techniques than open surgery and that one benefit of minimal-access surgery is that there will be less adhesion formation and therefore less risk of postoperative intestinal obstruction.

In animal studies, Fowler et al. [14] found a lower than expected adhesion rate after laparoscopic pelvic lymphadenectomy, and Tittel et al. [15] found less adhesions after laparoscopic bowel resections when compared to open bowel resections. In humans, Lundorff et al. [16] found less adhesion reformation at second-look laparoscopy after laparoscopic adhesiolysis when compared to open adhesiolysis. In two more recent animal studies, Marana et al. [17] and Perone [18] failed to find any difference in adhesion production between open and laparoscopic surgery at the site of surgery, but it was noted that less adhesions were formed to the wound after laparoscopic surgery [18].

The fibrinolytic activity of the peritoneum plays a key role in adhesion formation. Continued investigation of the pathogenesis of adhesion production is essential if an effective anti-adhesion agent is to be developed. As our understanding of adhesion development improves and the different mechanisms that produce different types of adhesions are clarified, it is essential that standard models for adhesion formation are developed and used to eliminate some of the disparity in published reports.

References

1. Raf LE (1969) Causes of abdominal adhesions in cases of intestinal obstruction. Acta Chir Scand 135: 73–76
2. Menzies D, Ellis H (1990) Intestinal obstruction from adhesions – how big is the problem? Ann R Coll Surg Engl 72: 60–63
3. Wiebel MA, Majno G (1973) Peritoneal adhesions and their relation to abdominal surgery. Am J Surg 126: 345-353
4. Myrhe-Jensen O, Larsen SB, Astrup T (1969) Fibrinolytic activity of serosal and synovial membranes. Arch Pathol 88: 623-630
5. Buckman RF, Buckman PD, Hufnagel HV, Gervin AS (1976) A physiologic basis for adhesion-free healing of de-peritonealized surfaces. J Surg Res 21: 67–76
6. Buckman RF, Woods M, Sargent L, Gervin AS (1976) A unifying pathogenetic mechanism in the etiology of intraperitoneal adhesions. J Surg Res 20: 1–5
7. Raftery AT (1981) Effect of peritoneal trauma on peritoneal fibrinolytic activity and intraperitoneal adhesion formation. Eur Surg Res 13: 397–401
8. Pennica D et al. (1983) Cloning and expression of human tissue-type plasminogen activator cDNA in E. Coli. Nature (Lond) 301: 214–221
9. Menzies D, Ellis H (1991) Adhesion formation – the role of plasminogen activator. Surg Gynecol Obstet 172: 362–366
10. Doody KJ, Dunn RC, Buttram VC (1989) Recombinant tissue plasminogen activator reduces adhesion formation in a rabbit uterine horn model. Fertil Steril 41: 926–929
11. Vipond MN, Whawell SA, Thompson JN, Dudley HAF (1990) Peritoneal fibrinolytic activity and intra-abdominal adhesions. Lancet 335: 1120–1122
12. Whawell SA, Vipond MN, Scott-Coombes DM, Thompson JN (1993) Plasminogen activator inhibitor 2 reduces peritoneal fibrinolytic activity in inflammation. Br J Surg 80: 107–109

13. Ellis H (1971) The cause and prevention of post-operative intra-peritoneal adhesions. Surg Gynecol Obstet 133: 497–511
14. Fowler JM et al. (1994) Pelvic adhesion formation after pelvic lymphadenectomy: comparison between transperitoneal laparoscopy and extraperitoneal laparotomy in a porcine model. Gynecol Oncol 55: 25–28
15. Tittel A et al. (1994) Laparoskopie versus Laparotomie. Eine tierexperimentelle Studie zum Vergleich der Adhesionsbildung im Hund. Acta Chir 379: 95–98
16. Lundorff P et al. (1991) Adhesion formation after laparoscopic surgery in tubal pregnancy: a randomised trial versus laparotomy. Fertil Steril 55: 911–915
17. Marana R et al. (1994) Laparoscopy versus laparotomy for ovarian conservative surgery: a randomised trial in the rabbit model. Am J Obstet Gynecol 171: 861–864
18. Perone N (1995) Is laparoscopy associated with a lower rate of postoperative adhesions than laparotomy? A comparative study in the rabbit. Aust NZ J Surg 65: 342–344

3.3 Role of Sutures and Suturing in the Formation of Postoperative Peritoneal Adhesions

D.P. O'Leary

Introduction

Peritoneal adhesions are abnormal fibrous connections between adjacent peritoneal surfaces. They are the commonest cause of small intestinal obstruction in developed countries [31, 45], a prominent reason for female infertility and a troublesome cause of abdominal or pelvic pain. When encountered by the surgeon, peritoneal adhesions make abdominal operations more difficult, hazardous and time-consuming.

Adhesions and Surgery

In the great majority of cases, peritoneal adhesions follow abdominal operations. In a prospective study of findings at laparotomy, Menzies and Ellis [24] observed that 93% of patients with peritoneal adhesions had a history of previous laparotomy. Conversely, 93% of patients who had previously undergone a laparotomy had adhesions, compared with 10.4% of those with no history of abdominal surgery. In an earlier study, among 1477 patients requiring surgery for adhesive small intestinal obstruction, 86% had previously undergone an abdominal operation, mostly an appendicectomy or gynaecological surgery [31].

Pathogenesis of Postoperative Adhesions

Factors which contribute to the formation of postoperative peritoneal adhesions include abrasive surgical trauma [4], the presence of blood clot or foreign materials in the peritoneal cavity [37, 38], peritoneal ischaemia [7] and infection [30]. Pathogenesis of adhesions appears to involve impairment of peritoneal fibrinolysis [4, 34, 48], leading to persistence of an early fibrinous inflammatory exudate, which is replaced by a chronic inflammatory response with fibrosis and established adhesions [26]. Loss or degradation of lubricating peritoneal phospholipids has recently been proposed as an additional factor promoting postoperative adhesions [43, 44].

Peritoneal Suturing and Adhesions

Suturing peritoneum introduces a foreign material and implies a degree of trauma and potential for peritoneal ischaemia, factors known to promote adhesion formation. This chapter reviews the evidence concerning the need to suture peritoneum and the potential for inducing adhesions under three headings:

1. Healing of peritoneal defects: sutured versus unsutured
2. Suturing the parietal peritoneum during abdominal wound closure
3. Incorporation of visceral peritoneum in suture lines

Healing of Peritoneal Defects: Sutured Versus Unsutured

Surgical interventions often cause defects in the parietal peritoneum or deperitonealization of viscera. Commonly quoted examples are the defects in the pelvic peritoneum after abdominoperineal resection of the rectum or pelvic exenteration. Traditionally, it has been assumed that peritoneal defects, like unsutured skin defects, heal from the edges inwards with fibrotic scarring and that this results in adhesions. Defects in parietal peritoneum have been sutured closed in the hope that this would reduce the likelihood of adhesions and the potential for small intestine obstruction due to herniation [42]. Indeed, Smith estimated that 2% of all postoperative deaths could be prevented by suturing peritoneal defects. Several current surgical texts perpetuate this approach by continuing to advise closure of peritoneal defects, e.g. after abdominoperineal resection [13, 53, 55].

In fact, healing of peritoneal defects is quite unlike healing of skin defects. More than a century ago, von Dembowski [6] reported that experimentally created parietal peritoneal defects left unsutured healed to form a smooth serosal layer without adhesions. This has since been confirmed by numerous researchers [7, 15, 35], and similar observations have been made concerning defects in visceral peritoneum [11, 32]. Although adhesions may form in relation to peritoneal defects, possibly due to injury to a second, contiguous, peritoneal surface [23], the predominant tendency is for peritoneal defects to regenerate a smooth serosa. Large defects heal as rapidly as small ones [8, 14, 15], suggesting that healing is not dependent on ingrowth from the peritoneal edges. The new mesothelium appears to be formed from primitive mesenchymal cells from the deeper layers or from the peritoneal cavity [8, 15, 33, 54]. In the case of parietal peritoneal defects, the new mesothelium is macroscopically indistinguishable from the surrounding serosa by 7 days [7, 15].

Contrasted with the healing of unsutured peritoneal defects, Thomas and Rhoads [47] and Singleton et al. [41] showed that suturing visceral peritoneal defects increased the incidence of adhesions. Later, in an elegant series of experiments, Ellis created defects measuring from 1×1 cm to 2×3 cm in the parietal peritoneum of dogs. Fifty-eight defects were left unsutured, of which 53 healed without adhesions within 1 week, only five (8.6%) forming adhesions. In contrast, of 19 similar defects sutured with fine silk, 16 (84.2%) formed adhesions [7]. Lengths of silk sutured loosely in the peritoneal layer did not promote adhesions, suggesting that adhesion formation resulted from suturing under tension rather than a reaction to the suture material. Ellis proposed that the adhesions were a response to ischaemia at the peritoneal edge [7]. Hubbard et al. [15], investigating the effects of different suture materials, reported that parietal peritoneal defects in dogs healed with a 40%–60% incidence of adhesions when left unsutured, compared with a 95%–100% incidence when sutured using chromic catgut or silk ($p < 0.001$). This group also found that unsutured visceral peritoneal defects created in small intestinal serosa healed with a 30% incidence of adhesions compared with 82% and 90% ($p < 0.001$) when sutured with silk or chromic catgut, respectively [15].

Clinically, in a prospective trial Irvin and Golligher [18] found no difference in the incidence of prolonged ileus or obstruction after rectal resection whether the pelvic peritoneum was sutured or left open. An earlier trial reported a higher incidence of small intestinal obstruction in patients in which the pelvic peritoneum was sutured (four out of 18) than in those in which it was left unsutured (none of 28) following abdominoperineal resection [49], i.e. exactly the reverse of what was predicted by Smith in 1895 [42]. The cause of such obstructions is usually adhesions to the suture line [51].

Conclusions

Despite recommendations to the contrary [13, 55], defects in visceral and parietal peritoneum are best left unsutured. This approach is based on sound experimental and clinical evidence and is advocated by increasing numbers of surgeons [3].

Suturing the Parietal Peritoneum During Closure of Abdominal Wounds

Although the parietal peritoneum is thin and weak, suturing it has long been considered an important part of abdominal wound closure. Indeed, as one author put it, "like eating peas off your knife, ... failure to close the peritoneum of an abdominal incision seems at first sight to be a gross deviation from what is right and proper" [1]. A recent questionnaire concerning surgeon's practice suggests that 86% of surgeons in the United Kingdom suture the peritoneal layer during closure of laparotomy wounds [40].

However, in patients who have previously undergone abdominal surgery, repeat laparotomy often reveals adhesions to the back of the scar. Among 210 patients undergoing repeat laparotomy, Menzies and Ellis [24] reported adhesions between the old scar and omentum is 81% and between the old scar and small intestine in 20%. Suturing peritoneal defects promotes adhesions, possibly because suturing under tension induces ischaemia [7]. However, it cannot be assumed that such a mechanism operates when incised peritoneum is sutured with less or no tension. These observations raise questions con-

Table 1. Results of prospective clinical trials on the necessity of closing parietal peritoneum after laparotomy

	Patients (n)	Dehiscence (%)		Hernia (%)	
		Sutured	Not Sutured	Sutured	Not Sutured
Mid-line and paramedian [9]	138 188	2.5	3.0	4.3	4.3
Mid-line [16]	185	0.0	1.0	1.0	1.0
Lateral paramedian [10]	152	0.0	0.0	0.0	1.3
Pfannenstiel [50]	333	0.0	0.0	0.0	0.0

No significant differences were observed between sutured or non-sutured groups in any of these studies.

cerning the need to suture the peritoneal layer during abdominal wound closure and about the possibility that this step may promote adhesions to the surgical scar.

Studies in animals have shown that suturing the peritoneum adds nothing to the strength of mid-line or paramedian wound closures (determined by the force necessary to disrupt the wound) [9, 19, 30]. In humans, the effects of peritoneal suturing on the healing of abdominal wounds have been evaluated in a number of prospective clinical trials (Table 1). In the first of these, Ellis and Heddle [9] observed no significant difference in wound dehiscence or incisional hernia rates between groups in which the peritoneum was sutured with chromic catgut or left unsutured during closure of paramedian and mid-line wounds. These observations were confirmed for mid-line wounds by Hugh et al. [16]. Similar findings have been reported for closure of lateral paramedian [10] and Pfannenstiel [50] incisions. In addition, Hugh et al. [16] demonstrated that peritoneal suture or non-suture produced no significant difference in postoperative pain scores or analgesic requirements. Long-term follow-up (beyond 1–2 years) and hence late incisional hernia rates are not reported in any of these studies, although delayed results are unlikely to be influenced by peritoneal suture [1].

Patients with ascites and patients undergoing peritoneal dialysis who undergo laparotomy require not only a strong, but also a leak-proof abdominal closure. Suturing the peritoneum may reduce leakage through the wound [50]. These groups represent a special case. Generally, however, the evidence suggests that suturing the peritoneum appears to be unnecessary during abdominal wound closure.

Table 2. Effect of suturing the parietal peritoneum on incidence of adhesions to the scar in animal models

Peritoneum sutured[a]		Peritoneum open		p value	Reference
Adhesions (n)	Total (n)	Adhesions (n)	Total (n)		
18	32	5	24	< 0.01	[5]
4	11	3	12	NS	[9]
8	10	2	10	< 0.05	[19]
6	12	1	11	< 0.05	[20]
11	15	6	15	0.07	[30]

NS, not significant.
[a]Suturing was performed using catgut.

Adhesions to the scar

Hubbard et al. [15] were probably first to suggest, with anecdotal evidence, that suturing the peritoneum during closure of a laparotomy wound might increase the incidence of adhesions compared with non-suture. The question was investigated formally by Conolly and Stephens [5] prompted by reports that suturing peritoneal defects causes adhesions. After mid-line laparotomy, they found adhesions to abdominal wounds in 18 out of 32 rats (56%) in which the peritoneum had been sutured with chromic catgut compared with only five out of 24 (21%) when the peritoneum was left unsutured ($p < 0.01$). Subsequent animal experiments (Table 2) have confirmed a trend to increased adhesion formation where the peritoneum was sutured which was statistically significant ($p < 0.05$) in three of five studies. Two animal studies have evaluated the effect of more or less reactive suture materials on adhesion formation. Although the numbers involved were small, the incidence of adhesions to the scar was not significantly different whether the peritoneum was sutured with catgut or nylon [19, 30].

Clinical studies of the effect of peritoneal suturing on adhesion formation are difficult to organize, being restricted to patients undergoing second laparotomies or "second-look" laparoscopy. Tulandi et al. [50] laparoscoped women who had previously undergone infertility surgery by laparotomy. Adhesions to the scar were noted in 14 out of 63 (22%) of those in whom the peritoneum had been sutured with catgut versus nine out of 57 (15.8%) where it had been left unsutured; however, the difference was not statistically significant.

Sepsis and Adhesion Formation

Suturing parietal peritoneum promotes a fibrinous inflammatory response [29] and perhaps increased adhesion formation [5, 19, 20]. In the presence of bacterial peritonitis, the fibrinous exudate may shield bacteria from host defences and administered antibiotics [36]. Surgical trauma and peritonitis each depress peritoneal fibrinolytic activity [4, 12, 52]. The net result of these interactions might be increased adhesion formation if the peritoneum is sutured in the presence of sepsis. This possibility was tested in rats undergoing laparotomy after intraperitoneal inoculation with bacterial cultures or saline. In ten animals that had received saline inoculum, the peritoneum was sutured with nylon and adhesions to the laparotomy scar formed in three animals. In contrast, in the presence of intraperitoneal infection, adhesions to the laparotomy scar formed in eight out of nine animals when the peritoneum was sutured with nylon but in only two out of ten when it was left unsutured ($p <$ 0.01) [30]. Intraperitoneal infection, independent of a particulate or chemical irritant, proved to be a potent cause of adhesions. Moreover, suturing the peritoneum and sepsis appeared to act synergistically to promote adhesions to the scar.

Conclusions

Suturing the peritoneal layer appears to add nothing to the strength of abdominal wound closure. In addition, the lowest incidence of adhesions to the scar is observed where the peritoneum is not sutured during abdominal wound closure, especially in the presence of peritonitis. Avoidance of this step should reduce operating times and costs.

Incorporation of Visceral Peritoneum in Suture Lines

Visceral peritoneum is invariably incorporated in sutured anastomoses involving the peritonealized parts of the gastrointestinal tract, e.g. gastric, biliary and intestinal anastomoses. Adhesions frequently form to these suture lines and may even be beneficial by providing an additional blood supply [7, 27] and perhaps by helping to contain minor leakage or sepsis.

Promotion of Adhesions

Experiments on the healing of peritoneal defects suggest that the incorporation of visceral peritoneum in suture lines promotes adhesions [41, 47]. In a limited number of instances, e.g. some ovarian operations, non-suture of visceral peritoneum may be practical and might result in a reduced incidence of adhesions. Thus Meyer et al. [25] observed that following cautery incisions in the ovary the degree of envelopment with adhesions, and their vascularity, was greater where the incisions had been sutured with polyglactin 910 than when they had been left unsutured.

More commonly, however, visceral peritoneum is sutured incidentally during closure or anastomosis of peritonealized viscera. Deliberate separation or avoidance of the peritoneal layer so as not to incorporate it in sutures is not generally considered desirable or practical. Indeed, the lack of a peritoneal layer may be one factor that contributes to the less reliable healing of oesophageal and low rectal anastomoses.

Influence of Choice of Suture Material or Technique on Adhesion Formation

Gastrointestinal surgeons differ widely in their choice of suture technique and suture material for anastomoses, but the effect of these differences on adhesion formation is largely unknown. The influence of suture material has been investigated by infertility surgeons. In a model using uterine horn repair to compare suture materials, Laufer et al. [21] observed adhesions in 11 out of 12 animals in which the repair was carried out with polyglactin 910 versus five out of 12 ($p < 0.01$) when polydioxanone was used. In contrast, Neff et al. [28], in a broadly similar model, found no difference in histological response or adhesion scores between these suture materials. The more reactive sutures are generally considered more likely to promote adhesions [39], but there is no solid evidence in favour of any particular material.

Additional Measures to Prevent Adhesions

Whereas adhesions related to suturing peritoneal defects or incised peritoneum may be largely avoided if the peritoneum is left unsutured, this option is not generally available when the visceral peritoneal layer is incorporated in sutures. Attention therefore switches to preventing adhesions to the suture line, rather than avoidance of suturing.

Given that factors promoting adhesion formation often work synergistically [30, 37], it would appear sensible to avoid other known provocative influences so as to minimize the effect of suturing, e.g. by using a gentle surgical technique and wet swabs to reduce peritoneal abrasion and removing all blood and clot at the end of abdominal operations. Use of omentum to wrap anastomoses may reduce the likelihood of adhesions to other viscera or to the laparotomy scar. In addition, in one experimental study omental wrapping provided an additional blood supply and reduced the leak rate from colorectal anastomoses [27]. Barrier methods of adhesion prophylaxis, e.g. expanded polytetrafluoroethylene (PTFE) membrane or oxidized cellulose (Interceed, Johnson and Johnson Patient Care Inc., New Brunswick, New Jersey, USA), appear to have a role in preventing adhesions after infertility surgery [17, 46, 54], although some experts remain to be convinced [2]. In gastrointestinal surgery, the potential efficacy of barriers in preventing adhesions would have to be weighed against the likely benefit that adhesions confer on anastomotic healing and containment of sepsis. Indeed, several foreign materials have been found to promote leakage from gastrointestinal anastomoses [22]. Use of phospholipids as peritoneal lubricants to restore a "physiological barrier" is an exciting new approach to preventing adhesions [43] (see also Chap. 18, this volume).

However, similar caveats apply with regard to healing of gastrointestinal anastomoses [43].

Conclusions

More research is needed into the effect of suture technique and suture material on adhesion formation following operations involving peritonealized viscera. Non-suture is not usually an option. Monofilament absorbables may have an advantage [21], and are currently recommended by some gynaecological experts [39] although the evidence is slight as yet.

Summary

Overall, suturing peritoneum appears to promote adhesions to the suture line. Defects in visceral or parietal peritoneum should heal and are best left unsutured to reduce the incidence of adhesions. With a few exceptions, the parietal peritoneal layer need not be sutured during closure of abdominal wounds. This approach does not compromise wound strength and may reduce the incidence of adhesions, especially in the presence of peritonitis. It should also reduce operating times and costs.

Incisions in visceral peritoneum may be best left unsutured, but it is impractical and undesirable to omit the visceral peritoneal layer from gastrointestinal anastomoses. Future research will need to be directed towards methods of preventing or controlling adhesions in relation to such suture lines. Meanwhile, every effort should be made to reduce to a minimum other factors known to promote adhesion formation.

References

1. Anonymous (1987) Leading article. Lancet 1: 727
2. Bowman MC, Cooke ID (1994) The efficacy of synthetic adhesion barriers in infertility surgery. Br J Obstet Gynaecol 101: 3–6
3. Bartolo DCC (1994) The rectum and anal canal. In: Keen G, Farndon JR (eds) Operative surgery and management, 3rd edn. Butterworth-Heinemann, Oxford, p 249
4. Buckman RF, Woods M, Sargent L, Gervin AS (1976) A unifying pathogenetic mechanism in the aetiology of intraperitoneal adhesions. J Surg Res 20: 1–5
5. Conolly WB, Stephens FO (1968) Factors influencing the incidence of intraperitoneal adhesions: an experimental study. Surgery 63: 976–979
6. von Dembowski T (1888) Ueber die Ursachen der peritonealen Adhäsionen nach chirurgischen Eingriffen mit Rücksicht auf die Frage des Ileus nach Laparotomien. Arch Klin Chir 37: 745–748
7. Ellis H (1962) The aetiology of post-operative abdominal adhesions. An experimental study. Br J Surg 50: 10–16
8. Ellis H, Harrison W, Hugh TB (1965) The healing of peritoneum under normal and pathological conditions. Br J Surg 52: 471–476
9. Ellis H, Heddle R (1977) Does the peritoneum need to be closed at laparotomy? Br J Surg 64: 733–736

10. Gilbert JM, Ellis H, Foweraker S (1987) Peritoneal closure after lateral paramedian incision. Br J Surg 74: 113–115
11. Glucksman DL (1966) Serosal integrity and intestinal adhesions. Surgery 60: 1009–1011
12. van Goor H, de Graaf JS, Grond J, Sluiter WJ, van der Meer J, Bom VJ, Bleichrodt RP (1994) Fibrinolytic activity in the abdominal cavity of rats with faecal peritonitis. Br J Surg 81: 1046–1049
13. Hawley PR, Thomson JPS (1987) Colonic surgery. In: Kirk RM, Williamson RCN (eds) General surgical operations, 2nd edn. Churchill Livingstone, Edinburgh, p 143
14. Hertzler AE (1919) The peritoneum. CV Mosby, St Louis
15. Hubbard TB, Khan MZ, Carag VR, Albites VE, Hricko GM (1967) The pathology of peritoneal repair: its relation to the formation of adhesions. Ann Surg 165: 908–916
16. Hugh TB, Nankivell C, Meagher AP, Li B (1990) Is closure of the peritoneal layer necessary in the repair of midline surgical abdominal wounds? World J Surg 14: 231–234
17. Interceed (TC7) Adhesion Barrier Study Group (1989) Prevention of postsurgical adhesions by INTERCEED (TC7), an absorbable adhesion barrier: a prospective randomized multicenter clinical study. Fertil Steril 51: 933–938
18. Irvin TT, Golligher JC (1975) A controlled clinical trial of three different methods of perineal wound management following excision of the rectum. Br J Surg 62: 287–291
19. Kapur BM, Daneswar A, Chopra P (1979) Evaluation of peritoneal closure at laparotomy. Am J Surg 137: 650–652
20. Kyzer S, Bayer I, Turani H, Chaimoff C (1986) The influence of peritoneal closure on formation of intraperitoneal adhesions: an experimental study. Int J Tissue React 8: 355–359
21. Laufer N, Merino M, Trietsch HG, DeCherney AH (1984) Macroscopic and histological reactions to polydioxanone, a new synthetic monofilament microsuture. J Reprod Med 29: 307–310
22. Laufman H, Method H (1948) Effect of absorbable foreign substances on bowel anastomoses. Surg Gynecol Obstet 86: 669–673
23. Menzies D, Ellis H (1989) Intra-abdominal adhesions and their prevention by topical tissue plasminogen activator. J R Soc Med 82: 534–535
24. Menzies D, Ellis H (1990) Intestinal obstruction from adhesions – how big is the problem? Ann R Coll Surg Engl 72: 60–63
25. Meyer WR, Grainger DA, DeCherney AH, Lachs MS, Diamond MP (1991) Ovarian surgery on the rabbit. Effect of cortex closure on adhesion formation and ovarian function. J Reprod Med 36: 639–643
26. Milligan DW, Raftery AT (1974) Observations on the pathogenesis of peritoneal adhesions: a light and electron microscopical study. Br J Surg 61: 274–280
27. McLachlin AD, Olssen LS, Pitt DF (1976) Anterior anastomosis of the rectosigmoid: an experimental study. Surgery 80: 306–311
28. Neff MR, Holtz GL, Betsill WL (1985) Adhesion formation and histologic reaction with polydioxanone and polyglactin suture. Am J Obstet Gynecol 151: 20–23
29. O' Leary DP (1984) Studies on the development of peritoneal adhesions. BSc dissertation, National University of Ireland
30. O' Leary DP, Coakley JB (1992) The influence of suturing and sepsis on the development of postoperative peritoneal adhesions. Ann R Coll Surg Engl 74: 134–137
31. Raf LE (1969) Causes of small intestinal obstruction; a study covering the Stockholm area. Acta Chir Scand 135: 67–72
32. Raftery AT (1973a) Regeneration of parietal and visceral peritoneum. Br J Surg 60: 293–299
33. Raftery AT (1973b) Regeneration of parietal and visceral peritoneum: an electron microscopic study. J Anat 115: 375–392
34. Raftery AT (1981) Effect of peritoneal trauma on peritoneal fibrinolytic activity and intraperitoneal adhesion formation: an experimental study in the rat. Eur Surg Res 13: 397–401
35. Robbins GF, Brunschwig A, Foote FW (1949) Deperitonealization; clinical and experimental observations. Ann Surg 130: 466–470

36. Rotstein OD (1992) Role of fibrin deposition in the pathogenesis of intraabdominal infection. Eur J Clin Microbiol Infect Dis 11: 1064–1068
37. Ryan GB, Grobety J, Majno G (1971) Postoperative peritoneal adhesions: a study of the mechanisms. Am J Pathol 65: 117–138
38. Saxen L, Myllarniemi H (1968) Foreign materials and postoperative adhesions. N Engl J Med 279: 200–202
39. Schwartz LB, Diamond MP (1993) Prevention of adhesion reformation. In: Sutton C, Diamond M (eds) Endoscopic surgery for gynecologists. Saunders, London, p 246
40. Scott-Coombes DM, Vipond MN, Thompson JN (1993) General surgeons' attitudes to the treatment and prevention of abdominal adhesions. Ann R Coll Surg Engl 75: 123–128
41. Singleton AO, Rowe EB, Moore RM (1952) Failure of reperitonealization to prevent abdominal adhesions in the dog. Am J Surg 18: 789–792
42. Smith JG (1895) Is the apposition of peritoneum to peritoneum a surgical error? Br Med J 1: 1–2
43. Snoj M, Ar' Rajab A, Ahren B, Bengmark S (1992) Effect of phosphatidylcholine on postoperative adhesions after small bowel anastomosis in the rat. Br J Surg 79: 427–429
44. Snoj M (1993) Intra-abdominal adhesion formation is initiated by phospholipase A_2. Med Hypotheses 41: 525–528
45. Stewardson RH, Bombeck CT, Nyhus LM (1978) Critical operative management of small bowel obstruction. Ann Surg 187: 189–193
46. Surgical Membrane Study Group (1992) Prophylaxis of pelvic sidewall adhesions with Gore-Tex surgical membrane: a multicenter clinical investigation. Fertil Steril 57: 921–923
47. Thomas JW, Rhoads JE (1950) Adhesions resulting from removal of serosa from an area of bowel; failure of oversewing to lower incidence in the rat and guinea pig. Arch Surg 61: 565–576
48. Thompson JN, Paterson-Brown S, Harbourne T, Whawell SA, Kalodiki E, Dudley HA (1989) Reduced human peritoneal plasminogen activating activity: a possible mechanism for adhesion formation. Br J Surg 76: 382–384
49. Trimpe HD, Bacon HE (1952) Clinical and experimental study of denuded surfaces in extensive surgery of the colon and rectum. Am J Surg 34: 596–602
50. Tulandi T, Hum HS, Gelfand MM (1988) Closure of laparotomy incisions with or without peritoneal suturing and second-look laparoscopy. Am J Obstet Gynecol 158: 636–637
51. Ulfelder H, Quinby WC (1951) Small bowel obstruction following combined abdominoperineal resection of the rectum. Surgery 30: 174–177
52. Vipond MN, Whawell SA, Thompson JN, Dudley HA (1994) Effect of experimental peritonitis and ischaemia on peritoneal fibrinolytic activity. Eur J Surg 160: 471–477
53. Williams NS (1993) Surgical treatment of rectal carcinoma. In: Keighley MRB, Williams NS (eds) Surgery of the anus, rectum and colon. Saunders, London, pp 1004–1005
54. di Zerega GS (1994) Contemporary adhesion prevention. Fertil Steril 61: 219–235
55. Zollinger RM, Zollinger RM (1988) Atlas of surgical operations, 6th edn. Macmillan, New York, p 150

3.4 Cytokine Response to Elective Surgery: A Possible Mechanism for Intraperitoneal Adhesion Pathogenesis

D.M. Scott-Coombes, J.M. Badia, S.A. Whawell, R.C.N. Williamson, and J.N. Thompson

Introduction

Cytokines are biologically active mediators of the immune and acute phase responses to inflammation [1]. The main actions of cytokines occur locally and influence a number of processes, including wound healing, debridement of dead tissues and control of infection, all of which may lead to subsequent scarring and adhesion formation. In addition, the local production of cytokines probably contributes to the systemic disturbance observed following surgery [2]. Within the peritoneal cavity, they are produced by mononuclear phago-cytes [3] and mesothelial cells [4]. Previous studies have measured cytokines in peritoneal fluid and plasma following surgery [5–8], but the correlation of systemic with intraperitoneal cytokine concentrations has been poorly docu-mented. The aim of this study was to investigate the intraperitoneal and sys-temic cytokine responses in patients undergoing elective laparotomy. The results of this study have been reported in brief elsewhere [7].

Patients and Methods

Patients

Six patients undergoing elective pancreatic surgery were entered into the study (cholangiocarcinoma, $n=1$; chronic pancreatitis, $n=2$; adenocarcinoma of pancreas, $n=3$). Peritoneal fluid was sampled via Silastic abdominal drains, and venous blood was aspirated from a central venous catheter. A blood sample was taken preoperatively. Samples of blood and peritoneal fluid were taken at 6, 8, 10, 12, 24, 36, 48 and 72 h from the beginning of the operation. All samples were centrifuged at 2500 g for 10 min at 4 °C, and the supernatant was stored at –80 °C until assay. This study was approved by the Ethical Committee of the Royal Postgraduate Medical School, and all patients gave informed consent.

Cytokine Assays

Interleukin-1β (IL-1β), interleukin-6 (IL-6) and tumour necrosis factor (TNF) were measured in plasma and peritoneal fluid using commercially available enzyme-linked immunosorbent "sandwich" assays (ELISA) (IL-1β from Cistron Biotechnology, Pine Brook, USA; IL-6 from Eurogenetics, Tessenderlo, Belgium; TNF from Biokine, T Cell Diagnostics, Teddington, UK). The minimum detectable concentrations were 20 pg/ml for IL-1β, 5 pg/ml for IL-6 and 1.5 pg/ml for TNF.

Statistical Analysis

Data are expressed as mean $\pm$ standard error of the mean (SEM). Data were analysed initially using analysis of variance (ANOVA) and then with paired t-tests when appropriate. The program StatView (Abacus Concepts, Inc, Berkley, USA) was used.

Results

Clinical Results

The operative procedures were pylorus-preserving proximal pancreatoduodenectomy ($n=5$) and choledochojejunostomy ($n=1$). The operative time was 5.3 $\pm$ 0.3 h. Intraoperative blood loss was 1700 $\pm$ 450 ml. There were no postoperative complications.

Cytokines

All peritoneal fluid samples had detectable TNF, IL-1β and IL-6. The first cytokine to reach peak concentrations was TNF, followed sequentially by IL-1β and IL-6 (Fig. 1). Maximal concentrations of TNF were reached at 8 h (298 $\pm$ 140 pg/ml) and were sustained during the first 12 h before falling to 43 $\pm$ 15 pg/ml at 24 h and 17 $\pm$ 3 at 48 h ($p < 0.05$). IL-1β rose to a peak (372 $\pm$ 142 pg/ml) at 12 h ($p < 0.05$), falling to 161 $\pm$ 50 pg/ml at 24 h and 81 $\pm$ 23 pg/ml at 48 h ($p < 0.05$). Thereafter, an increment was again seen at 72 h. IL-6 attained the highest concentrations of all three cytokines, being 72 $\pm$ 16 ng/ml at 6 h and increasing to a peak at 244 $\pm$ 59 ng/ml at 12 h ($p < 0.05$). Elevated IL-6 concentrations were more sustained compared with IL-1β and TNF, reaching a plateau between 24 and 72 h.

In plasma, IL-1β and TNF were below the level of detection at all time points. The preoperative IL-6 concentration was 0.03 $\pm$ 0.01 ng/ml; this increased to 0.54 $\pm$ 0.24 ng/ml at 6 h ($p < 0.05$) and reached a maximum value of 0.84 $\pm$ 0.55 ng/ml at 8 h. IL-6 concentrations were lower than corresponding peritoneal fluid concentrations by a factor of 300.

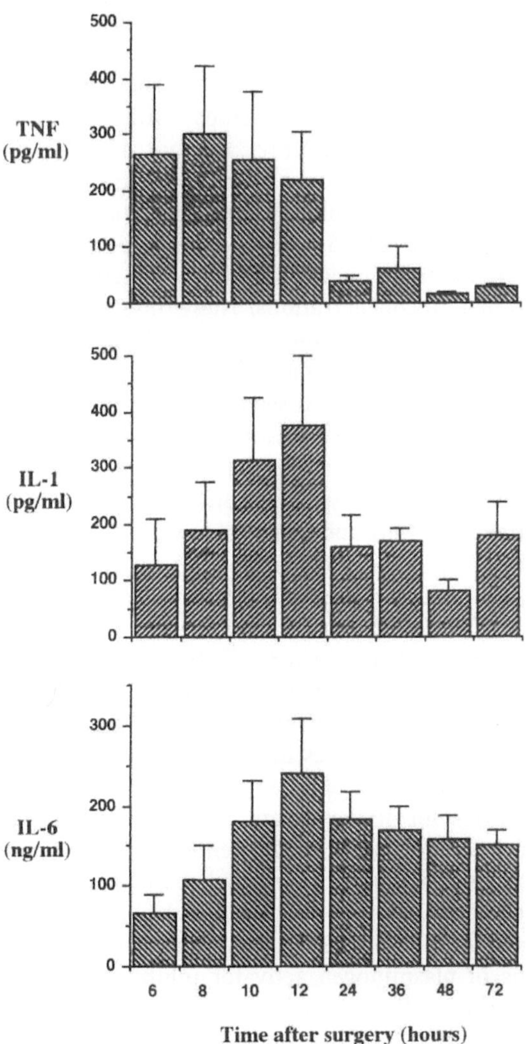

Fig. 1. Postoperative concentrations of cytokines within peritoneal exudate. *TNF*, tumour necrosis factor; *IL-1*, interleukin-1β; *IL-6*, interleukin 6

Discussion

The absence of IL-1β and TNF in plasma of patients undergoing elective surgery is in agreement with several previous reports [6, 10, 11], whereas IL-6 appears to be the cytokine which attains the highest postoperative plasma concentrations. Few reports have investigated the presence of cytokines within the peritoneal cavity. IL-6 has been reported to be a normal constituent of female pelvic peritoneal fluid and to be present in greater concentrations in patients with pelvic inflammatory disease [12], but the concentrations measured were far lower compared with our own results. Tsukada and colleagues [8] detected TNF, IL-1β and IL-6 within peritoneal exudate following laparotomy and demonstrated a correlation between cytokine concentration and the severity of surgical stress. In a pilot study, we demonstrated a similar sequential intraperitoneal cytokine response to this study, with IL-6 levels remaining elevated at 18 h, while interferon (INF)-γ was not detected [9]. Sequential assays of the systemic cytokine response to intravenous endotoxin injection in human volunteers have shown similar changes in plasma to those seen in the peritoneal fluid in our study [13–15]. Peak concentrations of TNF occurred between 1 and 3 h after endotoxin injection, whilst a reduction of this cytokine preceded maximal interleukin concentrations. These observations are consistent with TNF induction of IL-1β production [14, 16], and the similarity of our results suggests that these mechanisms may also operate within the peritoneal cavity. The high concentrations of IL-6 seen in postoperative fluid may result from complex amplification mechanisms involving TNF and IL-1β, both of which induce potent IL-6 responses in vivo [1, 16].

Sakamoto and colleagues [11] correlated cytokine concentrations at local and systemic levels in a single patient who underwent oesophagectomy; they found peak concentrations of IL-6 to be 100-fold greater in pleural fluid than in blood. The discrepancy between the cytokine concentrations measured in plasma and peritoneal fluid in our own study may be explained by a number of factors, including incomplete peritoneal absorption, dilution and first-pass hepatic metabolism. However, it seems likely that the systemic cytokine response is a secondary reflection of events largely within the peritoneal cavity.

Local cytokine production has important roles in the regulation of the inflammatory response, including neutrophil chemotaxis, activation of macrophages and initiation of processes for tissue repair and regeneration [1]. Peritoneal cytokines absorbed into the portal and systemic circulation may also stimulate the production of acute-phase proteins by hepatocytes [1].

We have previously reported a reduction in the functional fibrinolytic activity of postoperative peritoneal fluid following elective surgery secondary to increases in the concentrations of plasminogen activator inhibitors 1 and 2 [17], which may play a pivotal role in the formation of intra-abdominal adhesions [18]. In vitro studies have demonstrated increased plasminogen activator inhibitor-1 production by human mesothelial cells in culture following stimulation by TNF, IL-1β and IL-6, either alone or in combination [19]. Furthermore, a recent report has demonstrated a correlation between the concentrations of TNF in plasma and peritoneal exudate with the severity of intra-abdominal adhesions in an experimental study [20].

Conclusion

We have demonstrated a high-concentration, sequential, intraperitoneal cytokine response to elective surgery. The discrepancy between the cytokine concentrations in plasma and peritoneal fluid suggests that this response originates within the peritoneal cavity. Local intraperitoneal cytokine production probably modulates the intraperitoneal inflammatory response and may have important effects on the control of peritoneal fibrinolysis and adhesion formation. In addition, intraperitoneal cytokine production may generate secondary increases in systemic cytokine levels.

Summary

The aim of this study was to assess the intraperitoneal and systemic cytokine response in patients undergoing elective surgery. Six patients undergoing elective pancreatic surgery were studied (pancreatoduodenectomy, $n=5$; bypass, $n=1$). One venous blood sample was taken preoperatively. Peritoneal fluid and venous blood were sampled at 6, 8, 10, 12, 24, 36, 48 and 72 h after the beginning of surgery. IL-1β, IL-6 and TNF were measured in all samples using immunoassays.

All peritoneal fluid samples had detectable TNF, IL-1β and IL-6, with the following maximum values: TNF, 298 $\pm$ 140 (S.E.M) pg/ml at 8 h after beginning of operation; IL-6, 244 $\pm$ 59 ng/ml at 12 h; IL-1β, 372 $\pm$ 142 pg/ml at 12 h. Plasma IL-1β and TNF concentrations were very low or undetectable. Plasma IL-6 levels were 300-fold lower than peritoneal levels, with a maximum value of 0.84 $\pm$ 0.55 at 8 h.

There is a high-concentration, sequential, peritoneal cytokine response to laparotomy which is responsible for local inflammatory changes and probably also the inhibition of peritoneal fibrinolysis. This peritoneal response may also produce the secondary increases in systemic cytokine concentrations observed after operation.

Acknowledgement. J.M. Badia is the recipient of grant FISS 94/5024 from the Ministry of Health of Spain.

References

1. Van Deuren M, Dofferhoff ASM, van der Meer JWM (1992) Cytokines and the response to infection. J Pathol 168: 349–356
2. Molloy RG, Mannick JA, Rodrick ML (1993) Cytokines, sepsis and immunomodulation. Br J Surg 80: 289–297
3. Remick DG, Strieter RM, Lynch JP, Nguyen D, Eskandri M, Kunkel SL (1989) In vivo dynamics of murine tumour necrosis factor-alpha gene expression. Lab Invest 60: 766–771
4. Bejtes MGH, Tuk CW, Struijk DG, Krediet RT, Arisz L, Beelen RHJ (1993) Interleukin-8 production by human peritoneal mesothelial cells in response to tumour necrosis factor-alpha, interleukin-1 and medium conditioned by macrophages cocultured with Staphylococcus eidermidis. J Infect Dis 168: 1202–1210
5. Dinarello CA (1984) Interleukin-1 and the pathogenesis of the acute phase response. N Engl J Med 311: 1413–1418
6. Baigrie RJ, Lamont PM, Kwaitkowski D, Dallman MJ, Morris PJ (1992) Systemic cytokine response after major surgery. Br J Surg 79: 757–760

7. Scott-Coombes DM, Whawell SA, Thompson JN (1994) Peritoneal cytokine response in surgery. Br J Surg 81: 756
8. Tsukada K, Katoh H, Shiojima M, Suzuki T, Takenoshita S, Nagamachi Y (1993) Concentrations of cytokines in peritoneal fluid after abdominal surgery. Eur J Surg 159: 475–479
9. Badia JM, Whawell SA, Scott-Coombes DM, Abel PD, Williamson RCN, Thompson JN (1996) The peritoneal and systemic cytokine response to laparotomy. Br J Surg (in press)
10. Pullicino EA, Carli F, Poole S, Rafferty B, Malik STA, Elia M (1990) The relationship between the circulating concentrations of interleukin-6 (IL-6), tumour necrosis factor (TNF) and the acute phase response to elective surgery and accidental injury. Lymphokine Res 9: 231–238
11. Sakamoto K, Arakawa H, Mita S, Ishiko T, Egami H, Hisano S, Ogawa M (1994) Elevation of circulating interleukin-6 after surgery: factors affecting the serum level. Cytokine 6: 181–186
12. Buyalos RP, Watson JM, Funari VA, Martinez-Maza O, Azziz R (1992) Elevated interleukin-6 levels in peritoneal fluid of patients with pelvic pathology. Fertil Steril 58: 302–306
13. Martich GD, Danner RL, Ceska M, Suffredini AF (1991) Detection of interleukin-8 and tumour necrosis factor in normal humans after intravenous endotoxin: the effect of antiinflammatory agents. J Exp Med 173: 1021–1024
14. Cannon JG, Tompkins RG, Gefland JA, Michie HR, Stanford GG, van der Meer JWM, Endres S, Lonneman G, Corsetti J, Chernow B, Wilmore DW, Wolff SW, Burke JF, Dinarallo CA (1990) Circulating interleukin-1 and tumour necrosis factor in septic shock and experimental endotoxin fever. J Infect Dis 161: 79–84
15. Fong Y, Moldawer LL, Marano M, Wei H, Tatter SB, Clarick RH, Santhanam U, Sherris D, May LT, Sehgal PB, Lowry SF (1989) Endotoxemia elicits increased circulating beta 2 IFN/IL-6 in man. J Immunol 142: 2321–2324
16. Dinarello CA (1991) Interleukin-1 and interleukin-1 antagonism. Blood 77: 1627–1652
17. Scott-Coombes DM, Whawell SA, Thompson JN (1994) The human intraperitoneal fibrinolytic response to elective surgery. Br J Surg 81: 1472–1474
18. Vipond MN, Whawell SA, Thompson JN, Dudley HAF (1990) Peritoneal fibrinolytic activity and intra-abdominal adhesions. Lancet 335: 1120–1122
19. Whawell SA, Thompson JN (1995) Cytokine-induced release of plasminogen activator inhibitor-1 by human mesothelial cells. Eur J Surg 161: 315–317
20. Kaidi AA, Gurchumelidze T, Nazzal M, Figert P, Vanterpool C, Silva Y (1995) Tumour necrosis factor alpha: a marker for peritoneal adhesion formation. J Surg Res 58: 516–518

3.5 Prostaglandin Synthesis of Human Mesothelial Cells In Vitro Is Regulated by Transforming Growth Factor-β_1, Tumor Necrosis Factor-α, and Interleukin-1β

L. Tietze, T. Rütters, C. Schauerte, B. Amo-Takyi, B. Klosterhalfen,
K.-H. Treutner, C. Mittermayer, and S. Handt

Introduction

Inflammation is generally defined as a localized protective response elicited by injury or destruction of tissues which serves to destroy, dilute, or wall off both the injurious agent and the injured tissue. This complex, multicellular process is histologically characterized by a series of events including dilation of arterioles, capillaries, and venules with increased permeability and blood flow, exudation, and leukocytic migration into the inflammatory focus. This process may be understood as a concert of soluble and cellular components.

In the particular case of peritonitis, the early inflammatory response in the peritoneal cavity is regulated in part by the interaction of mesothelial cells and peritoneal macrophages. Peritoneal hyperemia, edema, and vasodilation may be caused by humoral factors, particularly prostaglandins (PG).

Clinically, the early phase of peritonitis is accompanied by an increased PG and cytokine concentration in the peritoneal cavity. During peritonitis in continuous ambulatory peritoneal dialysis (CAPD) patients, Steinhauer et al. [18] found an increased concentration of 6-keto-$PGF_{1\alpha}$, PGE_2, $PGF_{2\alpha}$ and thromboxane $B_2(TXB_2)$ with a predominance of vasodilative prostaglandins (6-keto-$PGF_{1\alpha}$ and PGE_2). This enhanced PG concentration is accompanied by an increased concentration of some macrophage-derived cytokines, particularly tumor necrosis factor (TNF)-α and interleukin (IL)-1β [2, 7].

In vitro studies demonstrated that mesothelial cells produce PGE_2 and PGI_2, but no lipoxygenase products [3, 4, 19]. Beside phospholipase A_2, which metabolizes cell membrane phopholipids to arachidonic acid, the key enzyme in PG synthesis is cyclooxygenase (COX), which converts arachidonic acid to PG H_2 (i.e., PG H_2 synthase) [5]. For many years, it was believed that PG were formed via the activity of a single enzyme, COX, which is present as a constituent in most cells; however, two isoforms of COX were recently identified. COX-1, which is constitutively expressed, and COX-2, which is inducible by a number of cytokines, in particular TNF-α and IL-1β [10, 13–15]. Transforming growth factor (TGF)-β, a potent cytokine released from activated macrophages and platelets, is known to augment mitogen-induced PG synthesis in swiss 3T3

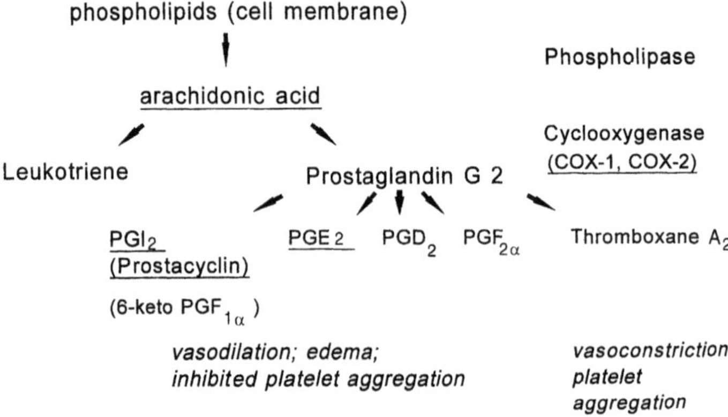

Fig. 1. Arachidinoic acid pathway; prostaglandin (*PG*) synthesis

fibroblasts and mouse embryo cells. Figure 1 shows a simplified scheme of arachidonic acid metabolism.

In the present study, we investigated the influence of the macrophage-derived cytokines TNF-α, IL-1β, and TGF-β1 on 6-keto-PGF$_{1\alpha}$ and PGI$_2$ production by human mesothelial cells in vitro. The results demonstrate that mesothelial PG production is increased by these cytokines, which in turn is partly caused by an induction of COX-2 de novo synthesis. This mesothelial cell response may contribute to the clinically observed increase in PG concentration in the peritoneal cavity and thus may contribute to vasodilation, edema, and hyperalgesia.

Materials and Methods

Materials

Tissue culture reagents were purchased from GIBCO (Karlsruhe, Germany). Human serum protein was obtained from a pool of at least 20 healthy donors.

Human recombinant TNF-α (1×10^8 U/mg) and IL-1β (ED$_{50}$, 0.1 ng/ml) were ordered from PBH (Hannover, Germany). TGF-β_1 was obtained from Boehringer (Mannheim, Germany).

Human Omentum Majus Mesothelial Cell Culture

Mesothelial cells derived from omentum majus were cultured according to the method described by Hinsbergh [9], with minor modifications and characterized as described in Chap. 10 (this volume).

All experiments were performed in 96-microtiter plates, which were precoated with 0.2% gelatine. A total of 20 000 cells/100 μl RPMI 1640 medium (GIBCO BRL, Life Technologies, USA) + 10% human serum protein were seeded into each well to establish a confluent monolayer. All experiments were performed 48 h after seeding without additional change of culture medium.

Cytokine Stimulation and Determination
of 6-Keto-Prostaglandin $F_{1\alpha}$ and Prostaglandin E_2

Culture medium was removed by aspiration, and the confluent monolayer was rinsed twice with serum-free RPMI 1640 (37 °C). Stimulation with TGF-β_1, IL-1β, and TNF-α was performed by adding these cytokines at different concentrations (0.001–10 ng/ml) in serum-free RPMI 1640 containing 1% human serum albumin. After 2, 6, 12, and 24 h, human omentum majus mesothelial cell (HOMC)-conditioned media were collected and centrifuged for 10 min (200 g). The supernatants were stored at –20 °C.

The immunoreactive 6-keto-$PGF_{1\alpha}$ and PGE_2 concentrations were determined using commercially available enzyme-linked immunosorbent assay (ELISA) kits (6-keto-$PGF_{1\alpha}$ and PGE_2 EIA Kit, PerSeptive Diagnostics, Cambridge, MA, USA). According to the manufactors description, cross-reactivity for the PGI_2 ELISA is 50% for PGE_1, 6% for PGA_1, and less than 2% for other arachidonic acid metabolites. Cross-reactivity of the 6-keto-$PGF_{1\alpha}$ ELISA for other prostaglandins than PG 6-keto-$PGF_{1\alpha}$ is less than 1%. The determined PG concentrations were related to the total protein concentration in each well (bicinchoninic acid, BCA, Pierce).

All experiments were performed at least three times in duplicate with HOMC from different donors.

Reverse Transcription Polymerase Chain Reaction Analysis of Cyclooxygenase-2 mRNA

For mRNA analysis, confluent HOMC were established in gelatine-precoated tissue culture flasks (75 cm^2, Falcon). At 72 h after the last cell culture medium change, the cells were rinsed twice with serum-free RPMI 1640 (37 °C). Stimulation was performed by adding recombinant IL-1β, TNF-α, and TGF-β1 (each 10 ng/ml in RPMI 1640 containing 1% human serum albumin). After 6 h, the medium was removed and the cells were detached by adding trypsin (0.125%). The cell suspension was washed once in phosphate-buffered solution (PBS) and centrifuged (10 min at 200 g), and the cell pellet was immediately frozen in liquid nitrogen and stored at –70 °C. Total RNA was extracted using a QIAGEN RNeasy Kit (Quiagen, Hilden, Germany) and stored at –70 °C.

Reverse transcription (RT) was performed with a first-strand cDNA synthesis Kit (Pharmacia Biotech, Freiburg, Germany) according to the manufacturer's instructions. Polymerase chain reaction, (PCR) for COX-2 and β-globin was performed in two 30-μl assays in BIOZYM 0.5-ml PCR tubes with 0.6 μl deoxynucleoside triphosphate (dNTP) mix each containing nucleotides deoxyadenosine (dATP), deoxycytidine (dCTP), deoxyguanosine (dGTP), and deoxythymidine triphosphate (dTTP) at a concentration of 10mM (mixed from Ultrapure dNTP Set 2DN5T, PHARMACIA BIOTECH), 0.75 units of Taq DNA polymerase, 3 μl tenfold concentrated PCR buffer (Boehringer, Mannheim, Germany), and 15 and 3 pmol β-globin and COX-2 sense and antisense primer, respectively (β-globin: sense primer, 5′-ATG GTG CAC ACT CCT GAG G-3′; anti-sense primer, 5′-GCC ATC ACT AAA GGC ACC GAG C-3′; fragment length, 225 bp, cDNA; COX 2: sense primer, 5′-AAC CCA CTC CAA ACA CAG-3′; antisense primer, 5′-CTG GCC CTC GCT TAT GAT CT-3′; fragment length, 411 bp, cDNA; GENSET SA, Paris, France). A total of 0.9 μl cDNA template was added to each tube, and PCR was performed in a thermocycler as follows: after 5 min denaturation at 95 °C, 28 cycles of 2-min annealing at 55 °C, a 2-min extension at 72 °C, and a 30-s denaturation at 95 °C were performed, followed by 5 min at 72 °C for final extension. Subsequently, 10 μl was mixed with 4 μl loading buffer, and electrophoresis was performed in 2% agarose gel (Gibco BRL Ultrapure Agarose Electrophoresis Grade). The molecular weight marker was pUC 19 DNA digested by Msp I (MBI Fermentas, Vilnius, Lithuania). Bands were stained with ethidium bromide, visualized under ultraviolet light and photographed.

Results

HOMC-conditioned media contained immunoreactive 6-keto-PGF$_{1\alpha}$ and PGI$_2$. After 24 h, the supernatants contained 4.525 pg 6-keto-PGF$_{1\alpha}$/μg cell protein ($n=3$; SEM, 0.7 pg/μg) and 0.51 pg PGI$_2$/μg cell protein ($n=3$; SEM, 0.2 pg/μg). During an incubation period of 24 h, we observed a continuous and a nearly linear accumulation of these PG. In all experiments, the immunoreactive 6-keto-PGF$_{1\alpha}$ concentration was about five- to tenfold higher than the determined PGE$_2$ concentration.

Incubation with TNF-α, IL-1β, and TGF-β_1 for 24 h caused an increase in the 6-keto-PGF$_{1\alpha}$ and PGI$_2$ concentration in a dose-dependent manner. After incubation with TNF-α, TGF-β_1, and IL-1β at a concentration of 10 ng/ml, at least a twofold increase of immunoreactive 6-keto-PGF$_{1\alpha}$ and PGE$_2$ was observed. Figures 2 and 3 show a representative experiment with a dose-dependent cytokine response of HOMC-conditioned supernatants and its effect on PG release.

This cytokine response was time dependent and showed a late onset. There was a significant increase in 6-keto-PGF$_{1\alpha}$ and PGE$_2$ concentrations after 6 h. Figures 4 and 5 are examples of time-dependent PG release after cytokine stimulation.

Preliminary results of mRNA analysis revealed an increased mRNA concentration for COX-2 mRNA after stimulation with TNF-α, IL-1β, and TGF-β1, but it should be noted that COX-2 mRNA was also detectable by RT-PCR in nonstimulated HOMC (Fig. 6).

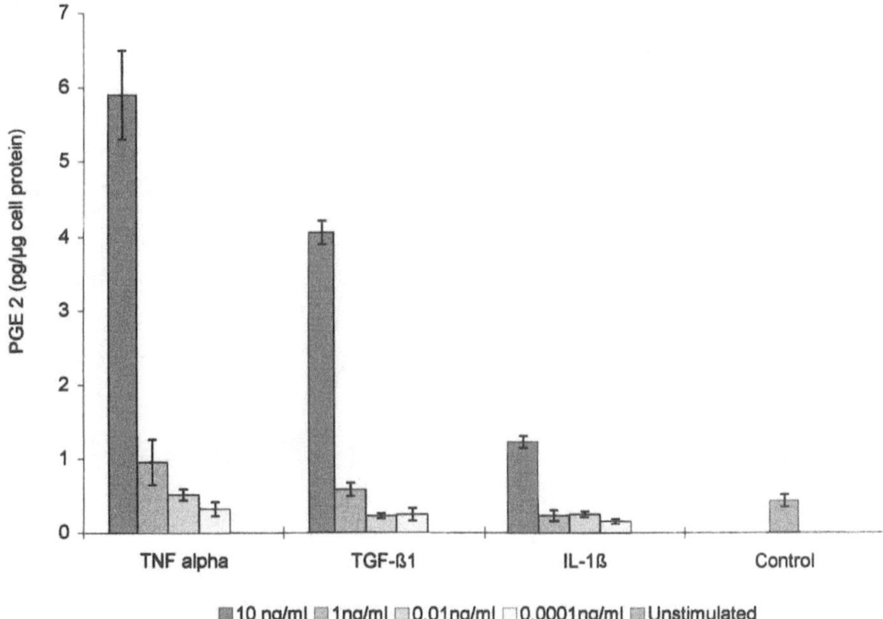

Fig. 2. Prostaglandin (*PG*) E_2 concentrations after incubation of human omentum majus mesothelial cells (HOMC) at different cytokine concentrations for a period of 24 h. *TNF*, tumor necrosis factor; *TGF*, transforming growth factor; *IL*, interleukin

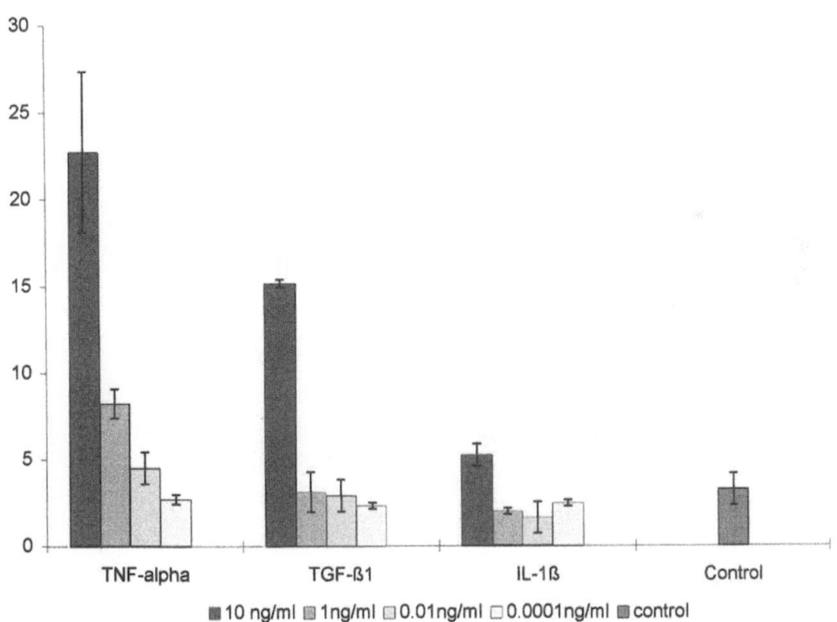

Fig. 3. 6-Keto-prostaglandin (*PG*) $F_{1\alpha}$ concentrations after incubation of human omentum majus mesothelial cells (HOMC) at different cytokine concentrations for a period of 24 h. *TNF*, tumor necrosis factor; *TGF*, transforming growth factor; *IL*, interleukin

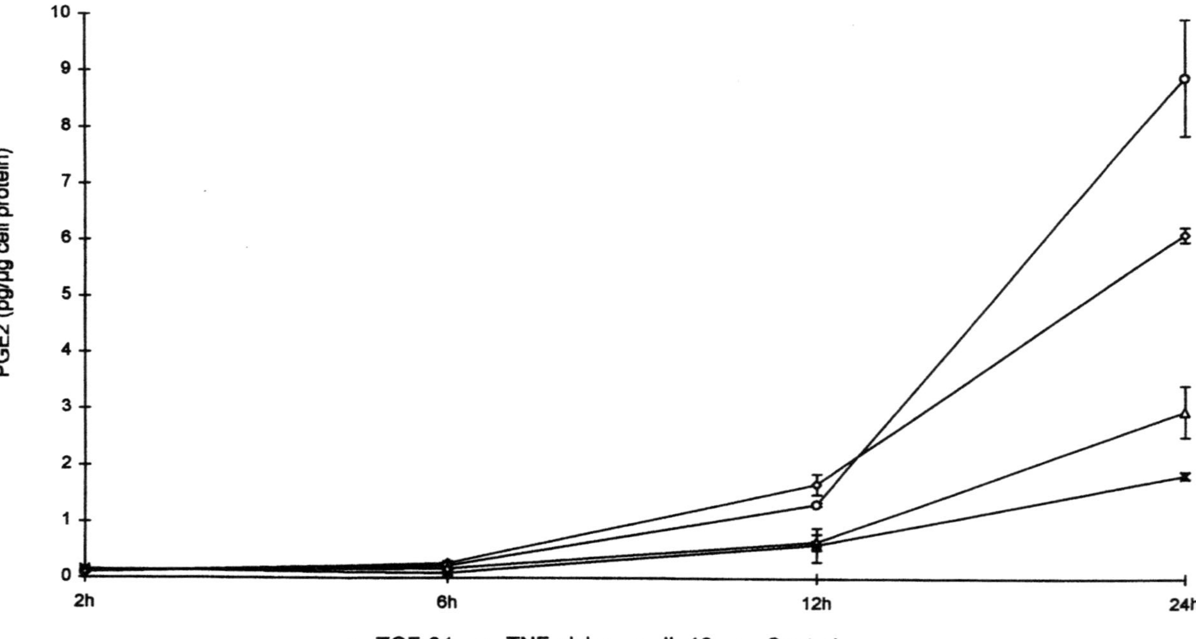

Fig. 4. Prostaglandin (*PG*) E_2 concentrations after 2, 6, 12, and 24 h of incubation with transforming growth factor (*TGF*)-β_1, tumor necrosis factor (*TNF*)-α, and interleukin (*IL*)-1β (each 10 ng/ml)

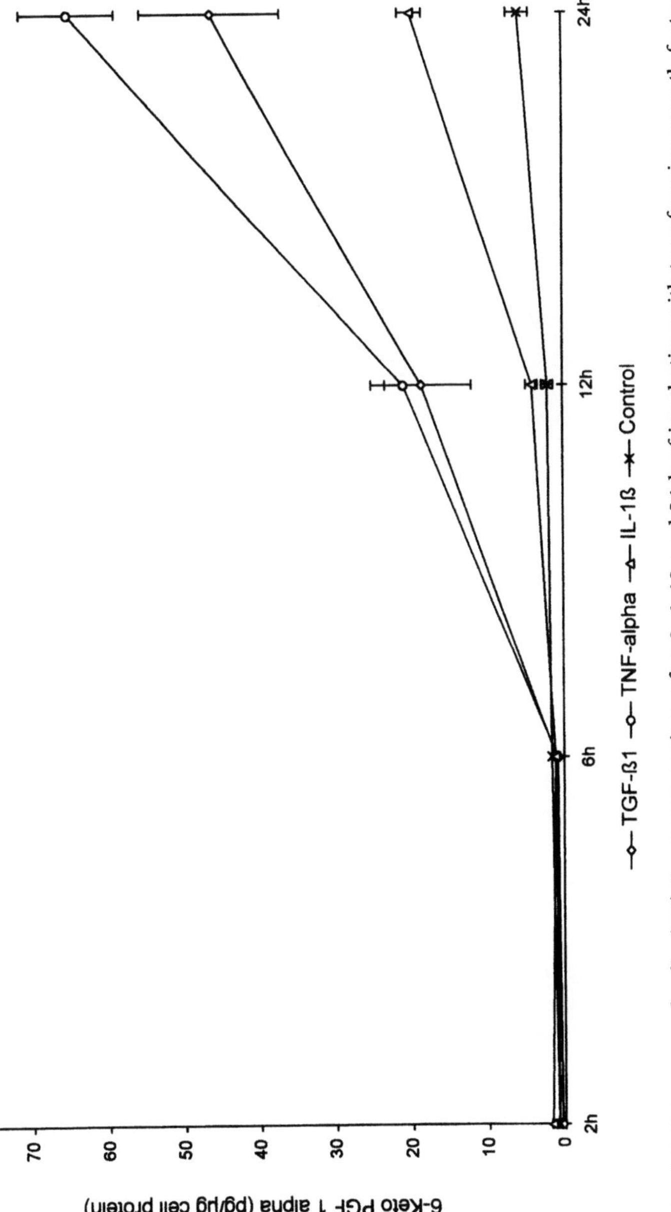

Fig. 5. 6-Keto-prostaglandin (*PG*) $F_{1\alpha}$ concentrations after 2, 6, 12, and 24 h of incubation with transforming growth factor (*TGF*)-β_1, tumor necrosis facor (*TNF*)-α, and interleukin (*IL*)-1β (each 10 ng/ml)

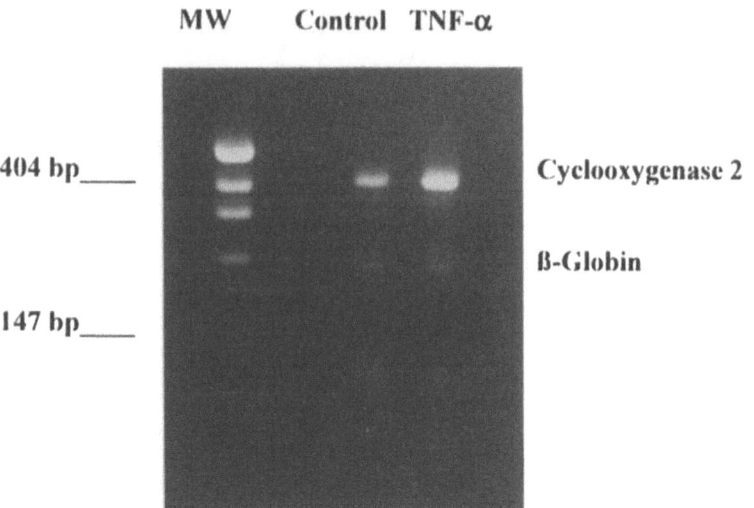

Fig. 6. Cyclooxygenase (COX)-2 mRNA analysis (reverse transcriptase polymerase chain reaction, RT-PCR) of human omentum majus mesothelial cells (HOMC) stimulated with tumor necrosis factor (*TNF*)-α (10 ng/ml; 6 h). β-Globin served as an internal standard for the quantity of extracted RNA

Discussion

Peritonitis is a complex, multicellular process involving mesothelial cells, the subserosal stroma, and inflammatory cells, particularly peritoneal macrophages and granulocytes. Histologically, the early inflammatory response is characterized by vasodilation with increased vascular permeability, leading to edema. These reactions are accompanied clinically by hyperalgesia. PG, such as PGE_2 and PGI_2, which are secreted by mesothelial cells [3, 4, 19, 21], are known to cause at least some of these tissue reactions, but the regulation of mesothelial PG production is not understood in detail. Inflammatory and macrophage-derived cytokines, such as TNF-α, IL-1β, and TGF-β_1, are known to increase PG synthesis in fibroblasts and glomerular mesangial cells [6, 8, 20].

The present study examines the role of these cytokines in PG production by human mesothelial cells in vitro.

The results demonstrate a time- and dose-dependent increase in 6-keto-$PGF_{1\alpha}$ and PGE_2 production by human mesothelial cells in vitro following incubation with these cytokines. These results are in agreement with the study by Topley [21], who demonstrated a dose- and time-dependent increase of PGE_2 and 6-keto-$PGF_{1\alpha}$ release by HOMC after incubation with peritoneal macrophage-conditioned media. Inhibition studies with anticytokine antibodies, IL-1 receptor antagonist (IL-1ra), and TNF-soluble receptors indicated that this stimulatory effect was partly related to the IL-1β and TNF-α content of the conditioned media, but inhibition with antibodies alone was not sufficient to inhibit the HOMC response completely. Our results suggest that TGF-β_1, which is secreted by activated macrophages, contributes to the HOMC response to macrophage-conditioned media. Preliminary studies on the mRNA level indicate that, under our culture conditions, COX-2 mRNA was detectable in small quantities in nonstimulated HOMC and that stimulation with TNF-α, IL-1β, and TGF-β_1 causes a stronger increase in the mRNA concentration for COX-2 and its metabolites, as reported by Topley et al. [21]. This discrepancy and the observation that even nonstimulated cells expressed COX-2 may indicate that, under our culture conditions, HOMC were not strictly growth arrested. Our results suggest that induction of COX-2 is at least augmented by TNF-α, IL-1β, and TGF-β_1 in proliferating mesothelial cells with a consecutive increase in the PGE$_2$ and 6-keto-PGF$_{1\alpha}$ concentrations.

Our results also confirm the observation that the increased PGE$_2$ and PGI$_2$ concentrations during peritonitis are caused partly by mesothelial cells, which respond to increased concentrations of inflammatory cytokines. This cytokine-mediated response is partly mediated by induction of COX-2 de novo synthesis.

PGE$_2$ and PGI$_2$ may exert cell-protective effects, as demonstrated in gastric mucosa cells. There is some evidence that this protective effect of PG may be mediated by the constitutively expressed COX-1, whereas the inflammatory reaction is mediated by COX-2 induction. Recent studies revealed selective COX antagonists which inhibit COX-2, but not COX-1 [11]. Besides a protective cell effect, PG may regulate the local peritoneal inflammatory response by inhibition of IL-1 secretion of macrophages [12]. Unfortunately, no information about the influence of these PG on the biology of mesothelial cells is yet available.

Further studies are required to elucidate mitogenic, cell-protective, and regulatory effects of PG on mesothelial cells in order to understand the role played by the inflammatory peritoneal PG response in the development of fibrous adhesions.

Summary

Serous body cavities are lined by mesothelial cells which participate in the regulation of inflammatory processes of serous membranes. The early peritoneal inflammatory response is accompanied by hyperemia, an increased peritoneal permeability and hyperalgesia. These effects may be caused by prostaglandins.

Here we describe the role of the macrophage derived cytokines TNF-α, TGF-β_1 and IL-1β on human mesothelial prostaglandin (PGE$_2$ and PGI$_2$) production. The results indicate that human mesothelial cells are an important source of intraperitoneal prostaglandins. The increased mesothelial PGE$_2$ and PGI$_2$ production after stimulation with TNF-α, TGF-β_1 and IL-1β may explain in part peritoneal hyperemia and the increased peritoneal permeability in the early phase of peritonitis.

Acknowledgements. The authors wish to thank Prof. Dr. Dr. med. h.c. V. Schumpelick and the members of the operation team of the surgical clinic of the RWTH Aachen for assisting with the collection of omentum majus specimens for mesothelial cell culture.

References

1. Baer AN, Green FA (1993) Cyclooxygenase activity of human mesothelial cells. Prostaglandins 46: 37–49
2. Brauner A, Hylander B, Wretlind B (1994) Inflammatory factors (TNF-α, IL-β, IL-1ra) during peritonitis in CAPD patients. Perit Dial Int 14: 48 (abstr)
3. Bult H, Coene MC, Rampart M, Hermann AG (1984) Complement derived factors and prostacyclin formation by isolated rabbit peritoneum and cultured mesothelial cells. Agents Actions 14: 237–247
4. Coene MC, Solheid C, Claeys M, Herman AG (1981) Prostaglandin production by cultured mesothelial cells. Arch Int Pharmacodyn Ther 249: 316–318
5. De Witt DL (1991) Prostaglandin endoperoxide synthase: regulation of enzyme expression. Biochim Biophys Acta 1083: 121–134
6. Elias JA, Lentz V (1990) IL-1 and tumour necrosis factor α stimulate fibroblast IL-6 production and stabilize IL-6 messenger RNA. J Immunol 145: 161–166
7. Fieren MW, van den Bemd GJCM, Bonta IL, Ben Efraim S (1991) Peritoneal macrophages from patients on continuous ambulatory peritoneal dialysis have an increased capability to release tumour necrosis factor during peritonitis. J Clin Lab Immunol 34: 1–9
8. Herschmann HR, Gilbert RS, Xie W, Luner S, Reddy ST (1995) The regulation and role of TIS 10 prostaglandin sythase-2. In: Samuelsson et al. (eds) Advances in prostaglandin, thromboxane, and leukotriene research, vol 23. Raven, New York, pp 23–28
9. Hinsbergh VWM, Kooistra T, Scheffer AA, van Bockel JH, van Muijen GNP (1990) Characterization and fibrinolytic properties of human omental tissue mesothelial cells. Comparison with endothelial cells. Blood 75: 1490–1497
10. Hla T, Nielson K (1992) Human cyclooxygenase-2 cDNA. Proc Natl Acad Sci USA 89: 7384–7388
11. Isakson P, Seibert K, Masferrer J, Salvemini D, Lee L, Needleman P (1995) Discovery of a better aspirin. In: Samuelsson et al. (eds) Advances in prostaglandin, thromboxane, and leukotriene research, vol 23. Raven, New York, pp 49–54
12. Knudsen PJ, Dinarello CA, Strom TB (1988) Prostaglandins post-transcriptionally inhibit monocyte expression of interleukin-1 activity by increasing intracellular cAMP. J Immunol 137: 3189–3194
13. Kujubu DA, Fletscher BS, Varnum BC, Lim RW, Herschman HR (1991) TIS10, a phorbol ester tumor promoter inducible mRNA from swiss 3T3 cells, encodes a novel prostaglandin synthase/cyclooxygenase. J Biol Chem 266: 12866–12872
14. Kujubu DA, Herschman HR (1992) Dexamethasone inhibits mitogen induction of the TIS 10 prostaglandin synthase/cyclooxygenase gene. J Biol Chem 267: 7991–7994
15. Kujubu DA, Reddy ST, Fletscher BS, Herschman HR (1993) Expression of the protein product of the prostaglandin synthase-2/TIS 10 gene in mitogen-stimulated swiss 3T3 cells. J Biol Chem 268: 5425–5430
16. Kumar V, Cotran RS, Robbins SL (eds) (1992) Basic pathology, 5th edn. Saunders, Philadelphia
17. Maher JF, Hirszel P, Lasrich M (1980) Modulation of peritoneal transport rates by prostaglandins. In: Sammuelsson RP, Paoletti RB (eds) Advances in prostaglandin and leukotriene research, vol 7. Raven New York
18. Steinhauer HB, Schollmeyer P (1986) Prostaglandin mediated loss of proteins during peritonitis in continuous ambulatory peritoneal dialysis. Kidney Int 29: 584–590
19. Stylianou E, Jenner LA, Davies M, Coles G, Williams JD (1990) Isolation, culture and characterisation of human peritoneal mesothelial cells. Kidney Int 37: 1563–1570

20. Topley N, Floege J, Wessel K, Hass R, Radeke HH, Kaever V, Resch K (1989) Prostaglandin E2 production is synergistically increased in human glomerular mesangial cells by combinations of IL-1β and tumour necrosis factor-α. J Immunol 143: 1989–1995
21. Topley N, Petersen MM, Mackenzie R, Neubauer A, Stylianou E, Kaever V, Davies M, Coles GA, Jörres A, Williams D (1994) Human peritoneal mesothelial cell prostaglandin synthesis: induction of cyclooxygenase mRNA by peritoneal macrophage-derived cytokines. Kidney Int 44: 900–909
22. Whatley RE, Satoh K, Zimmermann GA, McIntyre TM, Prescott SM (1994) Proliferation dependent changes in release of arachidonic acid from endothelial cells. J Clin Invest 94: 1889–1900

3.6 Peritoneal Fibrinolysis and Its Role in Adhesion Formation

J.N. Thompson, S.A. Whawell, D.M. Scott-Coombes,
and M.N. Vipond

Introduction

Adhesions are deposits of fibrous tissue which occur within body cavities such as the peritoneum, pericardium or pleura. They are the pathological result of injury to the lining membrane of such cavities. These abnormal deposits of fibrous tissue are a cause of major morbidity [1], being the commonest cause of small-bowel obstruction and secondary female infertility and representing a major risk factor for cardiac reoperation.

Pathology of Adhesion Formation

Histological studies of adhesion formation within body cavities clearly show a sequence of events starting with tissue inflammation and leading to fibrin deposition, within an inflammatory exudate, organisation of this fibrin with fibroblast invasion and collagen deposition, and later collagen maturation with the formation of permanent fibrous adhesions. A large number of experimental models of adhesion formation have been described using a variety of mechanisms of injury to the peritoneal membrane. Tissue ischaemia, bacterial or chemical peritonitis and mechanical injury all lead to a high incidence of fibrous adhesion formation [2]. In clinical practice, operative trauma is the commonest cause of adhesion formation, with up to 90% of patients developing intra-abdominal adhesions following laparotomy. Other causes include bacterial peritonitis, irradiation, allergic reactions and chemical and ischaemic injury.

Peritoneal Fibrinolysis

For many years it has been known that the peritoneum possesses fibrinolytic activity [3]. A number of experimental studies have demonstrated that injury to the peritoneum reduces its fibrinolytic capacity and that the same injuries are associated with later fibrous adhesion formation [4, 5]. These observations have led to the development of a hypothesis that normal peritoneal fibrinolytic

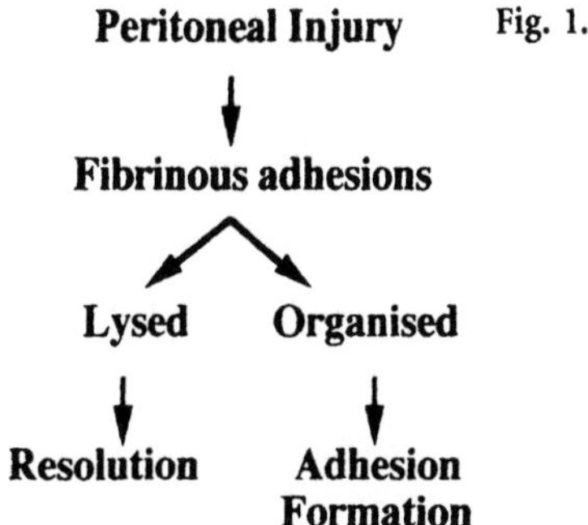

Fig. 1. The pathogenesis of permanent fibrous adhesions

activity prevents the formation of fibrous adhesions by lysing any fibrin deposits that may form within the peritoneal cavity (Fig. 1).

Our current understanding of the fibrinolytic system is shown in Fig. 2. Our early studies [6] of human peritoneum showed that normal tissue contained plasminogen-activating activity, and although there was considerable variation between patients, similar levels of plasminogen-activating activity were found in both visceral and parietal biopsies taken from different abdominal sites.

These studies also clearly showed a marked loss of peritoneal plasminogen-activating activity in the presence of bacterial peritonitis or tissue ischaemia (Figs. 3, 4). This finding supported previous experimental studies and was confirmed in human studies by Holmdahl et al. [7]. Antibody inhibition studies and subsequent antigenic immunoassays have shown clearly that tissue plasminogen activator (t-PA) is the major plasminogen activator in human peritoneal and pericardial biopsies [7–9]. However, the loss of peritoneal plasminogen-activating activity seen in patients with peritonitis was not as-

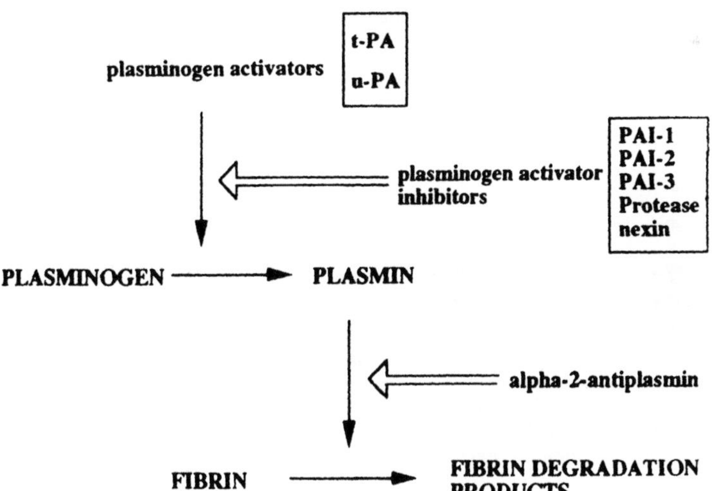

Fig. 2. The fibrinolytic system

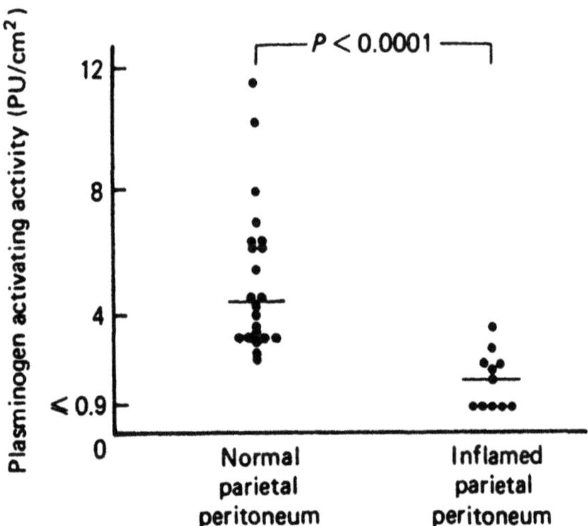

Fig. 3. The plasminogen activating activity of normal and inflamed human parietal peritoneum

sociated with a dramatic decrease in peritoneal t-PA levels, but with the production of inhibitors of t-PA, both plasminogen activator inhibitor (PAI)-1 and -2 being found in high concentrations in inflamed peritoneal tissue [8, 10].

The time course of changes in peritoneal fibrinolysis following a standardised peritoneal injury (i.e. elective laparotomy) was studied using samples of peritoneal cavity drain fluid. These studies [11] showed the rapid loss of

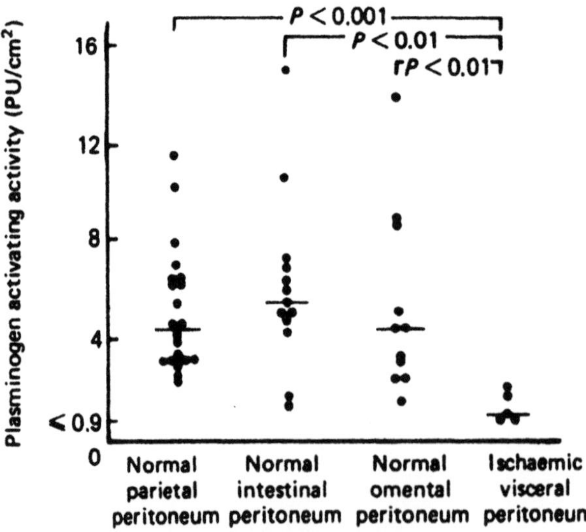

Fig. 4. The plasminogen activating activity of normal parietal, intestinal and omental human peritoneum compared with ischaemic visceral human peritoneum

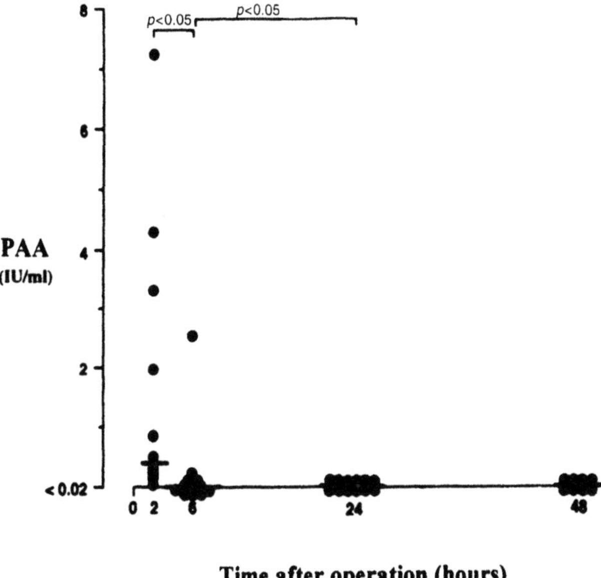

Fig. 5. Post-operative peritoneal fluid plasminogen activating activity (PAA)

peritoneal fluid plasminogen-activating activity during the first few hours following operation associated with concomitant rapid increases in the concentrations of both PAI-1 and -2 (Figs. 5–7). Experimental studies have also shown that, following peritoneal injury and the initial reduction in peritoneal

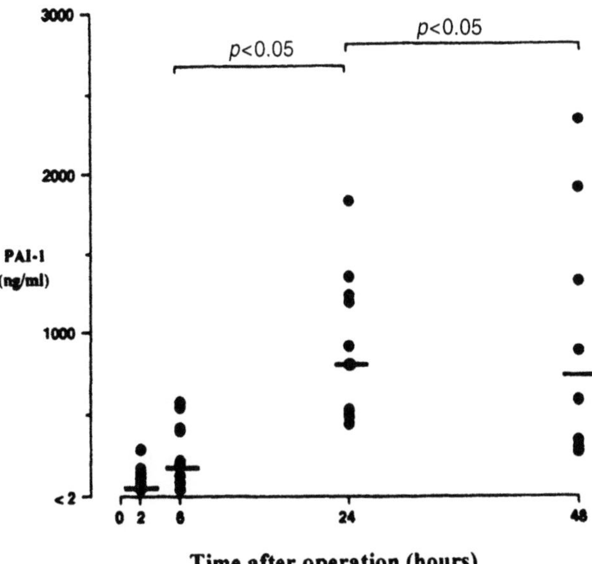

Fig. 6. Post-operative peritoneal fluid plasminogen activator inhibitor-1 concentrations

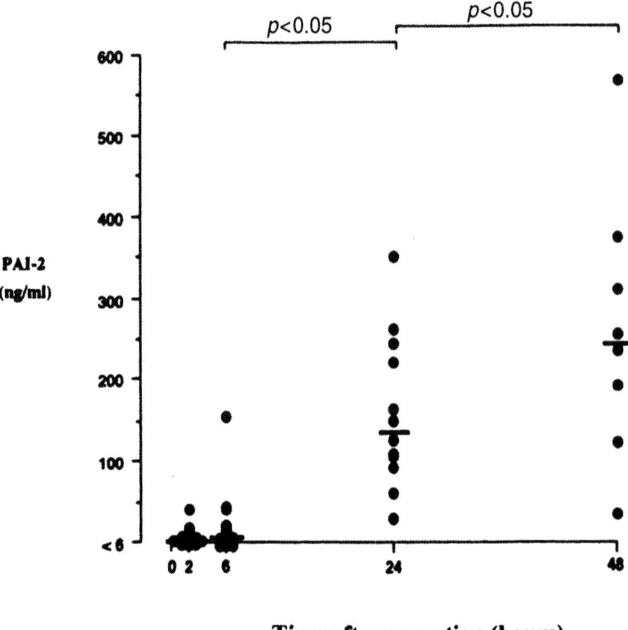

Time after operation (hours)

Fig. 7. Post-operative peritoneal fluid plasminogen inhibitor-2 concentrations

plasminogen-activating activity, there is a rebound period of increased fi-brinolytic activity [12]. Pathological studies have shown that collagen de-position occurs within 5 days of peritoneal injury, and thus it is likely that the duration of inhibition of peritoneal fibrinolysis is critical to the formation of permanent fibrous adhesions.

The localisation of the cell of production of PAI in inflamed human peri-toneum has been identified using in situ mRNA hybridisation for both PAI-1 and PAI-2 in inflamed human peritoneum. PAI-1 production was confined to the mesothelium and to endothelial cells lining submesothelial blood vessels [13]. By contrast, PAI-2 production was seen in mesothelium and in monocytes within the submesothelial tissues [14]. These studies confirm that the me-sothelium plays a critical role in the inhibition of peritoneal fibrinolysis that occurs following injury.

Peritoneal Cytokine Production and Its Effects on Fibrinolysis

We and others have studied peritoneal cytokine production following lapa-rotomy and in patients with bacterial peritonitis [15, 16]. These studies have shown a dynamic peritoneal cytokine response to injury in high concentra-tions. Badia et al. [15] found that the concentrations of the inflammatory cytokines tumour necrosis factor (TNF), interleukin-1 (IL-1) and interleukin-6 (IL-6) in postoperative peritoneal exudate were several hundred-fold higher than those found in the plasma of these patients. Similarly high levels of inflammatory cytokines are found in the exudate associated with acute bacterial peritonitis.

Studies of mesothelial cells either derived from human omentum [17] or from a human mesothelial cell line [18] have shown that the inflammatory cytokines TNF, IL-1 and IL-6 individually and synergistically stimulate mesothelial cells to produce PAI-1 in vitro (Fig. 8). This evidence, combined with the time course of peritoneal fluid cytokine and PAI production following surgery (Fig. 9), suggests that these inflammatory cytokines are probably the direct stimulus for PAI production and the subsequent loss of peritoneal fibrinolytic activity.

Summary

Human peritoneum possesses plasminogen-activating activity, which acts to prevent the deposition of intra-abdominal fibrin and its subsequent organisation into fibrous adhesions. This peritoneal plasminogen-activating activity is largely dependent on t-PA and is lost following peritoneal injury due to the production and release of high concentrations of PAI-1 and -2. Prolonged depression of peritoneal fibrinolysis allows organisation of fibrin deposits into permanent fibrous adhesions. PAI-1 is produced by both mesothelial cells and the endothelial cells lining submesothelial blood vessels. PAI-2 is produced by mesothelium and macrophages within peritoneal tissue. Inflamed human

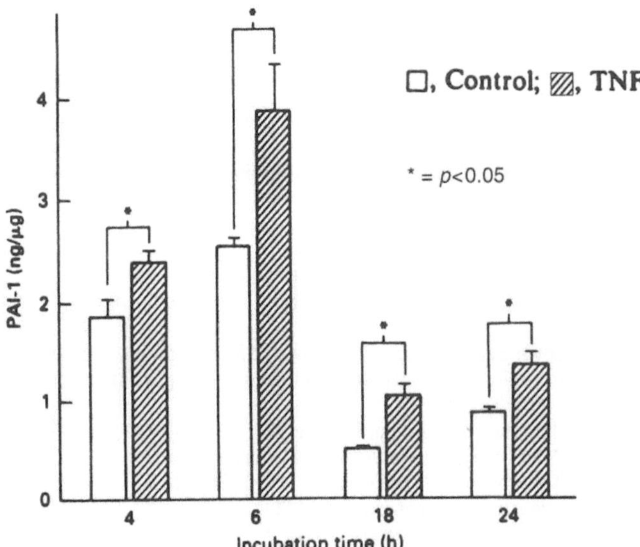

Fig. 8. The release of plasminogen activator-1 by human mesothelial cells in culture when stimulated by tumour necrosis factor alpha compared with control cultures

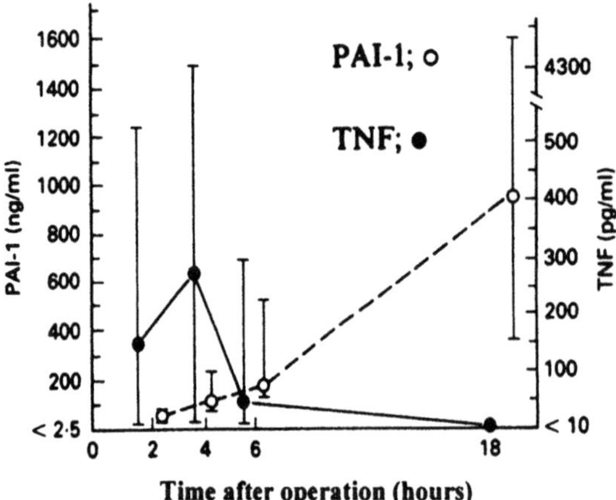

Fig. 9. The time course of post-operative peritoneal fluid tumour necrosis factor alpha and plasminogen activator inhibitor-1 concentrations

peritoneum (e.g. following operative injury or bacterial peritonitis) produces high concentrations of the inflammatory cytokines TNF, IL-1 and IL-6, which are released into the inflammatory peritoneal exudate. All three of these cytokines individually and synergistically stimulate human mesothelial cells in vitro to produce PAI-1. The time course of peritoneal exudate cytokine release following injury is consistent with these inflammatory cytokines being the major stimulus for PAI production, subsequent loss of peritoneal fibrinolytic activity and fibrous adhesion formation.

References

1. Thompson JN, Whawell SA (1995) The pathogenesis and prevention of adhesion formation. Br J Surg 82: 3–5
2. Ellis H (1982) The causes and prevention of intestinal adhesions. Br J Surg 69: 241–243
3. Porter JM, Ball AP, Silver D (1971) Mesothelial fibrinolysis. J Thorac Cardiovasc Surg 62: 725–730
4. Buckman RF, Buckman D, Hufnagel HB, Gervin AS (1976) A physiologic basis for the adhesion-free healing of the peritonealised surfaces. J Surg Res 21: 67–76
5. Raftery AT (1979) Regeneration of the peritoneum: a fibrinolytic study. J Anat 129: 659–664
6. Thompson JN, Patterson-Brown S, Harbourne T, Whawell SA, Kalodiki E, Dudley HAF (1989) Reduced human peritoneal plasminogen activating activity: a possible mechanism of adhesion formation. Br J Surg 76: 382–384
7. Holmdahl L, Eriksson E, Mohammed Al-Jabreen, Risberg BO (1994) Fibrinolysis in human peritoneum during surgery. Dept Surgery, University of Goteborg, Sweden
8. Vipond MN, Whawell SA, Thompson JN, Dudley HAF (1990) Peritoneal fibrinolytic activity and intra-abdominal adhesions. Lancet i: 1120–1122
9. Nkere UU, Whawell SA, Thompson JN, Thompson EM, Taylor KM (1992) Changes in pericardial fibrinolytic activity during cardiopulmonary bypass. Fibrinolysis 6 [Suppl 2]: 64

10. Whawell SA, Vipond MN, Scott-Coombes DM, Thompson JN (1993) Plasminogen activator inhibitor-2 inhibits peritoneal fibrinolytic activity in inflammation. Br J Surg 80: 107–109
11. Scott-Coombes DM, Whawell SA, Vipond MN, Thompson JN (1995) The human intraperitoneal fibrinolytic response to elective surgery. B J Surg 82: 414–417
12. Vipond MN, Whawell SA, Thompson JN, Dudley HAF (1994) Effect of experimental peritonitis and ischaemia on peritoneal fibrinolytic activity. Eur J Surg 160: 471–477
13. Whawell SA, Wang Y, Fleming KA, Thompson EM, Thompson JN (1993) Localisation of plasminogen activator inhibitor-1 production in inflamed appendix by in situ mRNA hybridisation. J Pathol 169: 67–71
14. Whawell SA, Thompson EM, Fleming KA, Thompson JN (1995) Plasminogen activator inhibitor-2 expression in inflamed appendix. Histopathology 27: 75–78
15. Badia JM, Scott-Coombes DM, Whawell SA, Abel PD, Williamson RCN, Thompson JN (1996) The dynamic peritoneal and systemic cytokine response to laparotomy. Br J Surg 83: 347-348
16. Tsukada K, Katoh H, Shiojima M, Suzuki T, Takenoshita S, Nagamachi Y (1993) Concentrations of cytokines in peritoneal fluid after abdominal surgery. Eur J Surg 159: 475–479
17. Van Hinsbergh VWM, Kooistra T, Schaffer MA, Van Bockel JM, Van Muijen GMP (1990) Characterisation and fibrinolytic properties of human omental tissue mesothelial cells. Comparison with endothelial cells. Blood 75: 1490–1497
18. Whawell SA, Scott-Coombes DM, Vipond MN, Tebbutt SJ, Thompson JN (1994) Tumour necrosis factor mediated release of plasminogen activator inhibitor-1 by human peritoneal mesothelial cells. Br J Surg 81: 214–216

3.7 Decreased Fibrinolytic Activity of Human Mesothelial Cells In Vitro Following Stimulation with Transforming Growth Factor-β_1, Interleukin-1β, and Tumor Necrosis Factor-α

L. Tietze, S. Handt, A. Ellbrecht, B. Klosterhalfen, B. Amo-Takyi,
K.-H. Treutner, and C. Mittermayer

Introduction

Mesothelial cells line serous body cavities as a simple squamous epithelium. These cells create a frictionless surface on the covered internal organs [4, 14] and are involved in the regulation of inflammatory and reparative processes in these cavities [18, 21, 28–30].

The importance of peritoneal adhesions as causes of chronic pain, intestinal obstruction, or infertility is well known, but the process of serosal wound healing, i.e., the inflammatory reparative response of the peritoneum is only partly understood.

Serosal wound healing is a complex, multifactorial process involving at least mesothelial cells, peritoneal macrophages, fibroblasts, and endothelial cells. This process is generally regulated by cell–cell interactions, extracellular matrix components, and humoral factors.

The early reparative response after peritoneal lesions is characterized by deposits of a fibrin-rich exudate and the presence of macrophages [5, 7, 33]. Gervin and Buckmann [1, 9] demonstrated that resolution of these fibrin deposits is a critical event in the process of tissue remodeling. A decreased serosal fibrinolytic activity, as observed after trauma, ischemia, and peritonitis [27], is accompanied by a high rate of fibrous adhesions. Augmentation of the fibrinolytic activity by intraperitoneal application of urokinase-type plasminogen activator was effective in preventing adhesions in 80% of experimental animals [9]. Therefore, the local regulation of plasminogen activator activity (PAA) seems to play a crucial role in tissue remodeling. Early resolution of the exudate may hinder the ingrowth of fibroblasts and capillaries, thus preventing the development of fibrous adhesions. The fibrinolytic activity of mesothelial cells is mediated by secretion of tissue-type plasminogen activator (t-PA), but not urokinase-type plasminogen activator, whereas the antifibrinolytic activity of mesothelial cells is regulated in part by secretion of plasminogen activator inhibitor (PAI) types 1 and 2 [15].

A decreased secretion of t-PA and enhanced secretion of PAI-1 and PAI-2 of human omentum majus mesothelial cells (HOMC) after stimulation with tumor necrosis factor (TNF)-α, as reported by Hinsbergh et al. [15], might explain in part the decreased fibrinolytic activity of serosal biopsies during peritonitis.

The influence of other cytokines secreted by activated peritoneal macrophages on mesothelial t-PA and PAI-1 production remains unclear. The effect of transforming growth factor (TGF)-β and interleukin (IL)-1 β on mesothelial cells was of particular interest in this study. TGF-β, described as an important factor for wound healing and tissue repair [10] which induces PAI-1 production in HT-1080 and endothelial cells [8, 20, 26] increased the severity of adhesion formation after intraperitoneal application in a rat model [34]. IL-1 seems to be a regulatory molecule for mesothelial cells which induce growth and cytokine secretion (IL-6, IL-8) [21, 28, 29].

In vivo fibrinolysis is characterized by the presence of mesothelial cells and fibrin. Fibrin increases the t-PA secretion of mesothelial cells [11], and the t-PA affinity to plasminogen is enhanced about 50 times in the presence of fibrin [16]. Cellular receptors participate in the regulation of plasmin activity, as was shown for endothelial cells [12].

In the present study, we investigated the influence of TGF-β_1, TNF-α, and IL-1β on the fibrinolytic activity of human mesothelial cells in the presence of fibrin using an in vitro cell/fibrin clot model. The results demonstrate that the fibrinolytic activity of HOMC in the presence of fibrin is decreased after incubation with TNF-α, TGF-β_1, and IL-1β. This antifibrinolytic effect is caused partly by a decreased t-PA secretion and an increased PAI-1 secretion, which may contribute to the decreased fibrinolytic activity of the peritoneum during peritonitis.

Materials and Methods

Materials

Tissue culture reagents were purchased from GIBCO (Karlsruhe, Germany). Human serum was obtained from a pool of at least 20 healthy donors.

Human recombinant TNF-α (1×10^8 U/mg) and IL-1β (ED_{50}, 0.1 ng/ml) were both acquired from PBH (Hannover, Germany). TGF-β_1 was supplied by Boehringer (Mannheim, Germany). Monoclonal antibodies against pancytokeratin, cytokeratin 8 and 18, CD14, and CD68 (clone PGM1) were ordered from DAKO (Hamburg, Germany).

Purified fibrinogen and plasminogen was purchased from American Diagnostica Inc. (Greenwich, CT, USA). Fibrinogen was purified further by dialysis at 4 °C to remove fibronectin, yielding a product with a clottability of 98%. Purified human thrombin was from Sigma (St. Louis, USA). Human recombinant t-PA (rt-PA) was generously donated from Genentech Inc. (San Francisco, CA, USA) (specific activity, 6×10^5 IU/mg).

Human Omentum Majus Mesothelial Cell Culture

Primary human mesothelial cells were derived from pieces of omentum majus according to the method of Hinsbergh et al. [15] with minor modifications. In brief, a fresh piece of omentum majus (roughly 5 × 5 cm), obtained from patients undergoing elective abdominal surgery, was transferred from the operation theatre in ice-cold buffer (10 mM hydroxyethylpiperazine ethane-sulfonic acid, HEPES; 140 mM NaCl; 4 mM KCl; 11 mM D-glucose; 1% human serum albumin; 100 IU penicillin; 0.1 mg/ml streptomycin). The tissue was rinsed three times in phosphate-buffered solution (PBS) at 37 °C. After digestion with 0.125% trypsin in PBS at 37 °C for 10 min, the tissue was removed and 20 ml RPMI 1640 medium (GIBCO BRL, Life Technologies, USA) containing 10% pooled human serum protein, L-glutamine, penicillin, and streptomycin was added. After centrifugation for 10 min at 200 g, the cells were washed in 20 ml PBS (37 °C). After further centriguation for 10 min at 200 g, the cells were resuspended in 10 ml RPMI 1640 containing 10% pooled human serum protein, L-glutamine, penicillin, and streptomycin and plated in a 75-cm^2 0.2% gelatin-coated tissue culture flask (Falcon, supplied by Becton Dickinson-Gambil, Heidelberg, Germany). The cell cultures were incubated at 37 °C in a humidified atmosphere of 5% CO_2 in air. Cells were passaged by incubating the monolayer with 0.125% trypsin for 2 min. After centrifuging the cells for 10 min at 200 g, they were washed in 20 ml PBS, centrifuged again for 10 min at 200 g, resuspended in 30 ml complete medium, and seeded as described above (splitting ratio, 1:3). Only cells from the first or second passage were used for the experiments described below.

All experiments were performed in 96-microtiter plates precoated with 0.2% gelatine. A total of 20 000 cells/100 µl were seeded into each well to establish a confluent monolayer. All experiments were performed 48h after seeding without changing the cell culture medium.

Immunofluorescence Microscopy

Immunofluorescence staining of mesothelial cells was performed on cell monolayers that had been grown on Labtek chamber slides (Nunc, Napperville, IL) coated with 0.2% gelatine. The monolayers were fixed in ethanol 80% (vol/vol) for 10 min at 4 °C, rinsed, and stored in PBS at 4 °C. Cells were incubated with various monoclonal antibodies for 30 min at room temperature and rinsed three times with PBS and subsequently incubated with fluorescein iso-thiocyanate (FITC)-labeled goat anti-mouse (1:50 in PBS; Dako). The cells were examined with a confocal laser scan microscope at a wavelength of 568 nm using a Zeiss LSM 410 equipped with an ArKr Laser.

Stimulation with Cytokines and Determination of Immunoreactive, Tissue-Type Plasminogen Activator and Plasminogen Activator Inhibitor Type 1

Confluent monolayers were established in microtiter plates as described above. After rinsing the monolayer twice with serum-free medium, the cells were stimulated by adding human recombinant TGF-β_1, TNF-α, and IL-1β in a concentration ranging between 0.1 and 10 ng/ml to serum-free medium which contained 1% human serum albumin. After 2, 6, 12, and 24 h, supernatants were collected, centrifuged and stored at –20 °C. t-PA and PAI-1 antigen concentrations were determined by enzyme-linked immunosorbent assay (ELISA) kits purchased from Biopool (Imulyse t-PA and PAI-1 respectively). Antigen concentrations were related to the total protein content in each well (bicinchoninic acid, BCA; Pierce).

In Vitro Human Omentum Majus Mesothelial Cells/Fibrin Clot Model

Confluent monolayers in 96-multiwell plates were prestimulated with TGF-β_1, TNF-α, and IL-1β (each 10 ng/ml) for 6 h. After collecting the supernatants, the cells were washed twice with serum-free medium. A fibrin clot was formed on the cells by adding a solution composed of fibrinogen (2 mg/ml), plasminogen (100 nM), and the cytokines indicated above in GBSH 5 buffer (121 mM NaCl, 0.8 mM Na$_2$HPO$_4$, 5.0 mM HEPES, 1.5 mM CaCl$_2$·2H$_2$O, 4.5 mM KCl, 0.2 mM KH$_2$PO$_4$, 1 mM MgCl$_2$·6H$_2$O, 0.6 mM MgSO$_4$·7H$_2$O, 4.5 g/l D-glucose). Fibrin formation was initiated by adding thrombin (1 U). The resulting clot volume per well was 65 μl.

Human rt-PA (0.5 nM) was added to the fibrin clot after 160 min to induce or augment clot lysis. Clot density was determined by measuring the optical density at 405 nm using a Microsoft Micro Plate Reader (Molecular Devices, Menlo Park, CA, USA). The experimental setup is illustrated in Fig. 1.

All experiments were performed at least three times in duplicate with HOMC from different donors.

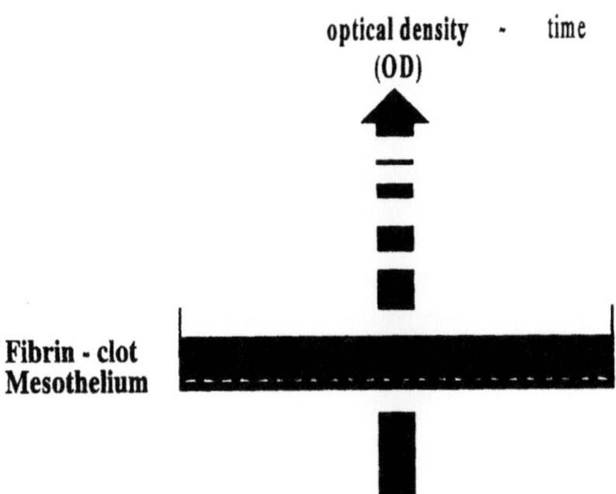

Fig. 1. Experimental setup of the mesothelial cell/fibrin clot model

Results

Characterization of Human Omentum Majus Mesothelial Cells

The mesothelial cell cultures were characterized by phase contrast microscopy, immunohistology, and electron microscopy. The obtained epitheloid cells grew as a monolayer, reaching confluence 4–10 days after initial seeding, and then showed a typical cobblestone-like growth pattern (Fig. 2). The cells were passaged up to five times, but after the third passage there was some transformation; the cell size increased and many cells were multinucleated.

Immunohistochemistry revealed a strong cytoplasmatic reactivity for pan-cytokeratin, cytokeratin 8 and 18, and vimentin, whereas the reaction to factor VIII antigen and *Ulex europaeus* was negative, indicating that no relavant contamination with endothelial cells had occurred.

Several antibodies against myelomonocytic-associated antigens were tested to determine the contamination with macrophages. In contrast to the macrophage populations, the obtained cells did not express CD14 or CD68.

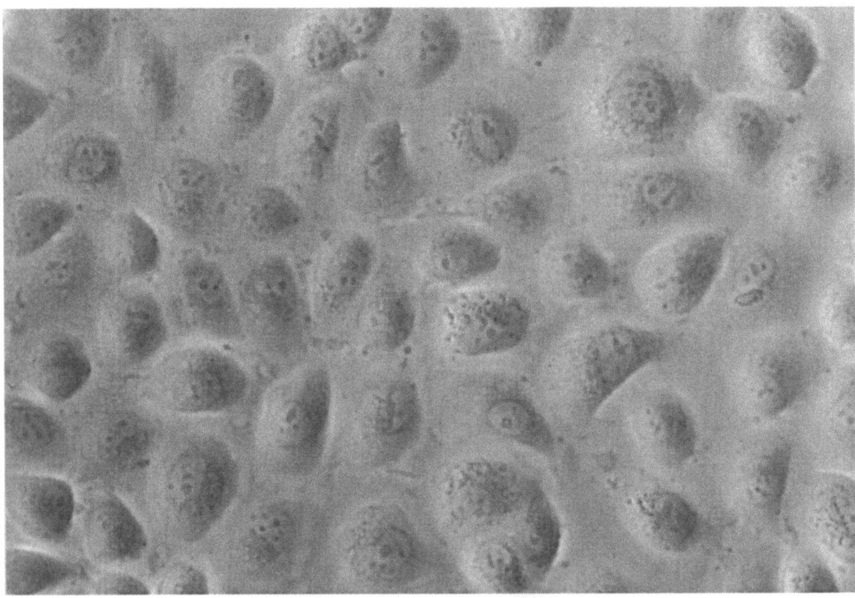

Fig. 2. Phase contrast micrograph of confluent human omentum majus mesothelial cells (HOMC)

Production of Tissue-Type Plasminogen Activator and Plasminogen Activator Inhibitor by Human Omentum Majus Mesothelial Cells

The t-PA secretion of HOMC from different donors was highly variable in the presence of 1% human serum albumin (HSA) and ranged from 24.52 to 107.66 ng/mg cell protein per 24 h, with an average of 56.15 ng/mg cell protein per 24 h (SD 32.53 ng/mg cell protein per 24 h; $n=9$).

The PAI-1 concentration in the supernatants ranged from 777 to 3294 ng/mg cell protein per 24 h, with an average of 1795 ng/mg cell protein per 24 h (SD 993 ng/mg cell protein per 24 h; $n=6$).

Stimulation with TNF-α and IL-1β caused a change in the morphology of HOMC with a shift from a polygonal toward a spindle cell-like appearance. Stimulation with TGF-β_1 did not induce this morphological response.

Stimulation of HOMC with TGF-β_1, TNF-α, and IL-1β caused at least a twofold decrease in the concentration of t-PA antigen after 24 h. The response was dose dependent at cytokine concentrations between 0.1 and 10 ng. There was a significant decrease in t-PA concentrations over a period of 12 h, showing a clear time dependency. These effects were not observed after heat inactivation of the cytokines (data not shown). Figures 3 and 4 show the t-PA antigen levels in the supernatants and their relationship to dosage and period of cytokine incubation in a representative experiment.

Incubation of HOMC with TGF-β_1, IL-1β, and TNF-α at a concentration of 10 ng/ml caused an at least 1.5-fold, time-dependent increase in the PAI-1 concentrations of the supernatants (24 h). The cytokine response for TNF-α and TGF-β_1 on PAI-1 concentrations was dose dependent, but a linear dose-response relationship for IL-1β was not reproducible. Figures 5 and 6 illustrate the relationships between PAI-1 concentrations and time and between PAI-1 concentrations and dosage of cytokines in a representative experiment.

In Vitro Clot Lysis in the Presence of Cytokine-Stimulated Human Omentum Majus Mesothelial Cells

In order to test the hypothesis that these cytokine effects on the antigen concentrations of t-PA and PAI-1 cause a decreased fibrinolytic activity of HOMC in the presence of fibrin, we modified an in vitro cell/fibrin clot model which had previously been used to measure the antifibrinolytic activity of human endothelial cells in vitro [13].

In nine out of 11 experiments with HOMC from different donors, no spontaneous fibrinolysis occurred. To investigate the influence of cytokines on antifibrinolytic properties of HOMC, we induced fibrinolysis by adding recombinant t-PA after 160 min. In contrast, spontaneous lysis occurred in two experiments under the same experimental conditions, but with HOMC from different donors. Cell passage rate did not influence the lysis time. In both spontaneous and induced fibrinolysis, stimulation with TGF-β_1 and TNF-α caused a marked delay in half lysis time, whereas stimulation with IL-1β induced a comparably low antifibrinolytic effect in the case of nonspontaneous

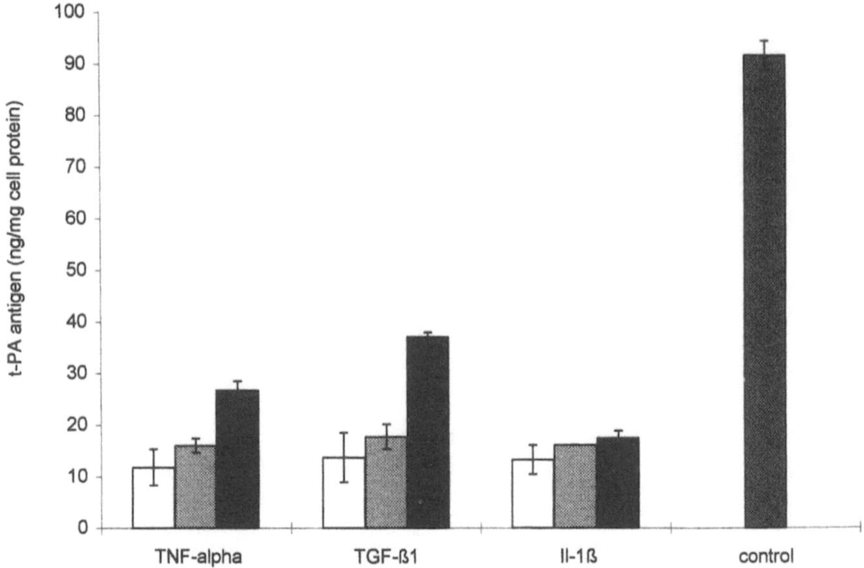

Fig. 3. Tissue-type plasiminogen activator (*t-PA*) concentrations after incubation with transforming growth factor (*TGF*)-β_1, tumor necrosis factor (*TNF*)-α, and interleukin (*IL*)-1β at different concentrations. *White bars,* 10 ng/ml; *shaded bars,* 1 ng/ml; *black bars,* 0.1 ng/ml. All supernatants conditioned for 24 h

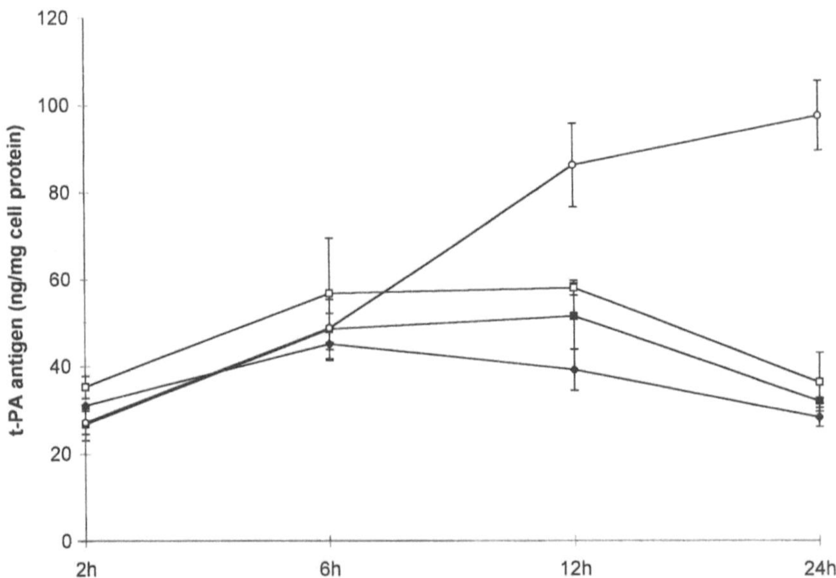

Fig. 4. Time and tissue-type plasminogen activator (*t-PA*) concentration curves of human omentum majus mesothelial cell (HOMC)-conditioned supernatants after incubation with transforming growth factor (*TGF*)-β_1, tumor necrosis factor (*TNF*)-α, and interleukin (IL)-1β (each 10 ng/ml) over a period of 24 h –□– TNF-alpha –■– TGF-β1 –●– IL-1 –○– control

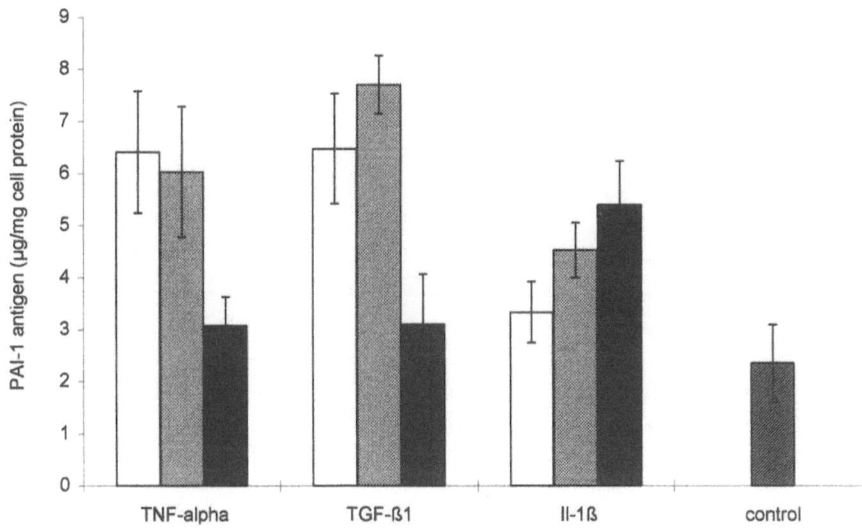

Fig. 5. Plasminogen activator inhibitor (PAI)-1 concentrations after incubation with transforming growth factor (*TGF*)-β_1, tumor necrosis factor (*TNF*)-α and interleukin (*IL*)-1β at different concentrations. *White bars*, 10 ng/ml; *shaded bars*, 1 ng/ml; *black bars*, 0.1 ng/ml. All supernatants conditioned for 24 h

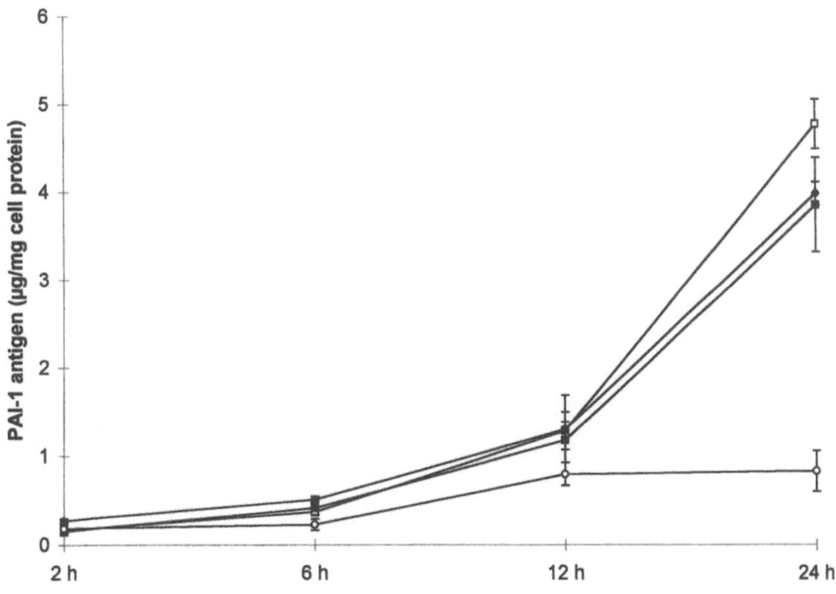

Fig. 6. Time and plasminogen activator inhibitor (*PAI*)-1 concentration curves of human omentum majus mesothelial cell (HOMC)-conditioned supernatants after incubation with transforming growth factor (*TGF*)-β_1, tumor necrosis factor (*TNF*)-α, and interleukin (*IL*)-1β (each 10 ng/ml) over a period of 24 h ···□··· TNF-alpha ─■─ TGF-β1 ·◆· IL-1β ···◇··· control

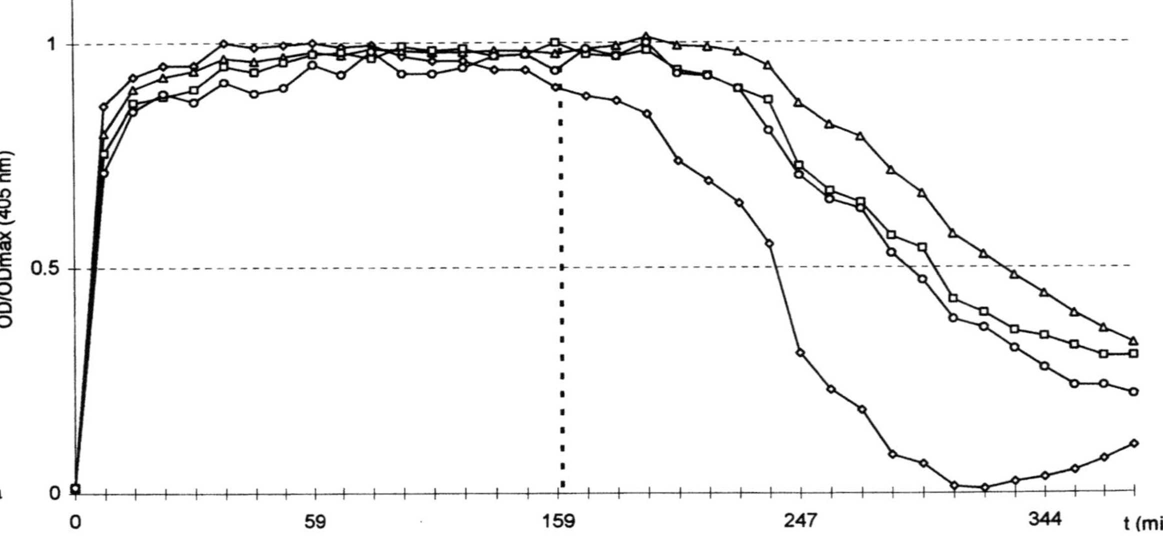

Fig. 7a,b. Kinetic profile of lysis experiments with unstimulated and cytokine-stimulated human omentum majus mesothelial cells (HOMC) in the presence of fibrin. *Diamonds*, control; *triangles*, transforming growth factor (TGF)-β_1; *squares*, tumor necrosis factor (TNF)-α; *circles*, interleukin (IL)-1β. Relative clot density is shown as optical density (*OD*) at 405 nm (OD/OD$_{max}$). Time of recombinant tissue-type plasminogen activator (rt-PA) administration (160 min) is indicated by a *vertical broken line*. **a** Cytokine response without spontaneous fibrinolysis **b** Response in an experiment with spontaneous fibrinolysis

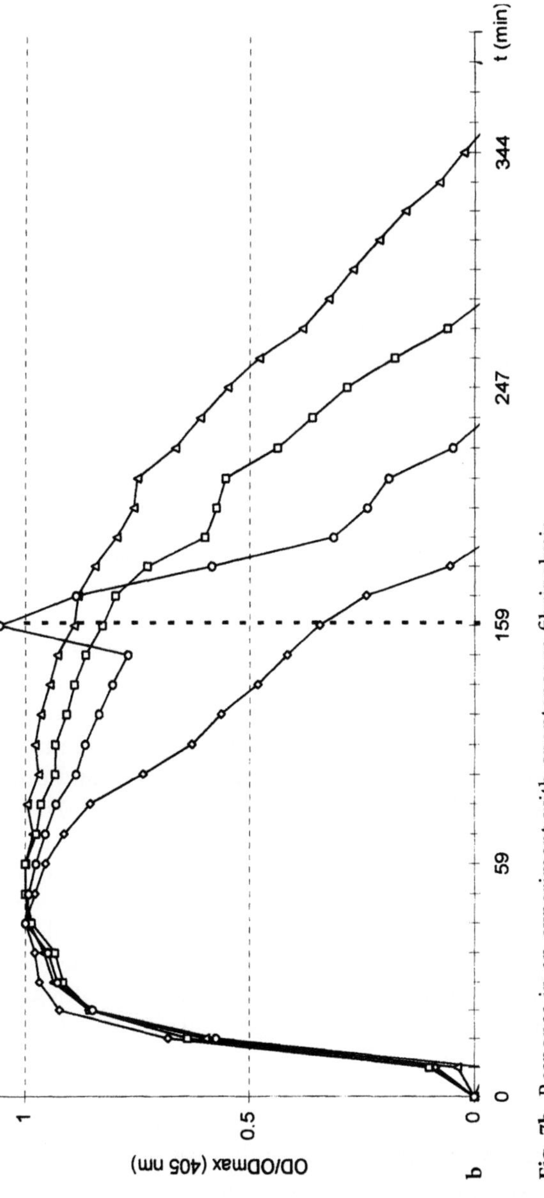

Fig. 7b. Response in an experiment with spontaneous fibrinolysis

lysis. The results from one in vitro lysis experiment with and one without spontaneous fibrinolysis are shown in Figs. 7a,b.

Discussion

Formation of peritoneal adhesions after trauma, peritonitis, ischemia, and radiation is a complex, multicellular process involving at least mesothelial cells, endothelial cells, fibroblasts, the extracellular matrix, and inflammatory cells, especially macrophages and their interaction. Although this process is not understood in detail, it is generally accepted that the early inflammatory reparative response is accompanied by deposition of a fibrin-rich exudate on the site of mesothelial injury [9, 19, 33].

According to a unified concept about the pathogenetic mechanism in the formation of peritoneal fibrous adhesions, decreased fibrinolytic activity of the serosa seems to be a major pathogenetic factor. This decreased fibrinolytic activity may cause a fibroblastic invasion with subsequent collagenous repair, resulting in the permanent adherance of two opposing serosal surfaces [1, 9]. A decrease in the fibrinolytic activity was observed following trauma, peritonitis, and ischemia [9, 27]. Exogenous augmentation of intraperitoneal fibrinolytic activity by administration of t-PA, urokinase-type plasminogen activator, or streptokinase was effective in preventing peritoneal adhesions in both a rat and a rabbit model [5, 9, 23, 24]. The reduction in peritoneal fibrinolytic activity observed after inflammation or the other conditions mentioned above may be caused by mesothelial cell injury, an altered balance between anti- and profibrinolytic properties of mesothelial cells or a combination of both [27]. The fibrinolytic activity of mesothelial cells is mediated by secretion of t-PA but not urokinase-type plasminogen activator, whereas the antifibrinolytic activity is regulated by secretion of PAI-1 and PAI-2 [15]. PAI-1 and PAI-2 were recently detected by mRNA in situ hybridization in mesothelial cells of inflamed peritoneum, but not in samples without peritonitis, suggesting an induction of PAI-1 m-RNA synthesis during peritonitis. Other sites of PAI-1 m-RNA induction were found to be endothelial cells and smooth muscle cells of vessel walls in the subserosal stroma [31, 32].

The influence of cytokines, which are found in increased concentrations during peritonitis or pleuritis, on fibrinolytic activity on mesothelial cells has only partly been investigated. We focused our attention on the influence of macrophage-derived cytokines, since the appearance of macrophages in the early phase of serosal wound healing seems to be crucial [33]. During peritonitis, increased concentrations of TNF-α and IL-1β were reported by Brauner et al. [2] and Fieren et al. [6]. IL-1 seems to be a regulatory molecule for mesothelial cells in the synthesis of cytokines [21, 28, 29].

TGF-β_1 is a protein which regulates the proliferation of epithelial cells, extracellular matrix formation, and the secretion of proteases which degrade extracellular matrix proteins [11]. TGF-β_1 induces an enhanced PAI-1 secretion in a variety of cell types, e.g., fibroblasts and endothelial cells [20, 22, 25, 26]. Our data indicate that TNF-α, IL-1β, and TGF-β_1, are potent regulators of the fibrinolytic activity of human mesothelial cells. This is in agreement with the published results mentioned above. The enhanced PAI-1 secretion and the decrease in t-PA secretion in the presence of TNF-α was reported in a similar manner by Hinsbergh et al. [15]. In contrast, Idell et al. [17] found an increase in t-PA production after stimulation with TGF-β_1 in human pleural mesothelial cells. These results were obtained from mesothelial cells derived from pleural exudates, perhaps indicating that these detached mesothelial cells express a t-PA secretion pattern which is different from HOMC. The increased rate of peritoneal fibrous adhesions after intraperitoneal application of TGF-β_1 [3] may be partly caused by the decreased fibrinolytic activity of mesothelial cells, as reported.

Summary

The decreased fibrinolytic activity of human mesothelial cells in vitro in the presence of TGF-β_1, TNF-α, and IL-1β may contribute in part to the decrease in the serosal fibrinolytic activity which was observed during peritonitis and may therefore be involved in the pathogenesis of fibrous adhesion formation. The demonstrated HOMC/fibrin clot model closely resembles the in vivo situation and allows further investigations of the influence of different cell types and agents in the regulation of fibrinolytic properties of human mesothelial cells.

The inflammatory-reparative response of serosal surfaces is a complex and multicellular process which is characterized by deposits of a fibrin-rich exudate and the local accumulation of inflammatory cells, particularly macrophages. Peritoneal fibrous adhesions may occur as a result of an insufficient lysis of the fibrin-rich exudate. Serosal hypofibrinolysis may be due to mesothelial cell death or an imbalance between pro- and antifibrinolytic factors produced by mesothelial cells. Mesothelial cells produce tissue-type plasminogen activator (t-PA) and plasminogen activator inhibitor Type 1 and 2 (PAI-1 and 2). Both the activator and inactivator activity is influenced by the presence of fibrin.

Here we describe a mesothelial cell/fibrin-clot model which closely resembles the in vivo situation. This model allowed the determination of pro- and antifibrinolytic effects of various agents and cells. The effects of the macrophage-derived cytokines TGF-β_1, TNF-α and IL-1β on the pro- and antifibrinolytic properties of mesothelial cells in this model are described in detail.

Acknowledgement. The authors wish to thank Prof. Dr. Dr. med. h. c. V. Schumpelick and the members of the operation team of the surgical clinic of the RWTH Aachen for assisting with the collection of omentum majus specimens for mesothelial cell culture.

References

1. Buckmann RF, Woods M, Sargent L, Gervin AS (1976) A unifying pathogenetic mechanism in the etiology of intraperitoneal adhesions. J Surg Res 20: 1–5

2. Brauner A, Hylander B, Wretlind B (1994) Inflammatory factors (TNF-α, IL-1β, IL-1ra) during peritonitis in CAPD patients. Perit Dial Int 14: 48 (abstr)

3. Chegini N, Gold LI, Williams RS, Masterson BJ (1994) Localisation of transforming growth factor beta isoforms TGF-β1, TRGF-β2, TGF-β3 in surgically induced pelvic adhesions in the rat. Obstet Gyn 83(3): 449–454

4. Dobbie JW, Lloyd JK (1989) Mesothelium secretes lamellar bodies in a similar manner to type II pneumocyte secretion of surfactant. Perit Dial Int 9: 215–219

5. Ellis M, Harrison W, Hugh TB (1965) The healing of peritoneum under normal and pathological conditions. Br J Surg 52: 471–476

6. Fieren MW, van dem Bemd GJCM, Bonta IL, Ben Efraim S (1991) Peritoneal macrophages from patients on continuous ambulatory peritoneal dialysis have an increased capability to release tumour necrosis factor during peritonitis. J Clin Lab Immunol 34: 1–9

7. Fotev Z, Whitaker D, Papadimitriou JM (1987) Role of macrophages in mesothelial healing. J Pathol 151: 209–219

8. Fujii S, Hopkins WE, Sobel BE (1991) Mechanisms contributing to increased synthesis of plasminogen activator inhibitor type 1 in endothelial cells by constituents of platelets and their implications for thrombolysis. Circulation 83: 654

9. Gervin AS, Puckett CL, Silver D (1973) Serosal hypofibrinolysis, a cause of postoperative abdominal adhesions. Am J Surg 125: 80–88

10. Gitelman SE, Derynck R (1994) Transforming growth factor-β (TGF-β). In: Nicola NA (ed) Cytokines and their receptors. Oxford University Press, Oxford, pp 223–226

11. Grulich-Henn J, Preissner KT, Müller-Berghaus G (1990) Heparin stimulates fibrinolysis in mesothelial cells by selective induction of tissue plasminogen activator but not plasminogen activator inhibitor synthesis. Thromb Haemost 64: 420–425

12. Hajjar KA, Jacovina AT, Chacko J (1994) An endothelial cell receptor for plasminogen/tissue plasminogen activator: identity with annexin II. J Biol Chem 269: 21191–21197

13. Handt S, Jerome WG, Braaten JV, Lewis JC, Kirkpatrick CJ, Hantgan RR (1994) PAI-1 released from cultured endothelial cells delays fibrinolysis and is incorporated into the developing fibrin clot. Fibrinolysis 8: 104–112

14. Hills BA, Butler BD, Barrow RE (1982) Boundary lubrication imparted by pleural surfactants and their identification. J Appl Physiol 53: 463

15. Hinsbergh VWM, Kooistra T, Scheffer AA, van Bockel JH, van Muijen GNP (1990) Characterization and fibrinolytic properties of human omental tissue mesothelial cells. Comparision with endothelial cells. Blood 75: 1490–1497

16. Hoylaerts M, Rijken DC, Lijnen HR, Collen D (1982) Kinetics of the activation of plasminogen by human tissue plasminogen activator. Role of fibrin. J Biol Chem 257: 2912–2919

17. Idell S, Zwieb C, Kumar A, Koenig KB, Johnson AR (1992) Pathways of fibrin turnover of human pleural mesothelial cells in vitro. Am J Respir Cell Mol Biol 7: 414–426

18. Jonjic N, Peri G, Bernasconi S, Sciacca FL, Colotta F, Pellici P, Lanfrancone L, Mantovani A (1992) Expression of adhesion molecules and chemotactic cytokines in cultured human mesothelial cells. J Exp Med 176: 1165–1174

19. Kumar V, Cotran RS, Robbins SL (eds) (1992) Basic pathology, 5th edn. Saunders, Philadelphia

20. Laiho M, Saksela O, Keski-Oja J (1987) Transforming growth factor-β induction of type-1 plasminogen activator inhibitor. J Biol Chem 262: 17467–17474

21. Lanfrancone L, Boraschi D, Ghiara P, Falini B, Grignani F, Peri G, Mantovani A, Pelicci PG (1992) Human peritoneal mesothelial cells produce many cytokines (granulocyte colony-stimulating factor [CSF], granulocyte-monocyte CSF, macrophyge-CSF, interleukin-1 [IL-1], and IL-6) and are activated and stimulated to growth by IL-1. Bood 80: 2835–2842

22. Lyons RM, Keski-Oja J, Moses HL (1989) Proteolytic activation of latent transforming growth factor beta is produced by cocultures of endothelial cells and pericytes. Proc Natl Acad Sci USA 86: 4544–4548

23. Menzies D, Ellis H (1989) Intra-abdominal adhesion formation and their prevention by topical tissue plasminogen activator. JR Soc 82: 534–535

24. Orita H, Fukasawa M, Girgis W, diZerga GS (1991) Inhibition of postsurgical adhesions in a standard rabbit model: intraperitoneal treatment with tissue type plasminogen activator. Int J Fertil 36: 172–177
25. Sato Y, Tsuboi R, Lyons RM, Moses H, Rifkin DB (1990) Characterization of the activation of latent TGF-β by cocultures of endothelial cells and pericytes in smooth muscle cells: a self-regulating system. J Cell Biol 111: 757–763
26. Schleef RR, Loskutoff DJ (1988) Fibrinolytic system of vascular endothelial cells. Haemostasis 18: 328–341
27. Thompson JN, Paterson-Brown S, Harbourne T, Whawell SA, Kalodiki E, Dudley HAF (1989) Reduced human peritoneal plasminogen activating activity: possible mechanism of adhesion formation. Br J Surg 76: 382–384
28. Topley N, Brown Z, Jörres A, Westwick J, Coles G, Davies M, Williams JD (1993) Human peritoneal mesothelial cells synthezise IL-8: synergistic induction by interleukin-1β and tumour necrosis factor alpha. Am J Pathol 142: 1876–1886
29. Topley N, Jörres A, Luttmann W, Petersen MM, Lang MJ, Thierauch KH, Müller C, Coles GA, Davies M, Williams JD (1993) Human mesothelial cells synthesize interleukin-6: induction by IL-1β and TNF-α. Kidney Int 43: 226–233
30. Topley N, Petersen MM, Mackenzie R, Neubauer A, Stylianou E, Kaever V, Davies M, Coles GA, Jörres A, Williams JD (1994) Human peritoneal mesothelial cell prostaglandin synthesis: induction of cyclooxygenase mRNA by peritoneal macrophage derived cytokines. Kidney Int 44: 900–909
31. Whawell SA, Thompson EM, Fleming KA, Thompson JN (1995) Plasminogen activator inhibitor-2 expression in inflamed appendix. Histopathology 27: 75–78
32. Whawell SA, Wang Y, Fleming KA, Thompson EM, Thompson JM (1993) Localisation of plasminogen activator inhibitor-1 production in inflamed appendix by in situ mRNA hybridisation. J Pathol 169: 67–71
33. Whithaker D, Papadimitriou JM (1985) Mesothelial healing: morphological and kinetic investigations. J Pathol 145: 159–175
34. Williams RS, Rossi AM, Chegini N, Schultz G (1991) Effect of transforming growth factor β on postoperative adhesion formation and intact peritoneum. J Surg Res 52: 65–70

4 Diagnostic of Peritoneal Adhesions

4.1 Value of Ultrasonography in Diagnosis of Peritoneal Adhesions

J. Conze, S. Truong, and V. Schumpelick

Introduction

Differentiation between interenteric adhesions and adhesions to the abdominal wall is a necessary prerequisite for evaluation of peritoneal adhesions by ultrasound. The two kinds of adhesions have different ultrasound criteria and show different ultrasonic signs. For that reason they will be explained separately.

Adhesions to the Abdominal Wall

Adhesions between the abdominal wall and the intestinum can be ultrasonographically detected by observation of the visceral movement in relation to the abdominal wall. This movement is called the visceral slide. There are two different types of visceral slide:

1. *Spontaneous* visceral slide, which is the visceral movement produced by the force of respiratory motion (Fig. 1).
2. *Induced* visceral slide, caused by manual ballottement of the abdomen. Adhesions between the abdominal wall and the intestinum can cause a restriction of the visceral slide (Fig. 2).

Patients and Method

The ultrasound examination is carried out with the patient in the supine position. We use a real-time ultrasound system with 3.5- and 7.5-MHz linear or curved transducers. To evaluate adhesions to the abdominal wall, we usually use a 7.5-MHz transducer. We prefer longitudinal scanning, because here spontaneous visceral slide is greater than in the transverse axis [1].

We start the examination by identifying the abdominal wall with its typical structures, i.e., the subcutaneous fatty tissue and the muscle layer. Underneath the abdominal wall, the intestinum is detected. By real-time ultrasound tracking of the varying echogenicity of the intestinum moving horizontally beneath the more stationary abdominal wall, the visceral slide can be identified. For measurement of the distance of the visceral slide, a focal area is

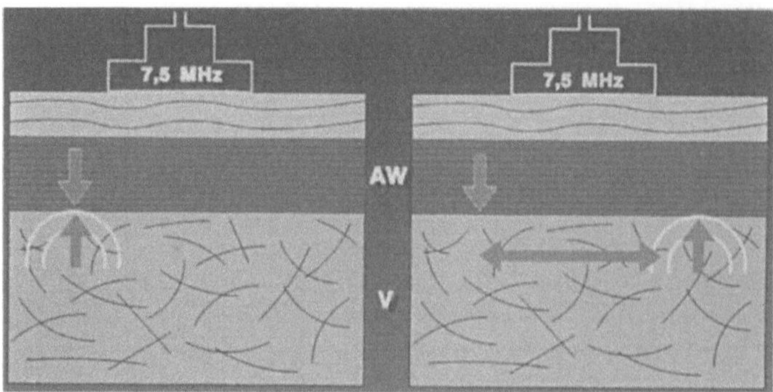

Fig. 1. 'Spontaneous viscera slide' (*AW*, abdominal wall; *V*, viscerum)

selected. A cluster of high- and low-echogenic structures near the surface of the moving viscera that move together through several respiratory cycles can be recognized [3]. The extend of the visceral slide can then be measured by the distance traversed by the focal area during one respiratory cycle.

During longitudinal scanning, the spontaneous visceral slide produced by regular respiratory movements ranges in distance from 2 to 5 cm [3]. In some patients, the normal respiratory motion is not very effective in producing visceral slide. In these cases, it is sometimes helpful to ask the patient to breathe more deeply and more intensely with a maximum of abdominal wall excursions. Longitudinal ultrasound scanning during these exaggerated re-spiratory movements usually reveals normal visceral slide.

If restricted spontaneous visceral slide was found, we applied a manual ballottement, a compression of the abdomen during longitudinal and trans-verse ultrasound scanning. This is called induced visceral slide [3]. The dis-tance horizontally traversed by induced visceral slide is usually less than the distance of spontaneous visceral slide.

Our criteria for establishing peritoneal adhesions to the abdominal wall are a spontaneous visceral slide of less than 1 cm or a spontaneous visceral slide of

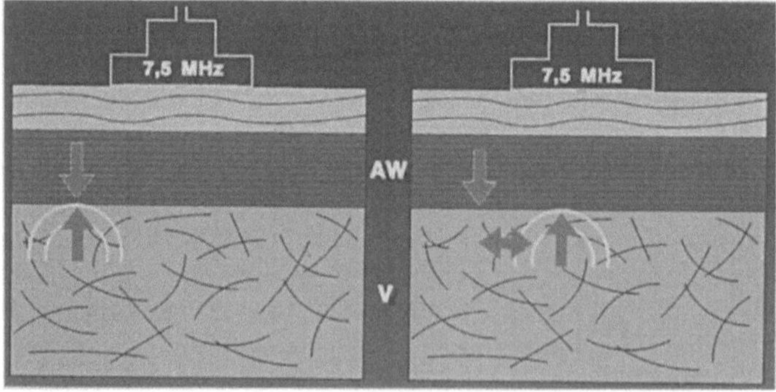

Fig. 2. 'Restricted viscera slide' (*AW*, abdominal wall; *V*, viscerum)

Table 1. Patient groups in a prospective study on 121 patients

Group	History	Patients	
		(*n*)	(%)
1	No previous abdominal surgery	97	80
2	Patients with previous peritonitis	8	7
3	Patients with previous operations	16	13

between 1 and 2 cm with an induced visceral slide of less than 1 cm. These criteria make it possible to detect and locate peritoneal adhesions.

In a prospective study on 121 patients, we compared the ultrasound findings with adhesions found intraoperatively. All patients came for an elective operation, such as cholecystectomy or fundoplication. In all cases a laparoscopic procedure was planned and performed. In the course of preoperative examinations, we always performed our own ultrasound examination. During this examination, we investigated the distance of spontaneous and induced visceral slide.

We divided our patients into three groups: group 1 comprised those patients with no previous abdominal surgery (80%); group 2 comprised those patients with a history of peritonitis or pancreatitis (7%); and group 3 comprised those patients with a history of previous abdominal surgery (13%). Of the 16 patients in the latter group, 11 had undergone only one previous operation and five patients more than one operation (Table 1).

Results

By means of our ultrasound examination, we were able to detect 14 patients who had the ultrasonic signs and fulfilled the criteria for peritoneal adhesions. In group 1, all patients had a visceral slide of more than 2 cm. In group 2, there were three patients with a spontaneous visceral slide of less than 1 cm, and two patients with one of less than 2 cm. When we performed ultrasound examination with manual ballottement, one of these patients showed a visceral slide of more than 1 cm. In group 3, we detected ten patients with peritoneal adhesions, three of whom had an induced visceral slide of less than 1 cm (Table 2).

Table 2. Results of ultrasound examination

Group	Patients (*n*)	Spontaneous visceral slide			Induced visceral slide		Adhesions
		> 2 cm	1–2 cm	< 1 cm	> 1 cm	< 1 cm	
1	97	97	–	–	97	–	–
2	8	3	2	3	1	1	4
3	16	4	5	7	2	3	10
Total	121	104	7	10	100	4	14

Table 3. Comparison between ultrasound and operative findings

Group	Patients (n)	Ultrasonic findings	Operative findings
1	97	0	1
2	8	4	6
3	16	10	11

Comparison of these data with the operative findings confirmed all ultrasonographically detected peritoneal adhesions.

However, we intraoperatively found four more patients with adhesions to the abdominal wall. These adhesions were located at the lateral sites of the abdominal cavity, and none of them caused any operative complications. (Table 3).

Discussion

In reviewing these results, we need to ask why ultrasound resulted in an incorrect diagnosis, i.e., why ultrasound examination failed to detect the other four patients with peritoneal adhesions to the abdominal wall. Possible reasons include the following:

1. Detection of single, dense adhesions or filmy adhesions without direct involvement of the bowel can be difficult.
2. In the lower abdomen, restricted visceral slide might be measured without adhesions, because in this area of the abdominal cavity the intestinum does not have as much mobility and flexibility of movement as in the middle abdomen (Fig. 3).
3. Restricted or reduced visceral slide can be caused by any disease associated with respiration. This includes any possible cause of inadequate respiratory movement with an impairment of respiratory excursions, e.g., chronic obstructive pulmonary disease, asthmatic or emphysematic disease.
4. Lack of compliance by the patient or impaired consciousness can result in impaired examination conditions. In such cases, all findings should be interpreted with caution.

Conclusion

Taking these possible mistakes into account, we can conclude that no peritoneal adhesions exist if visceral slide exceeds 2 cm. We found significant peritoneal adhesions to the abdominal wall when spontaneous or induced visceral slide was less than 1 cm.

It can be concluded that this method is very important in times of increasing use of minimally invasive surgery by laparoscopy, in order to provide surgeons

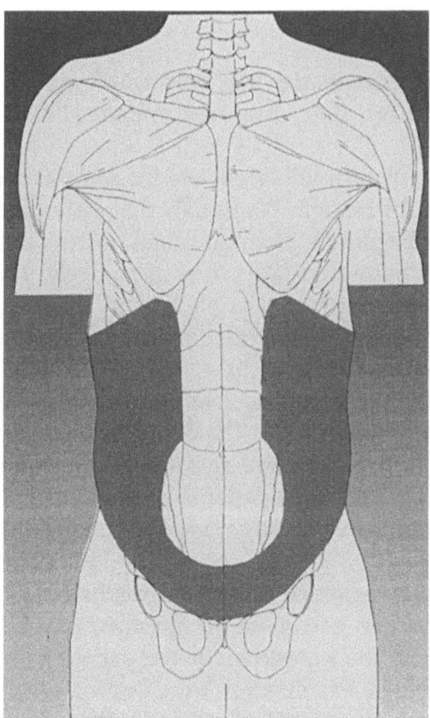

Fig. 3. Area of possible 'restricted viscera slide'

with better information for the selection of patients for operative procedures and for more precise guidance during the placement of the first trocar. It is helpful to know where to expect peritoneal adhesions to the abdominal wall so that surgeons can choose an alternative site for the first incision. A further advantage is the ease with which the method can be applied. Since most patients undergo a preoperative ultrasound examination, visceral slide can be assessed in the same session. It is absolutely noninvasive and is not time consuming.

Interenteric Adhesions

Interenteric adhesions are quite different from adhesions to the abdominal wall. They can cause an impairment of the intestinal passage with the clinical signs of intestinal obstruction. In a retrospective study we tried to estimate the value of ultrasound examination in the diagnosis of intestinal obstruction and investigated the possibility of differentiating between cause and site of the underlying problem.

Patients and Method

As already described above, ultrasound examination was performed with the patient in the supine position. We used a real-time ultrasound system with 3.5- and 7.5-MHz transducers.

The typical ultrasonic criteria for interenteric adhesions are the same as the ultrasonic signs of a mechanical bowel obstruction. We usually find distension of the small and/or large bowel. At the beginning of an intestinal obstruction, we often see pendular peristalsis, and later on peristalsis stops completely. The wall of the bowel is thickened. In many cases it is possible to find collapsed bowel behind the stenosis. In a profound intestinal obstruction, we also see free extraintestinal liquid between the intestinum (Figs. 4, 5).

In a retrospective trial we investigated the significance of ultrasound in the diagnosis of intestinal obstruction in 459 patients [4]. The data from a 5-year period were reviewed. In 459 patients in our clinic, we performed ultrasound examination as part of the diagnostic routine when patients showed acute or unclear abdominal complaints. Ultrasound was mostly done by the surgeons themselves.

After ultrasound examination, further radiologic diagnostic methods were applied, e.g., a plain abdominal film, barium enema, or an intestinal passage. Our ultrasound diagnosis was made with the knowledge of the patient's history, but before the results of the radiologic examination were known.

The ultrasound findings and diagnosis were verified either by the clinical course or by laparotomy.

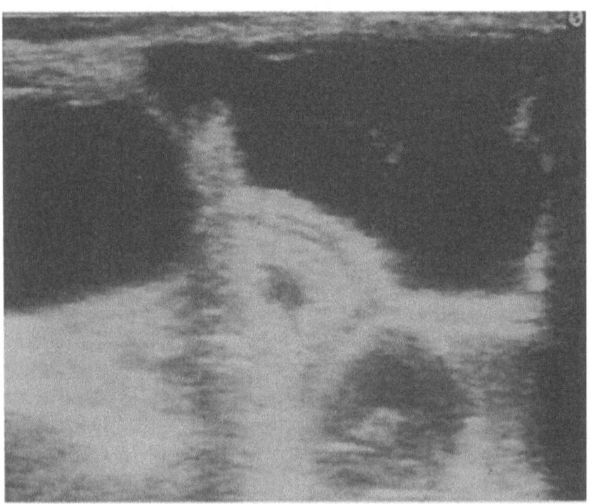

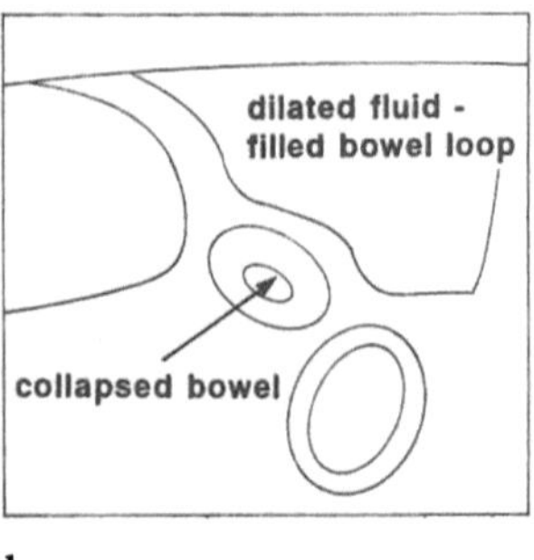

a   b

Fig. 4. a Ultrasound image and **b** diagram of a mechanical obstruction of the small bowel with distension of the liquid-filled bowel, thickening of the wall, and detection of collapsed bowel

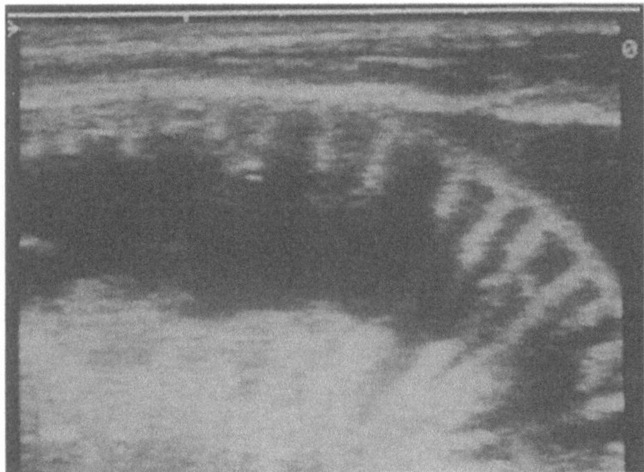

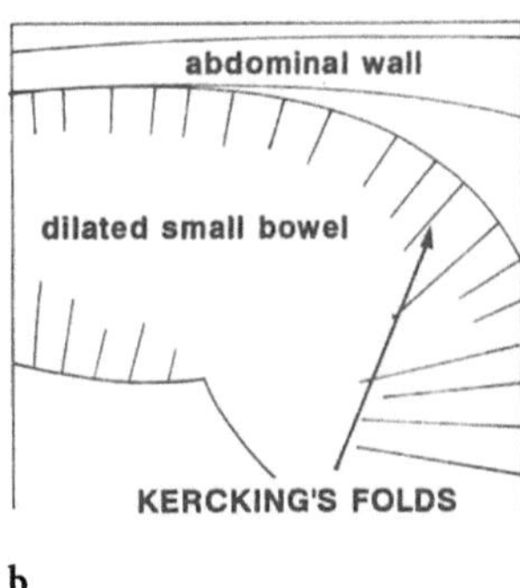

Fig. 5. a Ultrasound image and **b** diagram of a small-bowel obstruction, with echogenic structures of Kerckring's folds

Results

In 430 cases, we diagnosed an intestinal obstruction by ultrasound examination. In 29 patients, a clear ultrasound diagnosis could not be made, because of too much intestinal gas or too much abdominal pain in patients with peritonitis or acute pancreatitis. The overall sensitivity of ultrasound examination was about 93.7%. In paralysis, the correct diagnosis was obtained in 98% of patients.

By means of our ultrasound examination, we were able to identify mechanical obstruction in 91% of patients. However, only in 71% of the cases were we able to differentiate between small-bowel and large-bowel mechanical obstruction by ultrasound (Table 4).

There are many different causes of mechanical bowel obstruction. When we compared our ultrasound results with the operative results, we were only able to find the underlying cause of the mechanical bowel obstruction in 45%. The most common findings were large-bowel tumors, metastasis, or stenotic bowel inflammation, e.g., Crohn's disease, ulcerative colitis, or diverticulitis. Incarcerated hernia or invagination was observed less frequently.

Table 4. Localization of mechanical obstruction by ultrasound (US)

Obstruction	Patients (n)	Location small/large bowel		Accuracy of US (%)
		Correct	Incorrect	
Complete obstruction	116	97	19	84
Incomplete obstruction	188	120	68	64
Total	304	217	87	71

Table 5. Causes of intestinal obstruction and diagnostic results obtained by ultrasound (US)

Cause of obstruction	Patients (n)	Accuracy of US in detection of causes of obstruction (%)
Tumor	39	57
Inflammation	35	76
Hernia	13	72
Invagination	10	100
Band	136	0

In 136 patients, operation showed the underlying cause of the patient's complaints to be a mechanical obstruction by a band, which could not be demonstrated by ultrasound (Table 5).

Conclusion

On the basis of our experience, ultrasound has proven to be of significant importance in the diagnosis of intestinal obstruction. The underlying cause, however, can rarely be identified. With ultrasound, tumor, inflammation, and herniation can be seen, but not a band.

To evaluate adhesions to the abdominal wall, criteria concerning visceral slide make it possible to detect and locate abdominal adhesions. This method is helpful in planning laparoscopic operation to reduce the risk of bowel injury, especially in patients with a history of previous abdominal surgery. In over 700 laparoscopic cholecystectomies in our clinic, preoperative ultrasound scanning prevented an injury of the bowel by the first blind punction of the peritoneal cavity.

Summary

To evaluate peritoneal adhesions, one must differentiate between interenteric adhesions and adhesions to the abdominal wall. Adhesions between the abdominal wall and the intestinum can be ultrasonographically detected by observation of the visceral movement to the abdominal wall. This movement is called 'viscera slide'. It is produced by the force of respiratory motion (spontaneous 'viscera slide') or by manual ballottement of the abdomen (induced 'viscera slide'). Adhesions between abdominal wall and intestinum cause a restriction of the 'viscera slide'. In a prospective study we compared the ultrasound findings with the intraoperative adhesions.

Result.1: There are no adhesions when the spontaneous 'viscera slide' is > 2 cm.
     2: Significant adhesions could be observed when the spontaneous and induced 'viscera slide' is < 1 cm.

Intestinal obstruction can cause an impairment of the intestinal passage, with the clinical signs of intestinal obstruction. The ultrasonic criteria are a distension of the bowel, a thickening of the bowel wall, collapse of the bowel behind the stenosis and pendulum peristalsis. Free intra-abdominal liquid can be observed in profound obstruction.

In a retrospective trail we investigated the significance of ultrasound in diagnosis of intestinal obstruction in 459 patients. Mechanical obstruction was identified in 91%. In 71% of our patients ultrasound was successful in differentiating small bowel from large bowel obstruction. The underlying cause of ileus was yielded by ultrasound in 45% of the cases. There is no direct sonographic evidence of a band.

Conclusion. On the basis of our experience, ultrasound has proven to be of significant importance in the diagnosis of intestinal obstruction. The underlying cause can sonographically rarely be identified. To evaluate the adhesions to the abdominal wall, the criterion of the 'viscera slide' makes it possible to detect and locate abdominal adhesions. This method is helpful for the decision of laparoscopic operation and to reduce the risk of bowel injury by the first blind puncture with the trocar.

References

1. Kodama I, Loiacono LA, Sigel B et al. (1992) Ultrasonic detection of viscera slide as an indicator of abdominal wall adhesions. J Clin Ultrasound 20: 375–380
2. Link J, Marienhoff N, Benecke P et al. (1995) Die Bedeutung der Sonographie vor laparoskopischer Cholezystektomie. Fortschr Rontgenstr 162/1: 20–22
3. Sigel B, Golub RM, Laiocono LA et al. (1991) Technique of ultrasonic detection and mapping of abdominal wall adhesions. Surg Endosc 5: 161–165
4. Truong S, Arlt G, Pfingsten FP, Schumpelick V (1992) Die Bedeutung der Sonographie in der Ileusdiaganostik. Chirurg 63: 634–640

4.2 Conventional Radiography and Cross-sectional Imaging Modalities in the Diagnosis of Intestinal Adhesions

H.M. Klein, B. Klosterhalfen, C. Töns, G. Steinau,
and R.W. Günther

Introduction

Radiologists are able to visualize either structures of very different density or of different size. Their methods are limited to the determination of the thickness of the normal bowel wall or intramural gas collections and structures of 3–5 mm in thickness in a moving organ with peristaltic change of shape. It is not possible to visualize fibrous bands of less than 2 mm in thickness with a density that only differs by 5–10 HU from the surrounding enteric walls.

We cannot directly visualize peritoneal adhesions. Thus radiology has to restrict itself to the description of the functional deficits caused by adhesions and sometimes indirect signs such as adhesive compression or atypical positioning of bowel loops (Table 1). Nevertheless, diagnostic imaging methods have improved, and some of the new aspects are addressed here.

Conventional Radiography

Abdominal radiography is still the primary basic examination; it is easy to obtain and has low risk and discomfort for the patient. In the emergency situation of acute obstruction, it can often provide very helpful information about the diagnosis and sometimes even the location of the obstruction [3, 6, 12, 16].

Complete obstruction of the bowel is characterized by air–fluid levels and localized (prestenotic) dilatation. The sensitivity for detection of complete bowel obstruction is reported to be about 50% [6].

For incomplete obstruction, caused by peritoneal adhesions, the sensitivity is low. Meteorism and localized dilation of gas-filled loops may be vague signs of chronic incomplete obstruction. However, Kreitner and coworkers [10] reported on 253 patients under 31 years with nonspecific abdominal complaints which could be supposed to be caused partly by adhesive changes. They found radiographic images to be helpful in only 3.7% of cases, leading to a more strict indication of plain abdominal radiographs.

Table 1. Diagnostic value of imaging methods in bowel obstruction

Reference	Patients (n)	Radiography		Ultrasound		Fluoroscopy		CT	
		Sensitivity (%)	Specificity (%)	Sensitivity (%)	Specificity (%)	Sensitivity (%)	Specificity (%)	Sensitivity (%)	Specificity (%)
Frager et al. [3]	85	46	88	–	–	–	–	100	83
Gazelle et al. [4]	75	–	–	–	–	–	–	79	–
Megibow et al. [12]	167	25	–	58	–	85	–	94	96
Truong et al. [16]	459	90	–	93.8	–	–	–	–	–

CT, computed tomography.

Ultrasound

Sonographic examination is mandatory in patients presenting with abdominal complaints. The extensive study by Truong and coworkers [16] reported on 2581 patients, including 459 cases of surgically confirmed bowel obstruction. They found a sensitivity of 93.8% for the sonographic detection of bowel obstruction. The diagnosis of subclinical peritoneal adhesions is more difficult. The indirect sign of bowel loops fixed to each other or the abdominal wall is helpful and can be detected by the visceral slide technique [9, 14].

Contrast Examination

Small-Bowel Follow-Through. Fluoroscopic examinations after administration of iodine oral contrast agent are useful for the detection of a passage stop in acute bowel obstruction. This easy method can still be helpful in patients in which ultrasound demonstrates dilated loops and slow peristalsis, but the clinical signs are not specific. If a barium-containing agent is used, the better mucosal contrast provides a more subtle delineation of the bowel wall (Fig. 1). An advantage of this method is the combination of functional and morphological signs (band-like compresion of the bowel wall).

Double-Contrast Small-Bowel Follow-Through. The image quality of small-bowel follow-through can be improved by oral administration of acid-resistant coated effervescent agents [8] (Fig. 1).

Enteroclysis. The sensitivity of this invasive examination depends strongly on the experience of the radiologist and has been reported to be between 68% and 85% [11, 12]. The image quality is higher than in double-contrast small-bowel follow-through, but the positioning of the duodenal probe requires additional X-ray exposure and is inconvenient for the patient (Fig. 2).

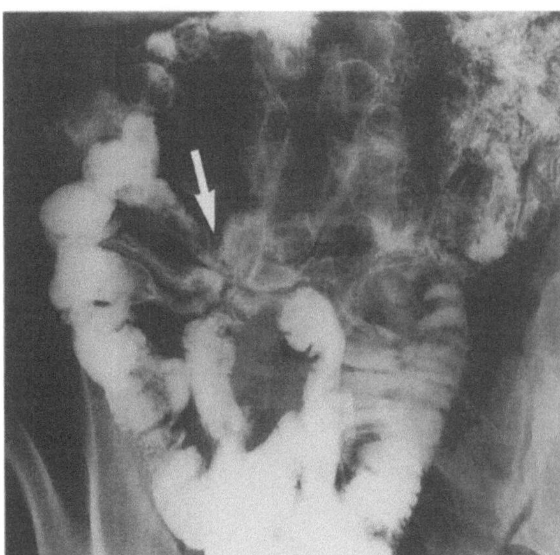

Fig. 1. Double-contrast small-bowel follow-through. Peritoneal adhesions with star-like convergence of ileum loops (*arrow*)

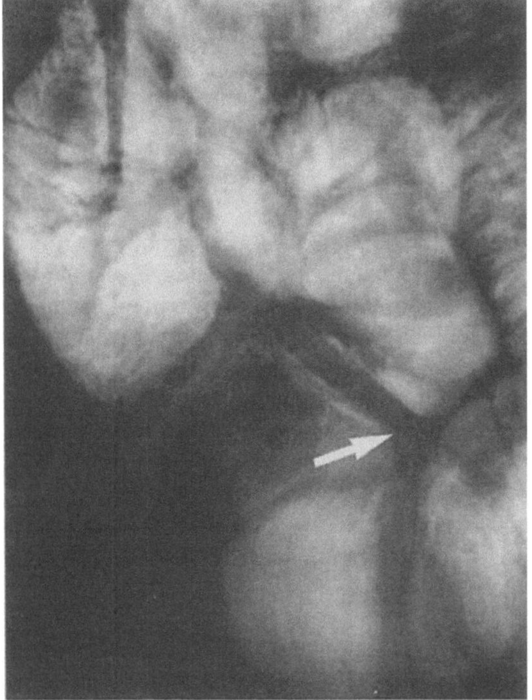

Fig. 2. Enteroclysis. Band-like compression of the bowel loops by adhesive fibrous strictures (*arrow*)

Table 2. Imaging signs of bowel obstruction [3, 4, 12, 16]

Sign	Radiography	Ultrasound	Fluoroscopy	CT
Dilatation	+	+	+	+
Air–fluid levels	+			+
Transition zone				+
Prestenotic dilatation	+		+	+
Wall thickening	(+)	+	(+)	+
Abnormal peristalsis		+	+	
Target sign (empty bowel distal to the obstruction)		+		+
Passage stop			+	
"String of beads" sign (gas between the enteric folds)		+		

CT, computed tomography

Computed Tomography

Attention has recently been focused on cross-sectional imaging of the gastrointestinal tract [1, 2, 4, 15, 17]. Computed tomography (CT) is a noninvasive, widely used method that can ascertain the status of the abdominal organs. Since the systems have been improved in terms of speed and spatial resolution, a subtle diagnostic workup of the gastrointestinal tract is now possible. Particularly with the use of the spiral CT technique, increasing accuracy in terms of spatial and time resolution can be expected [7]. Different authors have examined the diagnostic value of the method for bowel obstruction and reported a sensitivity of between 79% and 100% with a specificity of 83%–96% [3, 4, 11, 12] (Table 2, Fig. 3).

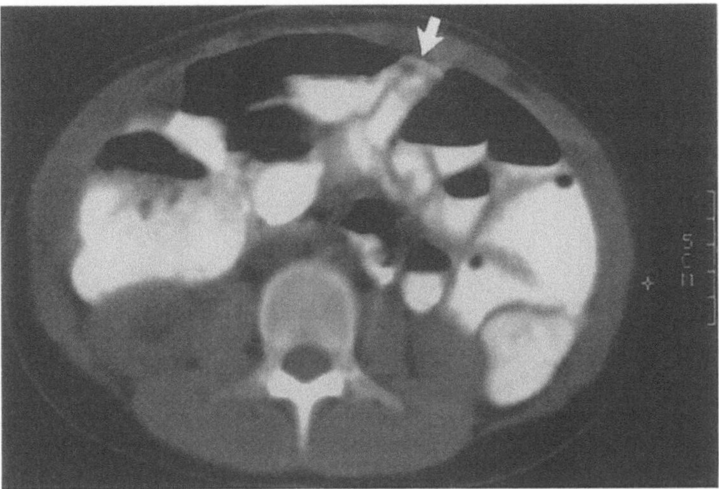

Fig. 3. Computed tomography (CT) enteroclysis. Adhesion of bowel loops to the abdominal wall after repeated surgery (*arrow*)

Zwaan et al. [17] and Thiele et al. [15] proposed a method of CT enteroclysis (Fig. 3). Gazelle and coworkers [4] have examined the diagnostic performance of abdominal CT with water as the distending agent (hydro-CT).

Magnetic Resonance Imaging

The experiences made with CT in the gastrointestinal tract have been applied to magnetic resonance imaging (MRI) [5]. The advantages of the method include the higher soft tissue contrast in MRI and the sensitive detection of bowel wall enhancement after i.v. administration of contrast agent. However, the low spatial and time resolution of the MRI systems presents a problem. Rapid technological progress is being made in this area, and contemporary systems now provide excellent image quality. The adequate intraluminal contrast agent may be water, mannitol solution, oral magnetite particles, or gadolinium diethylenetriaminopentoacetic acid (Gd-DTPA). The first studies with these agents are very promising (Fig. 4).

Conclusion

"The sun should never set on a small-bowel obstruction" is one of the rules of intestinal surgery. Radiologists can only provide help in the decision-making in cases in which the clinical situation allows a more sophisticated workup. The detection of peritoneal adhesions, in particular, requires all the diagnostic tools at our disposal. Progress is rapid, and it is not yet clear which imaging modality will be best suited for diagnosing chronic and acute adhesive disease. However, cross-sectional imaging will definitely play an important role. MRI

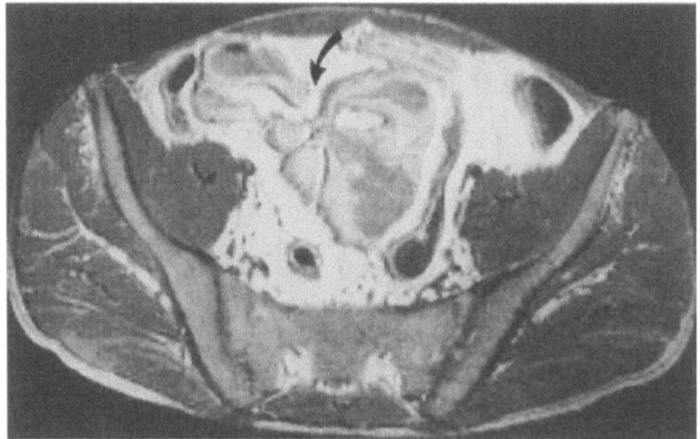

Fig. 4. Magnetic resonance imaging (MRI) of a patient with Crohn's disease; spin echo (SE), 15/600; 0.1 mmol gadolinium diethylenetriaminopentoacetic acid (Gd-DTPA)/kg; oral magnetite particles. Severe adhesive and inflammatory changes (*arrow*)

will certainly open up new possibilities, such as MR fluoroscopy and the highly sensitive detection of ischemic changes in strangulated bowel. The aim must be to provide a fast and reliable emergency diagnostic procedure and an efficient concept for chronic disease.

Summary

Diagnostic imaging of intestinal adhesions is mainly performed using ultrasound, considering the movement of the intestines relative to each other and to the abdominal wall. Conventional radiology can contribute to the diagnosis of acute obstructive disease, which is most frequently caused by adhesive bands. CT, and probably also MRI, will play a growing role in the future diagnostic work up of patients with abdominal disease. For adhesive changes, these methods provide all information of conventional imaging and add the demonstration of extraintestinal structures. The adequate imaging technique and the diagnostic performance (sensitivity/specificity) of these new concepts is the subject of ongoing clinical studies.

References

1. Balthazar EJ, Birnbaum BA, Megibow AJ, Gordon RB, Whelan CA, Hulnick DH (1992) Closed-loop and strangulating intestinal obstruction: CT signs. Radiology 185: 769–775
2. Faß J, Klose KC, Raguse T (1987) An evaluation of preoperative computed tomography for chronic inflammatory bowel disease. Coloproctology 4: 241–246
3. Frager D, Medwid SW, Baer JW, Mollinelli B, Freidman M (1994) CT of small-bowel obstruction. Am J Roentgenol 162: 37–41
4. Gazelle GS, Goldberg MA, Wittenberg J, Halpern EF, Pinkney L, Mueller PR (1994) Efficacy of CT in distinguishing small-bowel obstruction from other causes of small-bowel dilatation. Am J Roentgenol 162: 43–47
5. Goldberg HI, Thoeni RF (1989) MRI of the gastrointestinal tract. Radiol Clin North Am 27: 805–812
6. Gulliver DJ, Baker KA (1994) CT of the small bowel. Appl Radiol 11: 39–44
7. Kalender AW, Siessler W, Klotz E, Vock P (1990) Spiral volumetric CT with single breathhold technique, continuous transport and scanner rotation. Radiology 176: 181–183
8. Klein HM, Günther RW (1993) Double contrast small bowel follow-through with a new acid resistant effervescent agent. Invest Radiol 28: 581–585
9. Kolecki RV, Golub RM, Sigel R, Machi J, Kitamura H, Hosokawa T, Justin J, Schwartz J, Zaren HA (1994) Accuracy of viscera slide detection of abdominal wall adhesions by ultrasound. Surg Endosc 8: 871–874
10. Kreitner KF, Mildenberger P, Maurer M, Heintz A (1992) The value of imaging techniques in the diagnosis of non-specific abdominal pain in young patients. Aktuelle Radiol 1992: 234–238
11. Maglinte DDT, Gage SN, Harmon BH (1993) Obstruction of the small intestine: accuracy and role of CT in diagnosis. Radiology 188: 61–64
12. Megibow AJ, Balthazar EJ, Cho KC, Medwid SW, Birnbaum BA, Noz ME (1991) Bowel obstruction: evaluation with CT. Radiology 180: 313–318
13. Scholz FJ, Heiss FW, Roberts PL, Thomas C (1994) Diaphragmlike strictures of the small bowel associated with use of nonsteroidal antinflammatory drugs. Am J Roentgenol 162: 49–50

14. Sigel R, Golub RM, Ioiacono IA, Parsons RF, Kodama T, Machi J, Justin J, Sachdeva AK, Zaren HA (1991) Technique of ultrasonic detection and mapping of abdominal wall adhesions. Surg Endosc 5: 161–165
15. Thiele J, Kloppel R, Schulz HG (1993) CT-Sellink – Eine neue Methode zure Beurteilung der Darmwand. Fortschr Geb Rontgenstr 159(3): 213–217
16. Truong S, Arlt G, Pfingsten F, Schumpelick V (1992) Die Bedeutung der Sonographie in der Ileusdiagnostik. Chirurg 63: 634–640
17. Zwaan M, Gmelin E, Borgis KJ, Neubauer B (1991) Normale Wandstärke und tumoröse Wandveränderungen des Gastrointestinaltraktes in der Computertomographie. Fortschr Rontgenstr 155: 423–427

5 Complications of Peritoneal Adhesions

5.1 Adhesion Formation Following Incisional Hernia Repair: A Randomized Porcine Trial

P.M. Cristoforoni, Y.B. Kim, Z. Preys, R.Y. Lay, and F.J. Montz

Introduction

Incisional hernias remain a significant clinical problem in the modern era of surgery, occurring in up to 11% of laparotomy incisions [1, 2]. These hernias constitute an important source of operative related morbidity, with an impressive associated socio-economical impact [3]. The optimal method of management of large incisional hernias has yet to be described [3, 4]. Though selected individual patient variables (age, obesity, abdominal distention, etc.) increase the probability of failure, repair technique and choice of materials are prominent predictors of success or failure of attempted repair. Presently utilized techniques have significant associated rates of recurrence or complications which are related to the material used to repair the fascial defect (i.e., infection, foreign body reaction, adhesion formation with associated bowel obstruction) [5, 6]. In an attempt to minimize both rates of recurrence and negative side effects, new techniques and materials have been developed.

Recently many surgeons have advocated the use of prosthetic materials to facilitate closure, minimize suture line tense, and maximize the probability of successful repair [4, 7]. An ideal prosthetic material would allow for a massive fascial defect repair while assuring high tensile strength and low adhesion formation. One of the most promising of the newest materials is GoreTex Dual Mesh biomaterial, an expanded polytetrafluoroethylene (ePTFE) derived soft tissue patch [8]. One side of this patch has a pore size of less than 3 μm and is intended to result in minimal tissue ingrowth or attachment and therefore limit adhesion formation. The opposite surface has an open microstructure with an average pore size of 22 μm that allows for host tissue incorporation. A theoretically interesting improvement of this surgical patch would be the insertion of small holes or fenestrations. The purpose of adding these holes would be to facilitate fibroblast ingrowth and consequently improve the structural integrity and strength of the hernia repair. However, should an improvement in fibroblast integration lead to an increase in intraperitoneal adhesion formation, much of the advantages of this modification would be lost due to the potential risks of small bowel obstruction and other related complications.

We proposed to investigate, in a well standardized porcine model, the occurrence of intraperitoneal adhesion formation following repair of experimentally induced large fascial defects using commercially available surgical patches (Marlex and GoreTex Dual Mesh) and an experimentally modified GoreTex Dual Mesh produced by adding the above described fenestrations.

Methods

After obtaining approval from the UCLA Animal Research Committee, 60 female Red Durox hogs, each weighing 25 kg, were used for this investigation. The animals were housed at the UCLA Center for Health Sciences Vivarium. All animal procedures were performed in accordance with the standards described in the National Institute of Health Guide for the Care and Use of Laboratory Animals [9], in compliance with the Federal Animal Welfare Act.

Prior to surgery, the hogs were quarantined for a minimum of 10 days during which time they were allowed access to water and chow ad libitum. Animals were fasted for 12 h immediately prior to surgery. After induction of systemic analgesia (ketamine, 0.5 mg/kg) and general endotracheal anesthesia (halothane, 0.5 mg/kg; assisted volume-controlled ventilation with 40% O_2), the animals underwent exploratory celiotomy. They were placed in the supine position, prepped and draped using sterile technique. The creation of a large fascial defect, in an attempt to mimic an incisional hernia, and closure of the defect with either simple interrupted 0-Prolene sutures or with one of three synthetic surgical membranes (Marlex, Dual Mesh, and Dual Mesh with holes) undergoing evaluation was undertaken. The size of the fenestrations added to the Gore-DM "with holes" was 0.4 mm; the holes were evenly distributed on the full surface of the mesh, at 4 mm intervals. The abdomen was sharply opened via a 15 cm midline cutaneous incision beginning 5 cm below the costal margin and extending caudally. Following intraperitoneal exploration, a 6 × 4 cm section of the full thickness anterior abdominal wall, excluding the cutaneous surface, was resected en bloc using electrocautery. Due to the alleged adhesion preventive effect of the GoreTex Dual Mesh [8], we elected to evaluate its efficacy when placed in two different manners. Therefore, animals were randomly assigned to one of six different study groups, each including ten hogs. Group A underwent repair of the fascial defect by simple apposition of the two edges with interrupted 0-Prolene suture (Ethicon, Cincinnati, Ohio) in an inverted mattress technique, with sutures placed 1.5 cm from the fascial edge and 1 cm apart. Group B had repair effected by using an 8 × 6 cm piece of Marlex surgical membrane (Mx; C.R. Bard, Inc., Murray Hill, NJ), sutured in place using interrupted 0-Prolene sutures placed 1.5 cm from the wound edge and 1 cm apart. No attempt was made to over- or under-lay the Mx. Groups C and D had an 8 × 6 cm piece of GoreTex Dual Mesh (Gore-DM; W.L. Gore & Associates, Flagstaff, AZ) or GoreTex Dual Mesh with holes (Gore-DMH; W.L. Gore & Associates, Flagstaff, AZ, experimental only), placed in an overlay technique by means of interrupted 0-Prolene sutures placed 1.5 cm from the fascial edge and 1 cm apart. Group E and F were repaired using the same synthetic prosthetic materials as group C and D, respectively, but with the patches being placed in a intraperitoneal (underlay) position, with a 1.5 cm of the peritoneal edge underneath the edges of the patch (Gore DM-IP and Gore

DMH-IP). The side of the Gore-DM material presenting the closed micro-structure (i.e., anti-adhesion capacity) was placed toward the peritoneal cavity in all animals included in the Gore study groups. After assuring adequate hemostasis, the skin was closed using interrupted 2-0 Vicryl (Ethicon, Cincinnati, Ohio) in an inverted vertical mattress technique. The same senior surgeon personally performed all operations.

All animals were observed in the postoperative recovery area for 24 h after surgery and immediate recovery from general anesthesia. During that period, the animals were allowed access to water, but were withheld chow. Following the immediate postoperative recovery, the hogs were returned to the general animal run and allowed access to chow and water ad lib. All animals were observed on a twice daily basis. Abdominal incisions were evaluated for signs of bleeding, infection or breakdown; the animals were also observed for signs of gastrointestinal or urinary dysfunction.

Five weeks after the initial surgery the animals were killed using intravascular pentobarbital (100 mg/kg IV), explored, and adhesions scored. The anterior abdominal wall was entered in a U-shape manner 4 cm lateral and caudad to the margins of the pseudo-hernia repair. Adhesion appearance and tenacity were recorded and scored by the same investigator for all the animals, using a modification of a previously published method [10]. Unfortunately, due to the grossly different appearance of the primary Prolene suture and the Mx and Gore-DM synthetic prosthesis, a "blinded" scoring could not be performed. However, the investigator scoring the adhesions was unaware of whether Mx or Gore-DM was placed and, in the later instances, whether the materials were placed in an over- or under-lay technique or whether the Gore-DM was fenestrated. The technique employed for scoring quantifies adhesions by extent, type and tenacity to obtain a composite adhesion score for each animal (Table 1). Briefly, the adhesions were scored by evaluating: (a) the extent of abdominal wall, surface of the membrane, or suture lane involved in adhesion formation; (b) the type of adhesions gradated according to the most severe type present; and (c) adhesion tenacity based on resistance to gentle traction applied on the adhesion sites. The score assigned to each animal could range from 0 to 11.

Scores were reported as mean ± standard deviation (S.D.). The findings were analyzed by ANOVA or *chi* square analysis, as appropriate; $p < 0.05$ was selected for statistical significance.

Table 1. Adhesion scoring table (modified from [10])

Score	Extent (% of the surface)	Type (appearance)	Tenacity (resistance to lysis)
0	None	None	None
1	< 25	Filmy, transparent, avascular	Fall apart
2	< 50	Opaque, translucent, avascular	Lysed with traction
3	< 75	Opaque, translucent, capillaries	Sharp dissection required
4	> 75	Opaque, larger vessels present	–

Maximal score possible = 11.

Results

Three of the 60 animals died early in the postoperative period and therefore could not be evaluated for adhesion formation. One (Gore-DMH group) died in the immediate postoperative period while still in the recovery unit. A post-mortem examination was performed, and no abnormality was detected in the abdomen or the thorax. Presumed cause of death was respiratory failure. The second animal (Gore-DM) died 19 days after surgery because of a pulmonary infection. The third hog (Gore DMH-IP) died 13 days post-op with a small bowel obstruction associated with a diffuse purulent peritonitis. The animal had developed a massive subcutaneous abscess at the incision site, with the infection extending into the abdominal cavity despite aggressive antibiotic therapy. Thus, our results summarize data from a total of 57 hogs.

One animal (pig number 9, group Gore DM-IP) developed a large (reducible, and apparently asymptomatic) abdominal hernia at the side of repair. Because of the absence of apparent distress the study animal was followed and killed according to the scheduled plan. At time of the abdominal exploration at necropsy, the Gore-DM was found to be wrinkled and detached from the right caudal corner of the fascial defect. Extensive avascular adhesions originating from the lateral edges of the patch involved the omentum and the inferior margins of both liver and spleen.

The mean scores of the six study groups are as shown in Table 2. The animals in the control group, which were closed with interrupted stitches alone, developed significantly less adhesions than either Mx or Gore-DM (with or without holes) when these membranes were sutured in an overlying manner (Prolene vs Mx, $p < 0.0001$; vs Gore-DM, $p < 0.05$; vs Gore-DMH, $p < 0.01$). However, although the mean scores observed in the groups in which Gore-DM and DMH were placed intraperitoneally (5.6 ± 2.1 for Gore DM-IP and 5.8 ± 2.2 for Gore DMH-IP, respectively) were higher than those of the controls (4.1 ± 1.6), the differences were not statistically significant ($p = 0.08$ and 0.07, respectively). Marlex mesh induced significantly more severe adhesions than did Gore-DM when the membranes were placed with a similar (i.e., overlay) technique ($p < 0.001$).

The difference in adhesion formation which could be assigned to addition of holes was not statistically significant ($p = 0.20$ for the overlay technique and

Table 2. Adhesion scores of the 57 study hogs according to their group

Study group	Number of animals	Mean score	Standard deviation	Range	Intragroup variance
Control	10	4.1	1.6	3–8	2.54
Marlex	10	8.1	1.5	6–10	2.32
Gore DM	9	5.6	1.2	4–8	1.53
Gore DMH	9	6.7	2.2	4–10	4.75
Gore DM-IP	10	5.6	2.1	4–10	4.27
Gore DMH-IP	9	5.8	2.2	3–10	4.78

$p = 0.86$ for the intraperitoneal placement, respectively). The accurate intraperitoneal placement of the GoreTex patches did not significantly decrease their mean adhesion scores ($p = 0.96$ and $p = 0.40$ for DM and DMH, respectively) when compared to placing the same material in an overlay (i.e., extraperitoneal) fashion.

Discussion

The success of the repair of an incisional hernia is dependent on many factors, the most important apparently being the massive incorporation of healthy fascial tissue which is brought together under minimal tension [4–6].

In individual cases of incisional hernia repair, the size of the fascial defect and the condition of the actual fascia should dictate the selection of the most appropriate technique. The results of this experiment support the teaching that it would be preferable to simply close the defect by apposing fascial edges and suturing the wound in every hernia repair, assuming that minimal rates of hernia recurrence are guaranteed. This "prosthesis-free" approach would avoid the use of any unnecessary and potentially adhesion potentiating prosthetic materials. However, when the fascial defect is too large to allow a secure, tension-free, simple suture closure, the use of synthetic membranes is necessitated [3, 7].

The ideal prosthetic material for use in hernia repair should allow for maximal tissue incorporation while assuring high tensile strength. Numerous studies have reported the efficacy of selected synthetic prosthetic materials in the repair of large incisional hernias [7, 11, 12]. However, though hernia recurrence clearly indicates the failure of the repair, it must be stressed that a "successful" repair accompanied by severe intraperitoneal adhesions and associated bowel obstruction is far from desirable.

Marlex mesh, the knitted monofilament polypropylene patch first introduced in the early 1960s, is probably still the most widely used synthetic prosthesis for the repair of incisional hernias, although ePTFE is gaining popularity because of an apparent associated reduction in tissue reactivity and adhesion formation [3, 11].

Our experimental findings in this well standardized porcine model add credence to reports proposing a reduction in adhesion formation noticed when PTFE is compared to knitted polypropylene for the repair of fascial defects. Previous studies have demonstrated that ePTFE resulted in less adhesion to underlying organs than did Marlex mesh [13, 14]. This is presumably because of the limitation of fibroblast ingrowth into the small interfibrillar spaces of the ePTFE biomaterial [8]. If this is the case, the addition of microscopic fenestrations to an ePTFE biomaterial, with the proposed goal of enhancing tissue growth on the extraperitoneal surface of the mesh, could potentially result in an increased formation of intraperitoneal adhesions. Our study did not notice any statistically significant increase of adhesion formation when fenestrations were added to the Gore-DM. If the addition of such holes to the membrane would eventually prove to improve hernia repair rate and limit hernia recrudescence, a new Gore-DMH could offer a valid and even preferable alternative in the treatment of large incisional hernias.

The objective of our study was to evaluate the occurrence of intra-abdominal adhesions associated with the closure of incisional hernias. It is important to remember, however, that a number of other variables (i.e., repair failure and hernia recrudescence rate, postoperative febrile and infectious morbidity, postoperative pain) have an important role in the evaluation of any reparative technique. Should these other outcome parameters be equivalent, the prosthetic material of choice for the repair of incisional hernias too large to be simply closed with suture alone would be the one which induced the least amount of adhesion formation.

Acknowledgements. This study was supported in part by a grant from W.L. Gore and Associates, Inc., Flagstaff, Arizona. Dr. Cristoforoni is a fellow of the Associazione Italiana per la Ricerca sul Cancro, Milan, Italy.

References

1. Grace RH, Cox S (1976) Incidence of incisional hernia after dehiscence of the abdominal wound. Am J Surg 131: 210–212
2. Mudge M, Hughes LE (1985) Incisional hernia: a 10 year prospective study of incidence and attitudes. Br J Surg 72: 70–71
3. Santora TA, Roslyn JJ (1993) Incisional hernia. Surg Clin North Am 73: 557–570
4. Houck JP, Rypins EB, Sarfeh IJ et al. (1989) Repair of incisional hernia. Surg Gynecol Obstet 169: 397–399
5. George C, Ellis H (1986) The results of incisional hernia repair: a twelve year review. Ann R Coll Surg Engl 68: 185–187
6. Langer S, Christiansen J (1985) Long-term results after incisional hernia repair. Acta Chir Scand 151: 217–219
7. Larson GM, Harrower HW (1978) Plastic mesh repair of incisional hernias. Am J Surg 135: 559–563
8. Law NW (1994) Expanded polytetrafluoroethylene. In: Bendavid R (ed) Prostheses and abdominal wall hernias. RG Landes Company, Austin: p 290
9. Guide for the Care and Use of Laboratory Animals (1985) US Dept of Health and Human Services, Public Health Service, National Institute of Health, Bethesda
10. March CM, Boyers S, Franklin R et al. (1993) Prevention of adhesion formation reformation with the GoreTex Surgical Membrane. In: Diamond MP, diZerega GS, Linsky CB, Reid RL (eds) Gynecologic Surgery and Adhesion Prevention. Wiley-Liss, New York, pp 253–259
11. Bauer JJ, Salky BA, Gelernt IM et al. (1987) Repair of large abdominal wall defects with expanded polytetrafluoroethylene (PTFE). Ann Surg 206: 765–769
12. Tyrell J, Silberman W, Chandrasoma P et al. (1989) Absorbable versus permanent mesh in abdominal operations. Surg Gynecol Obstet 168: 227–232
13. Boyers SP, Diamond MP, DeCherney AH (1988) Reduction of postoperative pelvic adhesions in the rabbit with GoreTex Surgical Membrane. Fertil Steril 49: 1066–1070
14. Montz FJ, Monk BJ, Lacy SM (1993) Effectiveness of two barriers at inhibiting post-radical pelvic surgery adhesions. Gynecol Oncol 48: 247–251

5.2 The Role of Adhesion Formation in Gynecology and Reproductive Surgery

W. Schröder and W. Rath

Postoperative formation of intraperitoneal adhesions, a well-known frequent complication of intraabdominal surgery, also plays a key role in gynecological surgery, particularly in reproductive surgery. Large trials have demonstrated that more than 50% of all patients who undergo diagnostic laparoscopy do so in order to clarify adnexal factors for female infertility. Moreover, in another 33% of cases laparoscopy is performed because of clinical suspicion of adnexitis [1].

Prior surgery and inflammatory pelvic disease represent the most frequent causes of intraperitoneal adhesions which have to be focussed on from the gynecologist's point of view [2, 3]. Considering preventive as well as therapeutic aspects evaluation of the clinical consequences of adhesion formation in gynecology and reproductive surgery, particularly, is mandatory. Regardless of different initial steps of pathophysiology, which are broadly discussed in the other chapters of this book, there are four main clinical consequences of adhesions in gynecology:

- Postoperative complications after radical surgery
- Intraperitoneal therapy with antineoplastic agents
- Chronic pelvic pain
- Infertility

During the past decade operative concepts for gynecological cancers have drifted towards more radical procedures, especially for ovarian carcinoma. Recommendations for surgical treatment of this gynecological malignancy include removal of all grossly visible tumor as well as radical pelvic and para-aortic lymphadenectomy, which are also performed more often for cancers of the uterus. However, the increased frequency of radical surgical procedures is associated with a higher incidence of postoperative complications due to adhesions, such as bowel obstructions, lymph cysts or chronic pelvic pain [4]. Thus, reduction of those risks to the lowest achievable percentage requires that radical operations for gynecological cancers follow general surgical rules avoiding unneccessary trauma and bleeding. Moreover, especially for radical gynecologic operations prospective trials have demonstrated that the above-mentioned risks are markably reduced by leaving the peritoneum open (Table 1) [5–7].

Recently, intraperitoneal therapy of intraabdominal cancers with antineoplastic drugs has become more widespread. The different problems asso-

Table 1. Postoperative morbidity caused by adhesions after lymphadenectomy for gynecological cancer

Reference	Lymph cysts		Bowel complications	
	CP	OP	CP	OP
Pennehouat et al. [5]	36%	17%	–	–
Franchi et al. [7]	16%	16%	–	–
Benedetti-Panici et al. [6]	33%	15%	25%	6%

CP: closed peritoneum; OP: open peritoneum

ciated with these therapeutic procedures that may be related to adhesion formation will be discussed in detail (Chap. 7.3).

Chronic pelvic pain represents one of the major problems in gynecology. Although it is well documented that in 25%–30% of patients who undergo laparoscopy for chronic pelvic pain no anatomical or pathological correlate in the pelvis can be found, large trials have demonstrated that in 25%–50% or more of these cases, pain could be due to intraperitoneal adhesions [8–10].

Acute infections and/or postinflammatory adhesions are the most frequent cause of pelvic pain, accounting for 50% of cases [10]. However, after laparoscopically performed complete adhesiolysis, persistent or recurrent chronic pelvic pain was diagnosed in more than one third of cases (Table 2).

These data indicate that adhesions represent the major pathological findings in patients with chronic pelvic pain although a variety of psychosexual factors may play a role.

More than 50% of all patients who undergo diagnostic laparoscopy do so in order to clarify adnexal factors for female infertility [1]. In 40–50% of such cases adhesions are found as the primary cause demonstrating the predominant role of adhesions in reproductive surgery (Table 3).

During the past decades numerous adhesion classifications have been proposed, of which the modified Hulka score is the most widely used [11, 12]. The results of reproductive microsurgery are undoubtfully influenced by the extent and pattern of adhesions and tissue damages (Fig. 1, Table 4). As to whether the surgical approach, laparoscopy or laparotomy, has any influence on the incidence of adhesion reformation conflicting results have been obtained [13, 14].

Table 2. Follow-up of previously symptomatic patients after laparoscopic adhesiolysis (from [8])

	n	%
Disease-free	38	38.4
Improvement	20	20.2
Recurrent pain after disease-free interval	25	25.2
No change	16	16.2
Total	99	100

Table 3. Laparoscopic findings in patients with sterility (from [10])

| | Primary sterility | | Secondary sterility | |
	n	%	n	%
Normal	71	26	12	15
Acute/postinflammatory adhesions	106	39	43	52
Endometriosis	62	23	16	19
Myomas, polycystic ovary, ovarian cysts	31	12	10	12
Appendicitis	–	–	2	2
Ectopic pregnancy	–	–	–	–
Total	270	100	83	100

PREGNANCY RATE (%)

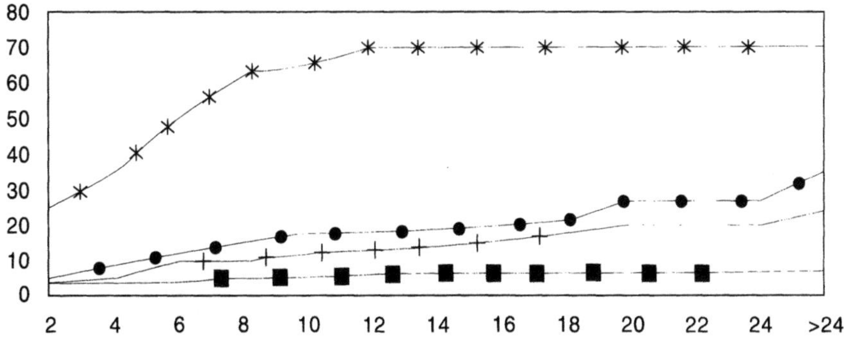

Fig. 1. Pregnancy rate after microsurgery for tubal problems ($n = 493$). (from [10])

Table 4. Pregnancy rate in relation to adnexal adhesions ($n=493$) (from [10])

Stage[a]	Ovario-salpingo-fimbriolysis + fimbrioplasty	Ovario-salpingo-fimbriolysis + salpingostomy
IA	54%	34%
IB	26%	19%
IIA	47%	25%
IIB	10%	9%

[a]I, >50% ovarian surface visible; II, < 50% ovarian surface visible; A, filmy/ avascular; B; thick/vascular

As a consequence of the challenge posed by the clinical problems of adhesions, considerable efforts in experimental and clinical research have been made in the field of adhesion prevention.

A variety of drugs, mainly corticosteroids, fibrinolytics, heparin and in particular, dextrans, have been instilled into the peritoneal cavity to prevent or at least reduce the reformation of adhesions after reproductive surgery [9–11]. However, these experimental and clinical studies have failed to demonstrate clear benefits [11]. Recently, the Nordic Adhesion Prevention Study Group reported that adhesion formation after microsurgical procedures was significantly reduced by application of an absorbable adhesion barrier (Interceed) to the adnexa [15]. Nevertheless, the problems associated with postoperative intraperitoneal adhesion formation, particularly after adnexal reproductive microsurgery, remain unsolved.

References

1. Schneider HPG, Karbowski B (1994) Endoskopische Diagnostik und Therapie der weiblichen Sterilität. In: Krebs D, Schneider HPG (eds) Endokrinologie und Reproduktionsmedizin III, 3rd edn. (Klinik der Frauenheilkunde und Geburtshilfe, vol III) Urban and Schwarzenberg, Munich, pp 103–118
2. Ellis H (1971) The cause and prevention of postoperative intraperitoneal adhesions. Surg Gynecol Obstet 133: 497–511
3. Grodstein F, Goldman MB, Cramer DW (1993) Relation of tubal infertility to history of sexually transmitted diseases. Am J Epidemiol 137(5): 577–584
4. Burghardt E (1993) Epithelial ovarian cancer: surgical treatment. In: Burghardt E (ed) Surgical gynecologic surgery. Thieme, Stuttgart, pp 459–467
5. Pennehouat G, Mosseri V, Durand IC et al. (1988) Lymphocèles et peritonisation après lymphadènectomies pour cancers de l'uterus. J Gynecol Obstet Biol Reprod 17: 373–378
6. Benedetti-Panici P, Maneschi F, Scotto di Palumbo V et al. (1995) Lymphadenectomy in gynecologic oncology: to drain or not to drain the retroperitoneum. Int J Gynecol Cancer 5 [Suppl 1]: 23
7. Franchi M, Zanaboni F, Beccaria C et al. (1995) Role of peritonealization in radical hysterectomy and node dissection (RHND): a multicenter randomized study. Int J Gynecol Cancer 5 [Suppl 1]: 24
8. Kolmorgen K, Schulz AM (1991) Ergebnisse nach per laparoscopiam ausgeführten Adhäsiolysen bei Patientinnen mit chronischen Unterbauchbeschwerden. Zentralbl Gynäkol 113: 291–295
9. Di Zerega GS, Rodgers KE (1992) The peritoneum. Springer, New York Berlin Heidelberg
10. Karbowski B, Schneider HPG (1994) Tubenfaktor der weiblichen Sterilität In: Krebs D, Schneider HPG (eds) Endokrinologie und Reproduktionsmedizin, Vol 3, 3rd edn. Urban and Schwarzenberg, Munich, pp 143–158
11. Gauwerky JFH, Kubli F (1986) Intraabdominelle Adhäsionen – Ursachen, Vorbeugung und Behandlung. Fertilitat 2: 125–134
12. Frantzen C, Schlösser HW (1984) Mikrochirurgie in der Gynäkologie. (Bücherei des Frauenarztes, vol 15) Enke, Stuttgart
13. Lundorff P, Hahlin M, Källfelt B et al. (1991) Adhesion formation after laparoscopic surgery in tubal pregnancy: a randomized trial versus laparotomy. Fertil Steril 55: 911–915
14. Operative Laparoscopy Study Group (1991) Postoperative adhesion development after operative laparoscopy: evaluation of early second look procedures. Fertil Steril 55: 700–704
15. Nordic Adhesion Prevention Study Group (1995) The efficacy of Interceed (TC7) for prevention of reformation of postoperative adhesions on ovaries, fallopian tubes and fimbriae in microsurgical operations for fertility: a multicenter study. Fertil Steril 63: 709–714

5.3 Causes of Intestinal Obstruction – A Retrospective Study of 550 Surgical Cases

K.-H. Treutner, P. Bertram, G. Lätzsch, and V. Schumpelick

Introduction

Intestinal obstruction is one of the predominant indications for emergency surgery. Despite the improvements in perioperative management and surgical technique, it still carries a significant risk of morbidity and mortality [3–6]. Our study was aimed at investigating the underlying causes of intestinal obstruction of patients who underwent surgery. The basic idea was that measures for prevention of intestinal obstruction and subsequent emergency surgery might be concluded from these data.

Patients and Methods

In a retrospective study, we evaluated the available and complete records of 550 patients operated on for intestinal obstruction at our department of surgery during the 22-year period from 1972 to 1993. The data regarding medical history, intraoperative findings, surgical procedure, and postoperative course were classified and evaluated by an electronic data base on a personal computer.

Results

The mean age of our group of 550 patients was 47.6 years, ranging from 0.1 to 93 years. The number of men (50.7%) and women (49.3%) was almost equal.

In 66.2% of patients, the small intestine was the site of obstruction, and in 33.8% the large bowel was affected. Adhesions and bands were the predominant cause (53.7%), followed by obstructing colonic carcinomas (13.1%), extraintestinal malignomas (12.9%), and inflammation (5.6%). All other diagnoses were below the 5% level (Table 1). In small-intestinal obstruction, the major causes were adhesions and bands (76.2%). In children below the age of 11 years, adhesions and bands (57.5%) and intussusceptions (31.1%) were the leading causes of intestinal obstruction. In the elderly patients (over 74 years), the major causes were malignant tumors (28.2%) and adhesions and bands (28.1%).

Table 1. Causes of intestinal obstruction in 550 surgical patients

Cause of obstruction	Incidence (%)
Adhesions/bands	53.7
Colonic carcinoma	13.1
Extraintestinal malignoma	12.9
Inflammation	5.6
Foreign bodies	4.8
Intussusception	4.2
Internal hernia	2.2
Volvulus	2.0
Intestinal ischemia	0.8
Inguinal and femoral hernia	0.7

In 94.5% of patients with intestinal obstruction due to adhesions and bands, there was a history of at least one previous laparotomy. The most common operations had been appendectomies (31.1%) and gynecologic procedures (15.3%). In the group of patients with a history of malignoma, 27.4% were now diagnosed with adhesive bowel obstruction, 32.3% suffered from primary or recurrent colonic carcinoma, and in 40.7% peritoneal carcinomatosis from various tumors was found.

The surgical procedure was restricted to the dissection of adhesions and bands in 25.8% of patients. In 28.2%, either ischemic lesions from strangulation, obstructive inflammation, or malignancy required bowel resection. In the group of patients with adhesions and bands as the causative factor, dissection was sufficient in 85.3%. In 11.8% and 2.9%, ischemia from strangulation required resections of the small or large bowel, respectively. In the whole group, a diverting or definitive ileostomy or colostomy was performed in 27.8%, either to protect a large-bowel anastomosis in the unprepared patient or for staged management. In those patients with irresectable malignomas, we preferred bypass procedures by interenteric anastomoses (8.4%) to avoid the inconveniencies of a stoma during the patients' limited life expectancy. The other operations mainly consisted in reposition and in reduction and repair of intussusceptions, volvulus, and hernias. Foreign bodies were mostly removed by simple enterotomy. Cases of gallstone ileus required the removal of the gall bladder as the underlying cause.

The postoperative course was uneventful in 56.7% of the patients. Besides a wound sepsis rate of 14.7%, the major complications were pneumonia (11.5%), renal insufficiency (9.6%), fistulous tracts (6.9%), cardiac insufficiency (4.4%), pancreatits (1.9%), peritonitis (1.8%), and pulmonary embolism (1.8%). During the hospital stay, the mortality rate was 18.2%, with cardiac failure as the leading course (49.2%). The other deaths were mostly attributed to sepsis and peritonitis (13.4%), pulmonary failure (11.0%), and pulmonary embolism (4.9%). The mortality rate in the subgroup of patients with adhesive obstruction was 15.3%. The mean age of those patients with a lethal outcome was 62.7 years (range, 2–93 years). In 32.1%, intestinal obstruction was caused by a malignoma.

Discussion

Intestinal obstruction is a frequently encountered problem in abdominal surgery. Despite all efforts to achieve an early diagnosis, rapid surgical intervention, and intensive care treatment, morbidity and mortality rates are still too high. A closer look at the underlying causes may initiate the search for and the application of methods to prevent at least some causes of intestinal obstruction.

For this purpose we evaluated the data of 550 patients who had been operated on for intestinal obstruction during a period of more than 20 years. The mean age of our group of patients (47.6 years) was lower than in a number of other studies. A more detailed analysis showed that 9.6% were younger than 11 years and 14.9% were older than 74 years of age. This reflects our broad range of patients from pediatric to geriatric surgery patients. Furthermore, as our department is a university hospital, a number of patients with serious concomitant disorders were referred to us.

In Western countries, the spectrum of intestinal obstruction has altered over the past few decades. Whereas 60 years ago strangulated hernias accounted for about 50% of cases, peritoneal adhesions are now the most common cause. Overall adhesive bowel obstruction is found in 20%–41%, and if we disregard colonic obstruction the figure rises to 54%–74% [1–3, 5–7]. These data support our findings of rates of 53.7% and 76.2% of obstruction with adhesions and bands as the causative factor in the whole group and in the subgroup of patients with small-intestinal obstruction, respectively.

In the current literature as in our study, colonic carcinoma is the second most common cause of intestinal obstruction [4, 5]. These advanced cases of obstructing and frequently incurable carcinomas are often found in elderly patients. In many of these cases, surgical therapy is therefore limited to resolving the obstruction by intestinal bypass procedures or abdominal stomas. Furthermore, advanced tumor stages, concomitant diseases, and prolonged bowel distension contribute to the poor prognosis of these patients. In our study, malignant tumors were found as the cause of intestinal obstruction in 28.2% of the patients over 74 years of age, and the mean age of those patients with a lethal outcome (62.7 years) was considerably higher than the mean age of the entire group (47.6 years).

An important finding was that, in subgroups of patients who either had a history of a malignant disease or were older than 74 years, adhesions and bands were found as the etiologic factor in intestinal obstruction in 27.4% and 28.1%, respectively. These patients were successfully treated by simple division of the adhesive bridges.

Conclusion

Peritoneal adhesions and colonic carcinoma are the most frequent causes of intestinal obstruction in Western industrialized countries. Hence there are two possible ways of reducing the incidence of intestinal obstruction, subsequent emergency surgery, and the resulting high rates of morbidity and mortality. Research must be aimed at the development of an agent to prevent postoperative adhesion formation, and screening for colonic adenomas and carcinomas must be carried out. Furthermore, neither knowledge of a previous malignant disease nor the mere fact of an advanced age should be regarded as reasons to deny surgery. In both cases, the intestinal obstruction can be expected to be treated by simple division of adhesions and bands in about 30% of patients.

Summary

We evaluated the records of 550 patients who underwent surgery for intestinal obstruction at our department of surgery from 1972 until 1993. The mean age of this group with about an equal number of male and female patients was 47.6 (0.1–93) years. The predominant site of obstruction was the small intestine (66.2%). The major causes were adhesions and bands (58.7%). Small intestinal obstruction was due to adhesions in 76.2%. Patients with adhesive bowel obstruction had a history of prior abdominal surgery in 94.5%. Even in the subgroups of patients with a history of a malignant disease or an age older than 74 years adhesions were the underlying cause in 27.4% and 28.1%, respectively. Obstructing colonic carcinoma was the second major cause of intestinal obstruction (13.1%). In the group of patients beyond 74 years of age, malignant tumors were the etiological factor in 28.2%. It can be concluded that the incidence of intestinal obstruction can be controlled by the prevention of postoperative adhesions and by screening examinations for colonic carcinoma or its precursor lesions.

References

1. Bevan PG (1984) Adhesive obstruction. Ann R Coll Surg Engl 66: 164–169
2. Cheadle WG, Garr EE, Richardson JD (1988) The importance of early diagnosis of small bowel obstruction. Am Surg 54: 565–569
3. Deutsch AA, Eviatar E, Gutman H, Reiss R (1989) Small bowel obstruction: a review of 264 cases and suggestions for management. Postgrad Med J 65: 463–467
4. Irvin TT (1989) Abdominal pain: a surgical audit of 1190 emergency admissions. Br J Surg 76: 1121–1125
5. McEntee G, Pender D, Mulvin D, McCullogh M, Naeeder S, Farah S, Badurdeen MS, Ferraro V, Cham C, Gillham N, Matthews P (1987) Current spectrum of instestinal obstruction. Br J Surg 74: 976–980
6. Mucha P (1987) Small intestinal obstruction. Surg Clin North Am 67: 597–620
7. Vick RJ (1932) Statistics of acute intestinal obstruction. Br Med J 2: 546–547

6 Peritonitis and Sepsis

6.1 The Peritoneal Cytokine Profile in Acute Peritonitis

J.M. Badia, S.A. Whawell, D.M. Scott-Coombes,
A.J. Waghorn, P.D. Abel, and J.N. Thompson

Introduction

Cytokines are polypeptides produced mainly by activated leukocytes in response to infection and injury, including surgical trauma. Within the peritoneal cavity they are produced by resident mononuclear phagocytes [1] and mesothelial cells [2]. Peritoneal cytokines mediate the local inflammatory changes that occur after surgery and are also partly responsible for the immunological and systemic acute phase responses to surgery [3].

In several reports, the cytokine levels in plasma after surgery or sepsis have been studied [4–6]. Others have demonstrated the presence of cytokines in the peritoneal fluid in different pathological conditions [7, 8]. The aim of this study was to assess level of cytokines in peritoneal fluid and systemic blood in patients with intra-abdominal infection.

Patients and Methods

Patients

Six patients undergoing emergency abdominal surgery were studied (five acute appendicitis, one diverticulitis). A venous blood sample was taken preoperatively. After gaining entry in the peritoneal cavity, 5ml of peritoneal fluid were sampled. All samples were centrifuged at 2500g for 10 min at 4 °C and the supernatant stored at –80 °C until assay. The study was approved by the Ethical Committee of the Royal Postgraduate Medical School and all patients gave informed consent.

Cytokine Assays

Interleukin-1β (IL-1β), interleukin-6 (IL-6) and tumor necrosis factor-α (TNF-α) were measured in plasma and peritoneal fluid using commercially available enzyme-linked immunosorbent "sandwich" assays (ELISA) (IL-1β from Cistron Biotechnology, Pine Brook, USA; IL-6 from Eurogenetics, Tessenderlo, Belgium; and TNF-α from Biokine, T Cell Diagnostics, Teddington, UK). The minimum detectable concentration was 20 pg/ml for IL-1β, 5 pg/ml for IL-6, and 1.5 pg/ml for TNF-α.

Statistical Analysis

Data are expressed as mean ± standard error of the mean (SEM). Data were analyzed using the Kruskal Wallis and Wilcoxon nonparametric tests. The program StatView 4.0 (Abacus Concepts, Inc., Berkeley, USA) was used.

Results

Operative procedures were five appendicectomies and one sigmoid colectomy. The duration of preoperative symptoms was 25 ± 3 h. The operative time was 42 ± 12 min. There was no postoperative complication.

In all six patients the microbiological swab taken from the peritoneal fluid during operation showed bacterial growth (four *E. coli*, two *B. fragilis* and one *Peptostreptococcus sp.*).

The mean cytokine levels in peritoneal fluid were: TNF-α, 33 ± 14 pg/ml; IL-1β, 432 ± 164 pg/ml; IL-6, 133 000 ± 52 000 pg/ml. Plasma IL-6 levels were substantially lower: 69 ± 24 pg/ml (Fig. 1). Plasma TNFα and IL-1β concentrations were very low or undetectable (<1.5 and <20 pg/ml, respectively).

Discussion

Several authors have reported low or undetectable postoperative plasma levels of TNFα, interferon(IFN)-γ and IL-1β [5, 9–11] and elevated IL-6 levels [5, 10, 11]. In sepis, systemic cytokine levels have been shown to be elevated [12, 13], although TNFα seems to not always be detectable [14, 15].

Few reports have analyzed the levels of cytokines in the peritoneal fluid. Buyalos et al. found a high IL-6 fluid concentration in female patients with pelvic pathology [7]. Tsukada et al. determined TNFα, IL-1β and IL-6 in peritoneal fluid after abdominal surgery, finding a correlation with the severity of surgical stress [8]. Scott-Coombes et al. found high levels of TNFα within 3 h of surgery for non-inflammatory conditions and elevated IL-1β and IL-6 levels until 18 h after the operation, while IFN-γ was not detected [16]. Sakamoto et al. found the peak concentration of IL-6 to be 100-fold greater in pleural fluid than in blood in one patient subjected to esophagectomy and thoracotomy [10].

In this study, a high concentration peritoneal cytokine response to acute abdominal inflammation was detected. Surgical injury to the peritoneal cavity results in the production of TNFα and IL-1β [4] by resident mononuclear phagocytes [1, 2]. These cytokines in turn stimulate the synthesis of IL-6[3]. Cytokines released into the peritoneum are then absorbed into the systemic and portal circulations, where they may initiate the production of acute-phase proteins by hepatocytes [3]. The imbalance between plasma and in-

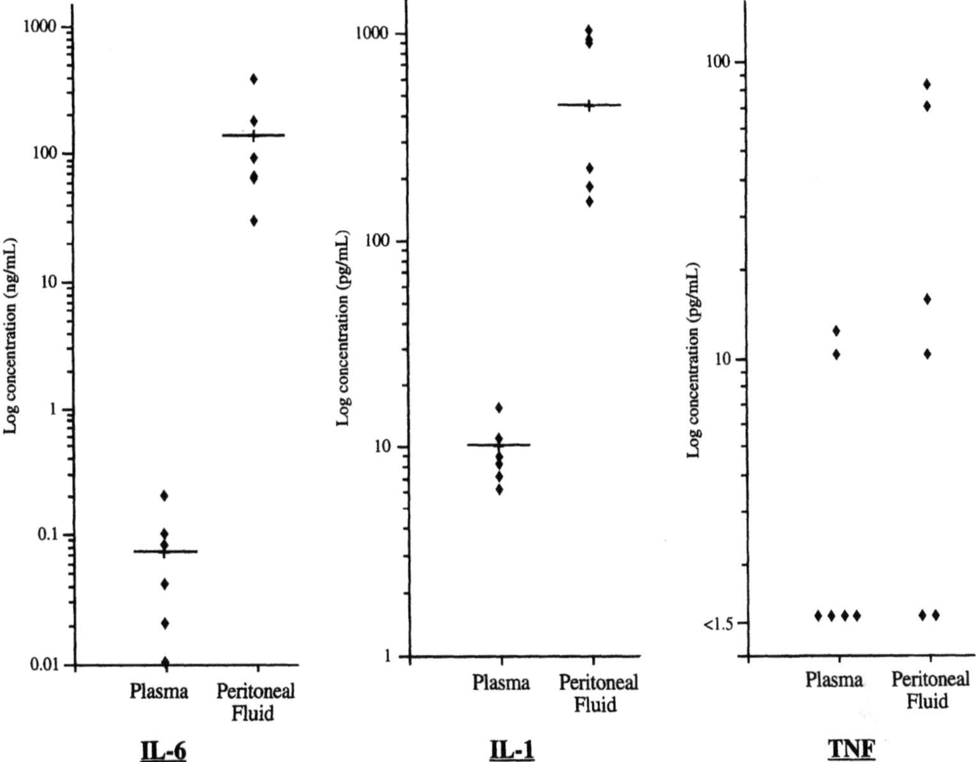

Fig. 1. Logarithmic scattergram for interleukin (IL)-1, IL-6 and tumor necrosis factor (TNF) in plasma and peritoneal fluid. Note that the concentration of IL-6 is expressed in ng/ml, whereas data from the rest of cytokines are in pg/ml

traperitoneal cytokine concentrations seen in this study may be explained by an incomplete absorption and rapid degradation of peritoneal cytokines, and their dilution in the plasma.

The concentration of intraperitoneal cytokines under normal conditions is not known. Control samples of peritoneal fluid are unobtainable, as the normal quantity of fluid is estimated to be less than 0.1 ml. It seems probable that, in the absence of an intraperitoneal stimulus such as infection or injury, IL-6 and other cytokines are undetectable in peritoneal fluid.

In some chronic pelvic conditions a low level of peritoneal fluid IL-6 has been described [7]. These levels are however, 100-fold lower than those seen in this study of acute peritoneal infection. Peritoneal fluid cytokines, especially IL-6, might be useful to differentiate acute inflammatory abdominal disease from other non-inflammatory causes of abdominal pain.

This study has shown a high concentration peritoneal cytokine response to acute abdominal infection. Cytokines mediate the local inflammatory changes in the peritoneum and may also contribute to the systemic response to intra-abdominal sepsis. In addition, they may be potentially useful as a diagnostic test of peritonitis.

Acknowledgement. Dr. JM Badia is the recipient of the grant 'Antoni de Gimbernat' 1993 from the City Council of Cambrils and the Catalan Society of Surgery, Spain.

References

1. Remick DG, Strieter RM, Lynch JP, Nguyen D, Eskandari M, Kunkel SL (1989) In vivo dynamics of murine tumor necrosis factor-alpha gene expression. Lab Invest 60: 766–771
2. Betjes MGH, Tuk CW, Struijk DG, Krediet RT, Arisz L, Hart M, Beelen RHJ (1993) Interleukin-8 production by human peritoneal mesothelial cells in response to tumor necrosis factor-alpha, interleukin-1, and medium conditioned by macrophages cocultured with Staphylococcus epidermidis. J Infect Dis 168: 1202–1210
3. Van Deuren M, Dofferhoff ASM, van der Meer JWM (1992) Cytokines and the response to infection. J Pathol 168: 349–356
4. Dinarello CA (1984) Interleukin-1 and the pathogenesis of the acute-phase response. N Engl J Med 311: 1413–1418
5. Baigrie RJ, Lamont PM, Kwiatkowski D, Dallman MJ, Morris PJ (1992) Systemic cytokine response after major surgery. Br J Surg 79: 757–760
6. Függer R, Zadrobilek E, Götzinger P, Klimann S, Rogy M, Winkler S, Andel H, Mittelböck M, Roth E, Schulz F, Fritsch A (1993) Perioperative TNF-alpha and IL-6 concentrations correlate with septic state, organ function, and APACHE II scores in intra-abdominal infection. Eur J Surg 159: 525–529
7. Buyalos RP, Watson JM, Funari VA, Martinez-Maza O, Azziz R (1992) Elevated inter-leukin-6 levels in peritoneal fluid of patients with pelvic pathology. Fertil Steril 58: 302–306
8. Tsukada K, Katoh H, Shiojima M, Suzuki T, Takenoshita S, Nagamachi Y (1993) Con-centrations of cytokines in peritoneal fluid after abdominal surgery. Eur J Surg 159: 475–479
9. Pullicino EA, Carli F, Poole S, Rafferty B, Malik STA, Elia M (1990) The relationship between the circulating concentrations of interleukin-6 (IL-6), tumour necrosis factor (TNF) and the acute phase response to elective surgery and accidental injury. Lymphokine Res 9: 231–238
10. Sakamoto K, Arakawa H, Mita S, Ishiko T, Ikei S, Egami H, Hisano S, Ogawa M (1994) Elevation of circulating interleukin-6 after surgery: factors influencing the serum level. Cytokine 6: 181–186
11. Ohzato H, Yoshizaki K, Nishimoto N, Ogata A, Tagoh H, Monden M, Gotoh M, Kishimoto T, Mori T (1992) Interleukin-6 as a new indicator of inflammatory status: detection of serum levels of interleukin-6 and C-reactive protein after surgery. Surgery 111: 201–209
12. Calandra T, Baumgartner JD, Grau GE, Mei-Miau W, Lambert PH, Schellekens J, Verhoef J, Glauser MP (1990) Prognostic values of Tumor Necrosis Factor/Cachectin, Interleukin-1, interferon-alpha, and interferon-gamma in the serum of patients with septic shock. J Infect Dis 161: 982–987
13. Ertel W, Morrison MH, Wang P, Ba ZF, Ayala A, Chaudry I (1991) The complex pattern of cytokines in sepsis. Association between prostaglandins, cachectin and interleukins. Ann Surg 214: 141–148
14. Groote A, Martin MA, Densen P, Pfaller MA, Wenzel RP (1989) Plasma tumor necrosis factor levels in patients with presumed sepsis. JAMA 262: 249–251
15. Debets J, Kampmeijer R, Van der Linden MPMH, Buurman WA, Van der Linden CJ (1989) Plasma tumor necrosis factor and mortality in critically ill septic patients. Crit Care Med 17: 486–494
16. Scott-Coombes DM, Whawell SA, Thompson JN (1994) Peritoneal cytokine response in surgery. Br J Surg 81: 756

6.2 Peritoneum and Sepsis: The Role of Sepsis in the Genesis of Peritoneal Adhesions

S. Bengmark

Introduction

The long list of prevention treatments (rather recently summarized by Christen and Buchmann [9]), underlines the fact that the pathophysiology of adhesion formation is, even today, not fully understood; neither is there a treatment that targets the cause of this problem. It is well documented that fibrin formation and lack of fibrinolysis are important ingredients in the formation of adhesions. This finding has, over the years, been the focus of an enormous amount of interest in the literature (see also this volume). Studies to identify the mechanisms of adhesion formation have, in the past, played an important role in furthering our understanding. Such studies will continue to be of great importance, more so as topical fibrin glues are increasingly used in abdominal surgery, especially in laparoscopic surgery. There have not been any studies to clarify if this will contribute to increased adhesion formation. Current information suggests that the fibrin glue can still be identified at the peritoneal surface after 3 weeks.

In the genesis of adhesions, the formation of the fibrin clot is, however, a secondary phenomenon, occurring when there is already a series of micro-injuries to the peritoneal membrane. The mesothelial cells per se, but also other cells abundant in the peritoneum, have the function of secreting many potent substances, which under certain circumstances can be noxious to the peritoneal membranes. Among these are various cytokines, leukotrienes, prostaglandins, lytic enzymes, lymphokinases, and oxidative free radicals.

As occurs at the mucosal membranes of the intestines, these substances are often released in response to physical, chemical, or microbial challenges. These changes are more pronounced in smokers, who are known to have permanent abnormal changes of the peritoneal membranes, including blebs and micro-villus-like structures of the mesothelial cell surface and, sometimes, perforated luminal membranes [25]. One can speculate that even individuals with low levels of antioxidants, such as the water-soluble molecule glutathione – the master antioxidant of the human body – and the "big three antioxidants" vitamin E, vitamin C and β-carotene, are more vulnerable to microinjuries of the peritoneal membranes and, as a consequence, adhesion formation. It is known, for example, that the lens of the eye, which is exposed to large amounts of light, needs 15–20 times more of these antioxidants to prevent oxidative injuries from occurring than the cells in the rest of the body. Similarly, the peritoneal cells exposed to the light of surgical lamps will also need a greater supply of antioxidants.

Influence of the Gut

It is well known today that translocation of bacteria and toxins to the peritoneum occurs early after trauma and that this plays an important role in determining outcome. Translocation occurs early – already during and immediately after surgery – especially in the intestinally starved patient. In a series of reviews, this important subject has been recently surveyed [4–8]. Trans-location of endotoxin, a key toxin, occurs almost immediately after major trauma and is likely to play an important role in the early stages of pathogenesis of peritonitis and also of peritoneal adhesions. Several substances active at the mucosal level reduce the risk of translocation and eventually also the degree of postoperative adhesion formation. These substances include surfactants made up of various glycolipids present as a thin fatty layer at the surface of the gastrointestinal mucosa. We found, in a series of studies, that pretreatment of the mucosa with a series of phospholipids and glycolipids not only prevented or reduced the extent of experimental peptic ulcer [11] and experimental ulcerative colitis [12]; it also prevented translocation from occurring [33]. As is shown in Table 1, pretreatment with phosphatidylcholine and phosphatidylinositol totally or almost totally prevented intestinal translocation from occurring 4 h after experimental subtotal liver resection. As is shown in Table 2, supply of natural surfactants together with fiber (β-glucans) and live lactobacilli prevented bacteremia [33]. Further studies in animals subjected to experimental peritonitis (Table 3) showed a pronounced reduction in bacteremia – at least to the same degree as after treatment with broad-spectrum antibiotics – but, and probably equally as important, a total prevention of the occurrence of endotoxin in the blood [24]. Although it has not been studied, it is likely that endotoxin is also prevented from occurring in the peritoneum. This could no doubt be of importance in preventing the subsequent development of adhesions.

Table 1. Translocation 4 h after 90% liver resection in rats and the influence of supplying phosphatidylcholine and phosphatidylinositol

	MLN	SC	PV
Sham	0/6	0/6	0/6
90% liver resection	10/10	10/10	2/10
90% liver resection + PC	1/6	1/6	0/6
90% liver resection + PJ	0/6	0/6	0/6

MNL, mesenteric lymph nodes; SC, central circulation; PV, portal veins; PC, phosphatidylcholine; PI, phosphatidylinositol.
After [33].

Table 2. Influence on translocation by oats (rich in natural surfactants and fiber, β-glucans) in combination with live lactobacilli (fermented) after 90% liver resection

	MNL	Liver
Sham operation + saline	0	0
90% liver resection + saline	10/10	5/6
90% liver resection + fermented oats	1/6	0
90% liver resection + unfermented oats	4/6	2/6

MNL, mesenteric lymph nodes.
After [33].

Table 3. Influence of supply of lactobacilli to rats after cecal ligation and puncture: comparison to untreated and broad spectrum antibiotic-treated animals

	Bacteremia	Leukocytes	Endotoxin
Untreated	22/36	2.3 ± 1.4	11.1 ± 5
Broad spectrum antibiotics	8/20	4.1 ± 2.3	1.5 ± 1.3
Lactobacilli	11/24	4.8 ± 1.8	0.0 ± 0

After [24].

It is well known that very early in the course of peritoneal sepsis, gut intramucosal pH decreases [26] and most likely, although this has not been studied, the pH at the peritoneal membranes, especially at the visceral peritoneum. It is further known that reduced gut intramucosal pH may lead to increased intestinal permeability [13, 18]. This relative ischemia is followed by release of toxic mediators and translocation of bacteria and endotoxins. Macrophages are important in producing – but also in preventing – adhesion formation. They seem to already be exhausted when there is a need for dissolutions of fibrin clots. My previous coworker Ar'Rajab, recently published [2] a study, in which macrophages were shown to play a key role in postsurgical peritoneal healing and adhesion formation. Battafarano et al. have recently described a dramatic increase in plasma tumor necrosis factor (TNF) after bacterial challenge [3]. This increase, as well as an increase in other important cytokines, is likely to also occur in the peritoneum.

Peritoneum and Peritoneal Surfactants

Like the peritoneum, the gastrointestinal mucosa is covered by a thin layer of surfacants, most often not more than 20–24 molecules thick, and organized in bilayers according to the hydrophilicity or hydrophobicity. The most frequent glycolipids in this membrane are phosphatidylcholine, phosphatidylethanolamine, phosphatidylinositol, and sphingolipids. Gangliosides are present in the outer layer in small quantities and regulate the fluidity and transport of substances through the membranes. These gangliosides also modulate activities of enzymes such as protein kinases. The surfactant layer is easily destroyed in connection with trauma, ischemia, and infection. It serves as a substrate for production of leukotrienes and prostaglandins, as arachidonic acids are released from these lipids. In patients with salpingitis, it has been observed that the concentration of leukotrienes and prostaglandins increase with the severity of infection [19]. As is known from earlier work, postoperative infertility rates correlate to the estimated severity of salpingitis. Thus, one might conclude that the activity of leukotrienes and prostaglandins in peritoneal fluids at the time of infection grossly reflects the risk of future adhesion formation. In local ischemia, and most importantly in infections, phospholipases eg., phospholipase A_2, are produced at the peritoneal surfaces. These enzymes have the ability to dissolve/destroy the surfacants. Uhl et al. have recently shown highly increased phospholipase A_2 activity in peritonitis, but not in severe trauma [31]. Such an increase is also likely to have an effect on the degree of adhesion formation. This is what led us early on to try using phospholipase inhibitors, substances which are often the same as calcium channel blockers. When these agents were tried in experimental models, we could reduce or prevent peritoneal adhesions from being formed. Similar studies have also been performed by Steinleitner et al. [30], who found a strong protective effect of verapamil, a calcium channel blocker, but also a phospholipase inhibitor. The treatment was found to be equally effective if the drug was administered subcutaneously or intraperitoneally. I personally am convinced that protection of the surfactants is the most important effect of this treatment.

Furthermore, in a series of studies with experimental adhesion models in rats, we could, by external supply of various glycolipids, reduce and prevent adhesion formation [1, 28, 29]. Important studies by Dr Treutner and Professor Schumpelick at the Chirurgische Klinik at the RWTH in Aachen have demonstrated the prevention of adhesions by external supply of glycolipids. These lipids constitute a positive development in the future prevention of adhesions. However, many studies remain to be done before the ideal lipid or combination of lipids is identified. I personally believe that this combination will probably include one or two key gangliosides as important ingredients.

Sepsis and Adhesion Formation

It is rather astonishing that little attention has been given to the role of infection in the genesis of adhesions. In report from 1992 [23], however, a mixture of intestinal bacteria was injected intraperitoneally in experimental animals. Laparotomy was performed 90 min later. Three groups were compared:

1. Controls: peritoneum sutured
2. Infected: peritoneum sutured, 4/0 monofilament nylon
3. Infected: peritoneum left unsutured

Of ten control animals, three developed adhesions and all to the sutured wound. The incidence of adhesions was higher in the infected groups, as eight out of nine and eight out of ten, respectively, developed adhesions. There were, however, significantly less incidences of adhesion to the wound in the non-sutured group, (two out of ten compared to eight out of ten), indicating even stronger adhesion formation when sepsis is combined with local ischemia, induced by suturing.

One could speculate that certain microbes are more deleterious to the peritoneal surfaces than others, as they are likely to produce enzymes more or less noxious to the membrane surfaces. Unfortunately, no such studies have been performed. Schoeffel et al. have, in a recent clinical study, described the correlation between the microbiology of the peritoneal exudate and the outcome of peritonitis [27]. This study gives the impression that the outcome, measured in mortality, is similar, irrespective of the inducing pathogen. It would be of great interest to determine if the degree of adhesions could be quantified months or years after recovery in such material.

Even if surfactants play the most important role in preventing early injuries to the peritoneal membrane, a well functioning subsequent fibrinolysis of formed clots is critical to avoid adhesions. Although the reasons for the poor fibrinolysis are not fully understood, it is clear, however, that peritoneal fibrinolysis is inhibited irrespective of the cause of injury – bacterial, chemical or ischemic [32].

Nutrition, Peritonitis and Adhesion Formation

It is increasingly clear that some nutrients play a key role in preventing infections, and eventually in preventing adhesion formation. Such a nutrient is arginine, which is known to regulate several important functions, including increased intestinal blood flow, and up-regulation of the local immune system [21]. It has recently been described [10] that ingested nitrate/nitrite, via production of NO in the stomach, stimulates visceral blood flow, mucus formation, bacteriostasis, and motility. Furthermore, it has been suggested [34] that, at least in septic shock, NO released by inducible enzymes has destructive effects, while NO released by constitutive enzymes is protective. There are indications that the effects are similar at the level of the colonic mucosa. It has been known for almost 10 years that arginine plays a key role in macrophage- and lymphocyte-mediated toxicity [20]. Furthermore, animals receiving arginine have a significantly increased ability to kill translocated organisms [15, 17] and an oral supply of arginine 3 days before induction of peritonitis increases animal survival [15, 22]. Gianotti et al. [16] compared diets with arginine, glycine, normal chow and AIN 76A. Arginine could totally or almost totally prevent translocation to the mesenteric lymph nodes, liver, and spleen. One can speculate that arginine also might have a preventive effect on adhesion formation. The importance of arginine is further supported by the finding that L-NAME, and NO synthetase inhibitor, increases mortality after intraperitoneal bacterial challenge [14].

Conclusion

For the postoperative outcome, it is essential that patients are fed enterally early on, preferably immediately. It is also essential to maintain low gastric pH by avoiding H_2-blockers and to early feed enterally. Furthermore, supply of NO-donating substances as well as surfactants and antioxidants seems essential. Such treatments will drastically reduce the incidence of postoperative and posttrauma sepsis, eliminate the need for stress ulcer prophylaxis, and very important, – shorten the hospital stay. It is likely, but unproven, that by these means the incidence of late complications, such as those induced by peritoneal adhesions, can be reduced.

References

1. Ar'Rajab A, Ahrén B, Rozga J, Bengmark S (1991) Phosphatidylcholine prevents postoperative peritoneal adhesions: An experimental study in the rat. J Surg Res 50: 212–215
2. Ar'Rajab A, Snoj A, Larsson K, Bengmark S (1995) Exogenous phospholipid reduces postoperative peritoneal adhesions in the rat. Eur J Surg 161: 341–344
3. Battafarano RJ, Dunn DL (1994) Contribution of local cytokine production to the systemic host septic response. Crit Care Med 22(1): 7–8
4. Bengmark S (1995) Econutrition and health maintenance: a new concept to prevent GI inflammation, ulceration and sepsis. An invited review. J Clin Nutr 15: 1–10
5. Bengmark S, Gianotti L (1995) Immunonutrition – a new aspect in the treatment of critically ill patients. In: Gullo A(ed) Intensive care, Apiche 1995. Springer, Berlin Heidelberg New York, pp 73–89
6. Bengmark S, Jeppsson B (1995) Gastrointestinal surface protection and mucosa reconditioning. J Parenter Enteral Nutr JPEN 19: 410–415
7. Bengmark S, Larsson K, Molin G (1995) Gut mucosa reconditioning with species-specific lactobacilli, surfacants, pseudomucus, and fibres – an invited review. Biotechnol Ther 5: 171–194
8. Bengmark S, Gianotti L (1996) Nutritional support to prevent and treat MOF. (1996) World J Surg 20: 474–481
9. Christen D, Buchmann P (1991) Peritoneal adhesions after laparotomy: prophylactic measures. Hepatogastroenterology 38(4): 283–286
10. Duncan C, Dougall H, Johnston P, Green S, Brogan R, Liefert C, Smith L, Golden M, Benjamin N (1995) Chemical generation of nitric oxide in the mouth from the enterosalivary circulation of dietary nitrate. Nature Med 1(6): 546–551
11. Dunjic BS, Axelson J, Ar'Rajab A, Larsson K, Bengmark S (1993) Gastroprotective capability of exogenous phosphatidylcholine in experimentally induced chronic ulcers in rats. Scand J Gastroenterol 18: 89–94
12. Fabia R, Ar'Rajab A, Willén R, Andersson R, Ahrén B, Larsson K, Bengmark S (1992) Effects of phosphatidylcholine and phosphatidylinositol on acetic-acid-induced colitis in the rat. Digestion 53: 35–44
13. Fink M, Antonsson J, Wang H, Rothschild H (1991) Increased intestinal permeability in endotoxic pigs. Mesenteric hypoperfusion as an etiologic factor. Arch Surg 126: 211–218
14. Fukatsu K, Saito H, Fukushima R, Inoue T, Lin Mt, Inaba T, Muto T (1995) Detrimental effects of a nitric oxide synthase inhibtor (N-omega-nitro-L-arginine methyl-ester) in a murine sepsis model. Arch Surg 130: 410–414
15. Gianotti L, Alexander JW, Fuskushima R, Pyles T (1993) Reduction of bacterial translocation with oral fibroblast growth factor and sucralfate. Am J Surg 165: 195–201
16. Gianotti L, Alexander JW, Pyles T, Fukushima R (1993) Arginine-supplemented diets improve survival in gut-derived sepsis and peritonitis by modulating bacterial clearance. Ann Surg 217(6): 644–654

17. Gianotti L, Munda R, Alexander JW, Tchervenkov JI, Babcock G (1993) Bacterial translocation: a potential source for infection in acute pancreatitis. Pancreas 8(5): 551–558
18. Haglund U, Bulkley G, Granger N (1987) On the pathophysiology of intestinal ischemic injury. Clinical Review. Acta Chir Scand 153: 321–324
19. Heinonen PK, Aine R, Seppälä E (1990) Peritoneal fluid leukotriene B_4 and prostaglandin E_2 in acute salpingitis. Gynecol Obstet Invest 29(4): 292–295
20. Hibbs JB, Vavrin Z, Taintor RR (1987) L-Arginine is required for expression of the activated macrophage effector mechanism causing selective metabolic inhibition in target cells. J Immunol 138: 550–565
21. Lieberman MD, Nishioka K, Redmond P, Daly JM (1992) Enhancement of interleukin-2 immunotherapy with L-Arginine. Ann Surg 215(2): 157–165
22. Madden HP, Breslin RJ, Wasserkrug HL, Efron G, Barbul A (1988) Stimulation of T Cell immunity by arginine enhances survival in peritonitis. J Surg Res 44: 658–663
23. O'Leary DP, Coakley JB (1992) The influence of suturing and sepsis on the development of postoperative peritoneal adhesions. Ann R Coll Surg Engl 74(2): 134–137
24. Nobaek S, Jeppsson B, Johansson ML, Marklinder I, Kasravi FB, Molin G, Bengmark S. Enteral Administration of Lactobacillus reuteri R2LC and oat fiber reduces the incidence of bacteremia in rats with experimental intraabdominal infection (submitted)
25. Pittilo RM, Nicholson LJ, Clarke NKF, Blow CM, Woolf N (1984) Cigarette smoke-induced injury of peritoneal mesothelial cells. Br J Exp Patho of 65: 365–370
26. Rasmussen I, Haglund U (1992) Early gut ischemia in experimental fecal peritonitis. Circ Shock 38(1): 22–28
27. Schoeffel U, Jacobs E, Ruf G, Mierswa F, von Specht BU, Farthmann EH (1995) Intraperitoneal micro-organism and the severity of peritonitis. Eur J Surg 161: 501–508
28. Snoj M, Ar'Rajab A, Ahrén B, Bengmark S (1992) Effect of phosphatidylcholine on postoperative adhesions after small bowel anastomosis in the rat. Br J Surg 79(5): 427–429
29. Snoj A, Ar'Rajab A, Ahrén B, Bengmark S (1993) Phospholipase-resistant phosphatidylcholine reduces intra-abdominal adhesions induced by bacterial peritonitis. Res Exp Med Berl 193: 177–122
30. Steinleitner A, Lambert H, Kazensky C, Sanchez I, Sueldo C (1990) Reduction of primary postoperative adhesion formation under calcium channel blockade in the rabbit. J Surg Res 48(1): 42–45
31. Uhl W, Beger HG, Hoffmann G, Hanisch E, Schild A, Waydhas C, Entholzner E, Müller K, Kellermann W, Vogeser M, Leskopf W, Zügel M, Busch EW, Büchler MW (1995) A multicenter study of phospholipase A_2 in patients in intensive care units. J Am Coll Surg 180(3): 323–331
32. Vipond MN, Whawell SA, Thompson JN, Dudley HA (1994) Effect of experimental peritonitis and ischaemia on peritoneal fibrinolytic activity. Eur J Surg 160(9): 471–477
33. Wang X-D, Soltesz V, Molin G, Andersson R (1995) The role of oral administration of oatmeal fermented by Lactobaccillus reuteri R2LC on bacterial translocation after acute liver failure induced by subtotal liver resection in the rat. Scand J Gastroenterol 30: 180–185
34. Wright CE, Rees DD, Moncada S (1992) Protective and pathological roles of nitric oxide in endotoxin shock. Cardiovasc Res 26: 48–57

6.3 Stage-Related Surgical Therapy of General Peritonitis

G.J. Winkeltau, P. Bertram, K.-H. Treutner,
and V. Schumpelick

Introduction

It was Martin Kirschner, from Heidelberg, who in 1926 was the first to describe the basic principles of surgical therapy of general peritonitis. Based on his prerequisites of: elimination of the infectious source, removal of toxic and infectious material from the peritoneal cavity, and prevention of systemic effects, the major elements in the so-called standard procedure became established: surgical removal of the infectious focus, intraoperative lavage, and drainage of the abdominal cavity [13]. This surgical procedure remains the gold standard for treating general peritonitis. Even the invention of antibiotic therapy has not altered this regimen, since antimicrobial agents have not been able to reduce the mortality rates significantly [7, 28]. Nonetheless, looking at the results, it was obvious that especially advanced stages of general peritonitis showed still unacceptably high mortality rates [7]. This initiated a search for more radical surgical procedures.

The first idea was to prolong the advantages of the intraoperative lavage during the early postoperative course [15, 17, 23]. The so-called continuous postoperative lavage (CPL) made it possible to wash out the toxic and infectious materials from the abdominal cavity for 72 h after the operation. Review of the experimental and clinical results found this therapy to be effective whenever the infectious source could thereby be eliminated.

For more advanced stages of general peritonitis in which complete elimination of the infectious source was not possible after 72 h, there seemed to be a need for more than one surgical intervention to bring the focus under control. For these cases, open abdomen management in combination with multiple re-explorations and intraoperative lavages was described in the early 1980s [21, 26, 30, 31].

However, the more aggressive the techniques became, the more complications appeared, and treating the still favorable stages of general peritonitis with highly aggressive surgical techniques exposed the patients to an unnecessary risk of a higher morbidity.

The solution to this problem is, in our opinion, a stage-related therapy of general peritonitis: Mild stages are excellently treated by the standard procedure, moderate forms can be handled by CPL, and advanced stages need multiple re-explorations and lavages. Therefore, we began a prospective protocol to review the effectiveness of stage-related treatment of general peritonitis.

Patients and Methods

Patients

From January 1992 to December 1994, 103 consecutive patients with the diagnosis of general peritonitis were treated in the surgical clinic of the RWTH Aachen. There were 34 female patients and 69 male patients. Their ages at the time of surgery ranged from 3 to 84 years (mean: 59 years).

Treatment Modalities

The prospective protocol included only patients with secondary general peritonitis (e.g., intestinal perforation, ascending peritonitis, postoperative peritonitis). Patients with localized peritonitis, intra-abdominal abscesses, or pancreatitis restricted to the bursa omentalis and the retroperitoneum were excluded.

All patients underwent median laparotomy. After the diagnosis was confirmed, further management corresponded to the protocol (Tables 1, 2).

After taking a swab for microbiological evaluations, antibiotic treatment was started. The abdominal cavity was cleaned and revised, and the infectious source was eliminated surgically. Afterwards an intraoperative lavage with 9–12 liters of Ringer's solution was performed and the intestinal tract decompressed by placement of a Dennis tube.

The severity of the peritonitis was scored intraoperatively by the Mannheim peritonitis index (MPI) (Tables [1, 3]). Using the MPI, three stages of the

Table 1. Prospective protocol of stage-related therapy of general peritonitis[a]

1. Median laparotomy
2. Swabs/cleaning
3. Complete revision of the abdominal cavity
4. Elimination of the focus
5. Intraoperative lavage (9–12 liters Ringer's solution)
6. Drainage
7. Classification of the stage according (Mannheim peritonitis index, MPI)[b]
8. Therapeutic regimen based on MPI stage
   Stage I (0–20 MPI points): four quadrant drainage; primary closure of the abdominal wall
   Stage II (21–29 MPI points): two inflow and two outflow catheters; postoperative lavage with 24–48 liters/24 h per 72 h
   Stage III (>29 MPI points): temporary closure with a mesh (e.g., Vicryl); open abdomen management and multiple re-explorations; secondary closure

[a]Chirurgische Klinik Aachen: January 1, 1992–June 30, 1994.
[b]See Table 2.

Table 2. Mannheim peritonitis index (MPI) and classification of disease stage

	Points[a]	Yes	No
Age > 50	5	( )	( )
Female	5	( )	( )
Organ failure	7	( )	( )
Neoplasm	4	( )	( )
Preoperative duration >24h	4	( )	( )
Focus other than large bowel	4	( )	( )
Diffuse spread	6	( )	( )
Exudation			
Clear	0	( )	( )
Suppurating	6	( )	( )
Fecal	12	( )	( )

Index = number of "Yes" answers.
[a]Maximum of 47 points.

underlying peritonitis were distinguished [8, 16, 29] (Table 4). Each stage was treated with a different therapeutic regimen.

There were 45 patients with stage I peritonitis (MPI score: 0–20) who were treated with the standard procedure, 34 stage II patients (MPI score: 21–29) were treated with CPL and 24 stage III patients (MPI score: >29) with the so-called Etappenlavage (multiple re-explorations and open abdomen management).

The standard procedure in stage I patients was finished after placement of a drain serving all four quadrants of the abdominal cavity and primary closure of the abdominal wall.

CPL was performed using the method described by McKenna [17]. Two inflow and two outflow catheters were placed and postoperative lavage with 24–48 liters of Ringer's solution per day was started immediately. The mean duration of the lavage was 48 h (range: 24–216).

Stage III patients were treated by open abdomen management, as described by Teichmann and Wouters [26, 31]. Whenever possible an absorbable Vicryl mesh was used for temporary closure of the laparostomy. Daily re-explorations (mean = 7; range: 5–12) and intraoperative lavage were performed until the infectious source was brought under control. The abdominal wall was closed secondarily (*n*=11) or left open (*n*=13).

Table 3. Prospective classification of treatment modalities according to the Mannheim peritonitis index (MPI)

Stage	MPI points	Therapy
I	< 20	Standard procedure
II	21–29	Continuous postoperative lavage (CPL)
III	> 29	*Etappenlavage*[a]

[a]Multiple re-explorations and open abdomen management.

Table 4. Classification of the stage according to
expected mortality rates

Peritonitis index[a]	Expected mortality (%)
0–20	0–6
21–29	20–30
> 29	75–100

[a]Based on the Mannheim peritonitis index.

Postoperative Course

The postoperative course on the ICU was evaluated by means of the APACHE
II score [14]. Statistical evaluation of the effectiveness of stage-related therapy
was performed by the MPI and the APACHE II scores. The statistically expected mortality was compared with the actual mortality in the treatment
groups.

Results

Mortality

The overall mortality was 16% (16/103) (Table 5). One 84-year-old patient died
due to myocardial infarction on the eighth postoperative day, which led to a
mortality of 2% (1/45) in stage I peritonitis. Mortality rates were 21% (7/34) in
stage II and 33% (8/24) in stage III patients.

The main causes of death were multiple organ failure (MOF) during the
course of the systemic inflammatory response syndrome (SIRS) (10 patients,
63%), and pneumonia by MRSA (3 patients, 19%). Other causes of death were
myocardial infarction (1), pulmonary embolism (1), and liver failure due to
alcoholic cirrhosis.

The statistically expected mortality rates were 37% according to the MPI and
32% according to the APACHE II score (Table 6). Therefore the actual mortality of 16% was more than 50% lower than statistically expected.

Table 5. Stage-related mortality rates (Chirurgische Klinik; January 1992–December 1994)

Stage	Treatment	Patients (*n*)	Mortality (*n*)	Mortality (%)
I	Standard procedure	45	1	2
II	Continuous postoperative lavage	34	7	21
III	Etappenlavage	24	8	33
Total		103	16	16

Table 6. Mortality rates according to the APACHE II score: comparison of statistically expected and actual mortality rates

APACHE II	Patients	Mortality (statistical)	Mortality (statistical)	Mortality (actual)	Mortality (actual)
< 10	10	–	–	–	–
11–15	10	1	13%	1	10%
16–20	34	6	18%	2	6%
21–25	25	9	36%	5	20%
> 25	24	17	71%	8	33%
Total	103	33	32%	16	16%

Morbidity

Some 69 common complications had to be treated in 45 of 103 patients (44%); these were mainly caused by hospital infections (pneumonia, urinary tract infections) or complications of the underlying SIRS (respiratory insufficiency, renal failure). The types and frequencies of these complications are displayed in Table 7.

The morbidity rates in the subgroups were 22% (10/45) in stage I, 47% (16/34) in stage II, and 79% (19/24) in stage III patients.

Complications related to the surgical technique were documented separately.

Complications of the postoperative lavage appeared in 17 of 34 stage II patients treated by CPL (50%). In 14 patients, significant fluid retention forced us to stop the lavage; in three patients (9%) there was a massive loss of potassium which had to be substituted.

Table 7. Morbidity (common postoperative complications)

Complication	n
Pneumonia	13
Pleural effusion	11
Atelectasis	4
Pulmonary edema	2
ARDS	2
Acute renal failure	9
Urinary tract infection	10
Liver failure	1
Pancreatitis	2
Phlebothrombosis	3
Embolism	1
Myocardial infarction	1
Cerebral infarction	1
Exogenous psychosis	5
Others	4

Complications of the implanted mesh occurred in nine of 24 stage III patients (38%). Minor tears were seen in six patients fistulas, in exposed small bowel loops appeared in three.

The abdominal drains caused relevant complications in four patients. Three showed a marked infection of the abdominal wall, one an intra-abdominal bleeding caused by an erosion of the drain.

Discussion

Due to the different outcomes associated with each stage (MPI) of general peritonitis, we recommend a stage-related therapeutic approach. Stage I is excellently treated by the standard procedure, stage II can be handled by CPL and stage III needs multiple re-explorations and lavages.

The criterion for defining the different stages of general peritonitis in our prospective study was the Mannheim peritonitis index. This scoring system is easy to handle and all needed information is available to the surgeon during the first operation. Therefore, the MPI can be used for a prospective protocol. The APACHE-II score is more differentiated, but the numerous data cannot be made available on the spot during an emergency operation. The score has been validated and was of high significance in predicting the outcome of a patient with general peritonitis treated at the ICU.

From January 1992 to December 1994 103 consecutive patients with general peritonitis were treated under the described prospective protocol. The 45 patients with stage I peritonitis were treated by the standard procedure, resulting in a mortality of 2% (1/45). Restricted application of this technique to patients with MPI <21 improves the effectiveness of this procedure in preventing therapy-related complications. It is assumed that the standard procedure is the appropriate regimen for 40%–60% of all patients admitted to hospital [29]. Medium and severe cases of general peritonitis have to be treated with more aggressive techniques.

CPL was shown to have a significant effect on mortality in animal experiments [3, 4, 9, 23, 24]. The analysis documented a highly effective elimination of contaminating substances such as blood, bacteria, endotoxins and inflammatory mediators in the abdominal cavity. Initial objections to the procedure have been rejected by international publications [19, 23, 25]. Prospective randomized studies showed mortality rates between 0% and 30%, but a review of these studies showed marked disadvantages (small patient groups, no classification of the severity of the underlying peritonitis, no score-related statistical evaluation) which revitalized the results. In nonrandomized studies from 1970 to 1983, the mortality rates varied between 0.6% and 43% [7, 15, 20]. The comparison of treatment groups with historical groups and the absence of exact statistical evaluations made those publications even more questionable.

In our patients with MPI scores between 21 and 29 who were treated with CPL, the mortality was 21%. The results documented that this procedure can be used to successfully treat peritonitis in medium stages in a high percentage of patients. However, the high rate of method-related complications e.g., fluid retention (14 patients; 41%) and massive loss of potassium (3 patients; 9%) are relevant side effects. Whether the results can be optimized by changing the treatment modalities needs to be considered.

The concept to open abdomen management and multiple re-explorations (Etappenlavage) fulfills the demand for a new, more aggressive therapy: scheduled relaparotomies make daily inspections of the abdominal cavity possible and lead to a reduction of abscess formations. Another major advantage of this method is the daily control of intestinal anastomoses. A review of the literature shows that, according to the severity of the underlying peritonitis, two to 13 re-explorations are necessary to get the infectious source under control [31], and average mortality rates differ between 19% and 62% [1, 2, 5, 22, 26, 27, 30].

In our group of patients the mortality rate was 33%. The limited use of Etappenlavage to patients with advanced cases of general peritonitis (MPI > 29) prevents the onset of method-related complications in patients with more favorable stages. Due to tears and pull-outs of the implanted mesh six patients (25%) had to be treated. In an additional three patients (13%), a fistula of the small bowel had to be operated on.

There is still a lack of criteria to determine whether an infection is definitely under control. Neither endotoxin nor inflammatory mediators like interleukin-6 have proven to be significant parameters. The surgeon's eye and experience are still necessary in the decision to end open abdomen management.

Despite these uncertainties a stage-related therapeutic approach is able to reduce the mortality rates in general peritonitis. In our group the overall mortality was 16% significantly better than statistically expected (37% according to the MPI and 32% according to the APACHE II score). A further reduction of the mortality rates can only be expected by progress in treatment of SIRS.

Stage-related therapy of general peritonitis seems to be able to reduce the overall mortality. Neither the exclusive use of the standard procedure nor the routine use of more aggressive therapies are able to reduce mortality and morbidity rates alone, and an individually based, stage-related approach should prove to be a welcome development.

References

1. Andrus C, Doering M, Herrmann VM, Kaminski D (1986) Planned reoperation for generalized intraabdominal infection. Am J Surg 152: 682–686
2. Arbogast R (1983) Erfahrungen der Würzburger Klinik mit der programmierten Lavage bei Peritonitis. In: Kern E (Hrsg) Die chirurgische Behandlung der Peritonitis. Springer, Berlin Heidelberg New York, pp 91–101
3. Artz CP, Barnett WO, Grogan JB (1962) Further studies concerning the pathogenesis and treatement of peritonitis. Ann Surg 155: 756–760
4. Cardis DT, Matheson NA (1968) Peritoneal lavage in peritonitis. Br Med J II: 219–224
5. Cuesta MA, Doblas M, Castaneda L, Bengoechea E (1991) Sequential abdominal re-exploration with zipper technique. World J Surg 15: 74–80
6. Dellinger EP, Wertz MJ, Meakins JL, Solomkin JS, Allo MD, Howard RJ, Simons RL (1985) Surgical infection stratification system for intraabdominal infection. Arch Surg 120: 21–29

7. Farthmann EH, Schöffel U (1990) Principles and limitations of operative management of intraabdominal infections. World J Surg 14: 210–217
8. Függer R, Rogy M, Herbst F, Schemper M, Schulz F (1988) Validisierungsstudie zum Mannheimer Peritonitis-Index. Chirurg 59: 598–601
9. Glover JL, Atkins P, Lempke RE (1969) Evaluation of peritoneal lavage therapy for peritonitis. J Surg Res 9: 531–535
10. Grund KE (1981) Chirurgische Probleme der Peritonitis. In: Behandlung der Peritonitis. In: Kempf P (Hrsg) W Zuckerschwerdt, München, S67–86
11. Herfarth CH, Heil TH (1980) Therapeutische Richtlinien bei postoperativer Peritonitis und Reintervention (Antibiotika, Drainage, Spülung). Langenbecks Arch Chir 352: 301–306
12. Kern E, Klaue P, Arbogast R (1983) Programmierte Peritoneal-Lavage bei diffuser Peritonitis. Chirurg 54: 306–310
13. Kirschener M (1926) Die Behandlung der akuten freien Bauchfellentzündung. Langenbecks Arch Klin Chir 142: 253–311
14. Knaus WH, Zimmermann JA, Wagner DP, Draper EA, Lawerence DE (1981) APACHE – acute physiology and chronic health evaluation: A physiologically based classification system. Crit Care Med 9: 591–597
15. Leibhoff AR, Soroff HS (1987) The treatment of generalized peritonitis by closed postoperative peritoneal lavage – a critical review of the literature. Arch Surg 122: 1005–1011
16. Linder MM, Wacha H, Wesch G, Striefendsand RA, Gundlach E (1987) Der Mannheimer Peritonitis-Index. Ein Instrument zur intraoperativen Prognose der Peritonitis. Chirurg 58: 84–92
17. McKenna JP, Currie DJ, MacDonald JA, Mahoney LJ, Finlayson DC, Lanskail JC (1970) The use of continuous postoperative therapy of late peritoneal sepsis. Surg Gynecol Obstet 130: 254–258
18. Meakins JL, Solomkin JS, Allo MD, Dellinger P, Howard RJ, Simmons RL (1984) A proposed classification for intra-abdominal infections. Arch Surg 119: 1372–1378
19. Neugebauer R, Wolter D, Claes L, Bültmann B (1979) Die Bauchdeckenersatzplastik durch ein unbeschichtetes Kohlenstoffasergewebe. Eine tierexperimentelle Untersuchung am Kaninchen. Langenbecks Arch Chir 350: 83–93
20. Oguz M, Bektemir M, Dülger M, Yalin R (1988) Treatment of experimental peritonitis with intraperitoneal povidone-iodine-solution. Can J Surg 31: 169–176
21. Pichlmayr R, Lehr J, Pahlow J, Guthy E (1983) Postoperative kontinuierliche offenen dorso-ventrale Bauchspülung bei schweren Formen der Peritonitis. Chirurg 54: 299–305
22. Schein M, Saadia R, Jamieson JR, Decker GAG (1986) The "sandwich technique" in the management of the open abdomen. Br J Surg 73: 369–370
23. Schumer W, Lee DK, Jones B (1964) Peritoneal lavage in postoperative therapy of late peritoneal sepsis. Surgery 55: 841–846
24. Sleeman HK, Diggs BW, Hayes DK, Hamit HF (1969) Value of antibiotics, corticosteroids, and peritoneal lavage in the treatment of experimental peritonitis. Surgery 66: 1060–1066
25. Stephen M, Loewenthal K (1978) Generalized infective peritonitis. Surg Gynecol Obstet 147: 231–235
26. Teichmann W, Wittmann DH, Andreone PA (1986) Scheduled reoperations (etappenlavage) for diffuse peritonitis. Arch Surg 121: 147–152
27. Walsh GL, Chiasson P, Hedderich G, Wexler MJ, Meakins JL (1988) The open abdomen. The marlex mesh and zipper technique: a method of managing intraperitoneal infection. Surg Clin North Am 68: 25–40
28. Winkeltau GJ, Winkeltau GU, Klosterhalfen B, Niemann H, Treutner KH, Schumpelick V (1992) Differenzierte chirurgische Therapie der diffusen Peritonitis. Chirurg 63: 1035–1040
29. Wittmann DH (1986) Intraabdominelle Infektionen. Analysieren und gezielt behandeln. Hoechst Monographie "Aktuelles Wissen Hoechst". Reihe Antibiotika
30. Wittmann DH, Aprahamian C, Bergstein JM (1990) Etappenlavage: Advanced diffuse peritonitis managed by planned multiple Laparotomies utilizing zippers, slide fastener, and Velcro Analogue for temporary abdominal closure. World J Surg 14: 218–226
31. Wouters DB, Krom RAF, Sloof MJH, Kootstra G, Kuijjer PJ (1983) The use of marlex mesh in patients with generalized peritonitis and multiple organ system failure. Surg Gynecol Obstet 156: 609–614

7 Peritoneal Drainage and Chemotherapy

7.1 Effects and Side Effects of Abdominal Drainage

V. Zumtobel, R. Ernst, and M. Senkal

After about 30 experiments in animals Yates [7] concluded that most of the serous exudate of an abdominal drain is caused by its own foreign-body reaction, that there is draining inward as well as outward, and that abdominal drains usually will seal off within 24 h. In 1905 he wrote: "There is probably no detail in modern surgical pathology that deserves more thorough comprehension, but which is less definitely understood by the average teacher, practitioner, and student than the nature of the reaction of the peritoneum to drainage". Meanwhile modern and well-tolerated materials should reduce the foreign-body effect and allow better drainage function.

In two prospective randomised clinical trials we tested the efficiency of silicone tube drains in patients undergoing cholecystectomy. Despite ultrasonographically controlled good position of the drains, fluid retention was found in 41% and 32% of cases. There was no difference in fluid retention between the groups of patients with drainage and those without drainage. The retained fluid was resorbed in the following days without any complications [5, 6]. In another clinical trial, Hagmüller et al. [3] found similar results in patients undergoing resection of the colon, with a higher incidence of complications in the group of patients with drainage.

Material and Methods

We felt it might be instructive to observe the effects of several types of drains commonly used to drain fluid appearing in the abdomen subsequent to surgery of the colon. Three drains were tested: Penrose drains, single-lumen silicone tubes, and single-lumen rubber tubes, all with one or two side holes. Under intravenous anaesthesia, two small segments of the transverse colon at least 15 cm apart were resected in mongrel rabbits and two anastomoses were performed using standardized one-layer suture lines. One of the two anastomoses was drained; the other remained nondrained. Another drain of the same type was placed into the lower abdomen. To prevent dislocation the drains were fixed at the intraperitoneal tip and at the peritoneum near the separate insertion stab incision by suture.

To prevent exogenous infection the extraperitoneal tips of the drains were placed in a closed subcutaneous pocket. Thus each animal served as its own control concerning the healing of an anastomosis with or without local drain-

Table 1. Adhesions in the lower abdomen caused by different types
of drains (% of surface of drain)

Drain	Circular adhesions	Total adhesions
Penrose ($n=10$)	8	21
Silicone tube ($n=10$)	1	5
Rubber tube ($n=10$)	2	2

age and also concerning the effects of drains placed at an anastomosis or free
in the lower abdominal space. The animals were not given perioperative antibiotics and were reoperated 7 days after surgery.

Results

Drainage of the lower abdomen was well tolerated. Penrose drains showed few
adhesions at the suture fixation and at the uncovered parts of gauze. Silicon
tube and rubber tube drains showed only a few adhesions at the suture fixation
and at the entrance into the peritoneum (Table 1).

Much greater effects could be seen from drainage of the anastomosis.
Penrose drains led to broad adhesions between the drain itself and the anastomosis and also between the drain and other neighbouring organs. Silicone
drains were mostly adherent around the fixing sutures, and rubber drains
induced intensive tissue reaction over the whole length of contact to the
anastomosis (Table 2). In the case of leakage of the anastomosis, all types of
drains became completely surrounded with strong adhesions and effectively
isolated from the peritoneal cavity. The incidence of leakage from the drained
suture lines of the colon was 40%, with no difference between the different
types of materials used, whereas the leakage rate from undrained suture lines
was only 12% (Table 3).

Microscopic studies revealed varying degrees of wound healing. At the
position of the drain there was extended inflammation with high percentage of
fibrin and intensive infiltration from granulocytes, histiocytes and lymphocytes
in the serosa of the suture line. Opposite the drain, much less reaction was
found on the same suture line. The least inflammation of the serosa developed
in the nondrained anastomoses (Table 4).

Table 2. Adhesions at the anastomosis site caused by different types
of drains (% of surface of drain)

Drain	Circular adhesions	Total adhesions
Penrose ($n=10$)	65	75
Silicone tube ($n=10$)	35	35
Rubber tube ($n=10$)	65	70

Table 3. Adhesions at the anastomosis site (% of circumference) and occurrence of anastomotic leaks with and without drainage

	Adhesions	Leakages	
Penrose ($n=10$)	84	4	
Silicone tube ($n=10$)	61	5	(40%)
Rubber tube ($n=10$)	52	3	
No drainage ($n=30$)	42	5	(17%)

Table 4. Increased inflammatory reaction at the anastomosis and histological findings in the serosa

	Fibrin/granulocytes (%)	Histiocytes/lymphocytes (%)
Drain position	60	68
Opposite side	25	24
No drainage	8	15

Discussion

In our experimental series in rabbits we found only little reaction of the peritoneal cavity to Penrose, silicone tube and rubber tube drains if infection and local organ injury were absent. There were only small fibrinous adhesions localized at the sutures for fixation or at uncovered parts of Penrose gauze caused by local ischaemia or mechanical irritation. Placed to an anastomosis of the colon, drains increased the development of inflammative reactions and augmented the rate of suture line leakage to 40% by preventing omentum or other organs from sealing the leak, while the leakage rate from undrained anastomosis was only 12%. No fatal peritonitis was observed in our series. Berliner et al. [2] performed two anastomoses of the left colon in dogs. One of the anastomoses was drained by placing a half-inch rubber tube at the suture line. Leakage was found from ten of the drained suture lines and from three of the nondrained suture lines.

Three dogs died from diffuse peritonitis secondary to leakage from drained anastomoses, while leakage of undrained anastomoses was not fatal. Manz et al. [4] reported similar results from their experimental studies.

On the other hand functional longevity of intraperitoneal drains seems to be incomplete and of only short duration [3, 5, 6]. Agrama et al. [1] inserted various types of drains into the peritoneal cavity of 28 dogs. After 1–7 days, all drains failed to show the presence of 200 cm^3 coloured fluid injected intraperitoneally. On autopsy, all tubes were surrounded and occluded by omentum.

Conclusion

Projecting these experimental results to humans, the routine use of "prophy-lactic" drains should be limited to operations with a high likelihood of drain-age, such as operations on the oesophagus, biliary tract and pancreas. Drains with contact to an anastomosis or suture line may increase local inflammation and support the development of suture leakage with further complications. Therefore, if no drainage of intestinal liquids occurs, the drain should be removed within 24–48 h.

References

1. Agrama HM, Blackwood JM, Brown CS, Machiedo GW, Rush BF (1976) Functional long-evity of intraperitoneal drains. Am J Surg 132: 416–421
2. Berliner SD, Burson LC, Lear PE (1964) Use and abuse of intraperitoneal drains in colon surgery. Arch Surg 89: 686–690
3. Hagmüller E, Lorenz D, Werthmann K, Trede M (1990) Nutzen und Risiken einer Drainage nach elektiven Colonresektionen. Chirurg 61: 266–271
4. Manz W, La Tendresse C, Sako Y (1970) The detrimental effects of drains on colonic anastomoses. Dis Colon Rectum 13: 17–25
5. Schäfer K, Wedmann B, Finke U, Börsch G, Brand J (1988) Efficiency of drainage after cholecystectomy. Dig Surg 5: 18–23
6. Wiemer C, Ernst R, Wedmann B, Zumtobel V (1991) Die problemlose Cholezystektomie mit oder ohne Wunddrainage. In: Zumtobel V, Schäfer K (eds) Wunddrainage in der Elektiv- und Notfallchirurgie. Pabst, Lengerich, pp 41–50
7. Yates JL (1905) An experimental study of the local effects of peritoneal drainage. Surg Gynecol Obstet 1: 473–492

7.2 Influence of Different Abdominal Drainages on the Bioelectrical and Motor Activities of the Small Bowel

P. Klever, C. Töns, G. Arlt, A.P. Oettinger, and V. Schumpelick

Introduction

Drainage of the abdominal cavity is sometimes necessary after abdominal surgery, and several materials are used as drains [10]. Whether drains are even necessary after surgery is often controversial [2, 3, 8]. One problem in the use of drains is that biomaterials in the peritoneal cavity disrupt the physiology of the host and may cause bacterial translocation [1, 6]. Another problem is the irritation or evisceration of anastomosis and bowel in the early postoperative period [7, 9].

Methods

In an experimental study we investigated the influence of drains on the restitution of small bowel motility in general in the early postoperative period. In addition, we examined the influences of the use of different materials or different shapes, on the motor activity of the small bowel.

We tested three different drains made up of two different materials (Table 1, Fig. 1). The Easy-Flow is a silicone drain with a rectangular cross-section which works by capillary and gravity forces. The Jackson-Pratt is also a silicone drain but its cross-section changes from rectangular to circular. In the rectangular part there are also additional sideholes. This drain works mainly with suction. The third drain was a rubber-tube made of latex with a circular cross-section. The rubber-tube is rather rigid, the Jackson-Pratt is soft, and the Easy-Flow is very soft.

A total of 16 mongrel dogs underwent a median laparotomy under general anesthesia. In four dogs each, the three different drains were placed from the left paracolic space to the Douglas pouch, where they were fixed. For the registration of slow waves, spike activity and motor activity a bipolar serosal EMG electrode was fixed to the small bowel 50 cm apart from the ligament of Treitz. A serosal microballoon catheter was placed into the small bowel wall next to the EMG electrode. In the control group an upper median laparotomy was performed without implantation of drains. The registration of slow waves, spike activity and motor activity was started 24 h after laparotomy and was carried out daily under standardized conditions until the seventh postoperative

                                                                P. Klever et al.

Table 1. Types of drains and materials

	Material	Shape	Principle	Rigidity
Easy-Flow	Silicone	Rectangular	Capillary gravity	Very soft
Jackson-Pratt	Silicone	Rectangular to circular	Capillary suction/gravity	Soft
Rubber tube	Rubber	Circular	Tube	Rigid

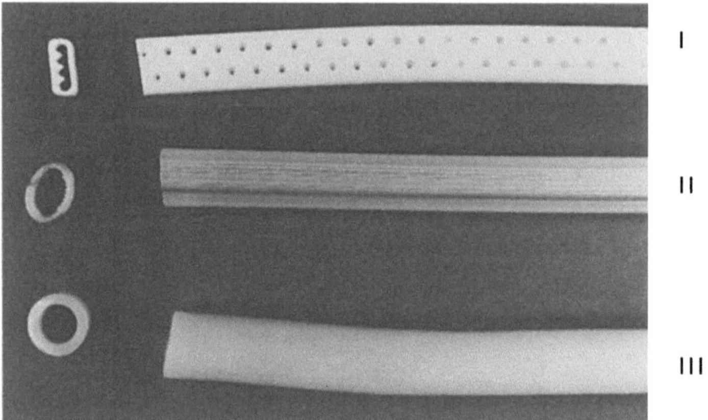

Fig. 1. Three different drains. *I*, Jackson-Pratt; *II*, Easy-Flow; *III*, rubber tube

day. After relaparotomy on the eighth day the peritoneal reaction was examined histologically and the extent of adhesion formation was analysed quantitatively using a digitizer tablet and a microcomputer.

Results

Slow Waves

The frequency of slow waves did not show significant differences between the groups and the controls (Table 2). On the first 2 days, the value of the slow wave frequency (swf) (cycles/min) was about 16.9 and 19.8 in all of the groups. On the seventh day, the swf value was between 17.3 (control) and 17.5–18.9 in the drain groups. Only the Jackson-Pratt group showed a slightly higher swf, but without any statistical significance.

All drains had some influence on the restoration of spike activity of the small bowel (Table 3). In the control group spike activity was normalized after 2 days; the index of spike activity (SA), measured in percent, was 59.5 ± 14.8. In the Easy-Flow group spike activity was normalized after 2 days as well (SA 52 ± 12.7). In the Jackson-Pratt group spike activity returned to normal after

Table 2. Slow waves, frequency (cycles/min)

	Postoperative day				
	1	2	3	4	7
Easy-Flow	16.8 ± 3.8	17.6 ± 3.5	17.6 ± 2.2	16.8 ± 1.7	17.5 ± 1.8
Jackson-Pratt	19.7 ± 1.08	19.8 ± 1.04	20.3 ± 0.8	19.3 ± 1.8	18.9 ± 0.5
Rubber tube	18.2 ± 1.1	19.2 ± 0.3	18.3 ± 0.5	18.2 ± 0.6	17.7 ± 1.1
Control	17.5 ± 4.9	17.6 ± 2.5	18.1 ± 2.1	17.9 ± 2.1	17.3 ± 3.4

Table 3. Index of spike activity (%)

	Postoperative day				
	1	2	3	4	7
Easy-Flow	32.3 ± 3.4	31.2 ± 19.8	52 ± 12.7	57.1 ± 14.4	54.9 ± 8.1
Jackson-Pratt	15 ± 12.4	6.9 ± 3.2	11.1 ± 5.6	39.5 ± 22.2	48.2 ± 2.8
Rubber tube	24 ± 7.3	42.4 ± 26.1	42.4 ± 16.1	45.3 ± 11.3	47.9 ± 14.8
Control	33.8 ± 15.4	28.6 ± 2.6	59.5 ± 14.8	55.9 ± 1.9	47.2 ± 1.4

3 days (SA 39.5 ± 22.2) and in the rubber tube group after 4 days (45.3 ± 11.3). After 7 days there were no further differences between the groups. Due to the large interindividual variations this tendency of delayed restoration of spike activity in the rubber tube group and the Jackson-Pratt group did not reach statistical significance.

Motor Activity

The measurements of motor activity, measured in mm Hg, showed that the Jackson-Pratt group had a delayed recovery to normal values (Table 4). In this group, motor activity started with 8.3 ± 6.7 on the first postoperative day and was normalized on the fourth day with a value of 28.9 ± 9.4; this was not statistically significant ($p > 0.05$). After 4 days the amplitude of type III waves were equal in all four groups.

Table 4. Motor activity amplitude of type III waves (mm Hg)

	Postoperative day				
	1	2	3	4	7
Easy-Flow	19.2 ± 11.6	26.3 ± 3.2	25.8 ± 3.9	31.5 ± 7.4	34.8 ± 2.2
Jackson-Pratt	8.3 ± 6.7	6.8 ± 2.1	10.8 ± 6.5	28.9 ± 9.4	32.9 ± 8.2
Rubber tube	17.9 ± 0.9	24.9 ± 12.7	26.9 ± 2.2	28 ± 8.1	33.4 ± 6.4
Control	18.2 ± 8.6	25.6 ± 2.7	29.9 ± 11.2	30 ± 4.6	28 ± 6.3

Table 5. Histology results

	Inflammation (n)
Easy-Flow	2/4
Jackson-Pratt	4/4
Rubber tube	4/4

Histology

Histologic examination of the peritoneum near the tip of the drains showed signs of moderate inflammation in all animals in the rubber tube and Jackson-Pratt groups. The degree of inflammation was higher for the rubber tube out of four dogs with an Easy-Flow drain had no peritoneal reaction at all (Table 5). Fig. 2a shows a peritoneal imprint of the rubber tube group which shows some erythrocytes, desquamated mesothelial cells and PMNs (polymorphonuclear neutrophil leukocytes), indicating acute inflammation. Figure 2b shows a peritoneal imprint of the Easy-Flow group without signs of inflammation.

Adhesion

After relaparotomy on the eighth day, the extent of adhesion formation was analysed quantitatively using a digitizer tablet and a microcomputer. Adhesion

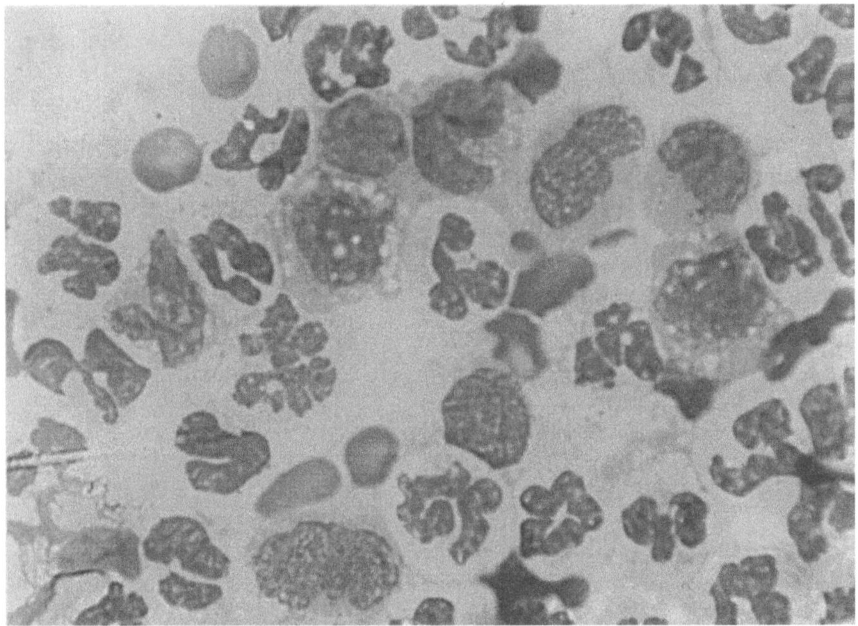

Fig. 2a,b. Peritoneal imprint, **a** with signs of acute inflammation (rubber tube group) and **b** without signs of inflammation (Easy-Flow group)

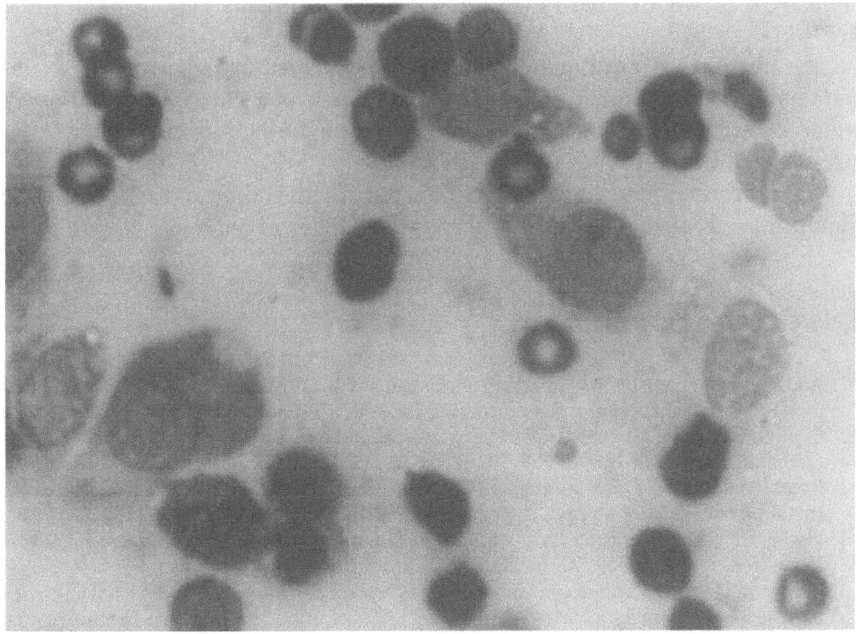

Fig. 2b

formation was highest in the rubber tube group with a surface area of 6148 mm^2 (range 3250–9600) (Table 6). In all other groups adhesion formation was less and similar to the control group. The difference however was not statistically significant, probably because of the large interindividual differences and the small number of animals.

Discussion

Based on our examination we conclude that the use of drains seems to influence motor activity of the small bowel and the integrity of the peritoneal cavity. This influence is caused both by the drain material and by its shape and function.

In general, the Easy-Flow drains, made of silicone, had the least influence on the motor activity of the small bowel, but the difference with the Jackson-Pratt

Table 6. Adhesions

	Surface area (mm^2)
Easy-Flow	4900 (range 3000–6540)
Jackson-Pratt	5100 (range 3250–6710)
Rubber tube	6148 (range 4790–9600)
Control	5063 (range 3400–6280)

drain, also made of silicone, was not statistically significant. Other investigations have shown a higher rate of fluid drainage using the Jackson-Pratt drain [10, 4].

The histological examination after 8 days showed a higher degree of inflammation for the rubber drains. These results are in accordance with those of other investigators [5, 6]. In addition adhesion formation after 8 days was pronounced in the rubber tube drain group.

The differences described here although indicative, did not reach statistical significance, probably because of the small number of animals.

References

1. Andersson R, Jeppson B, Holmberg A, Bengmark S (1990) Implantable drainage after major abdominal surgery in compromised patients. HPB Surg 2(4): 261–264
2. Bona S, Gavelli A, Huguet C (1994) The role of abdominal drainage after major hepatic resection. Am J Surg 167(6): 593–595
3. Brewster NT, King PM, Cunningham C, Adam RD, Griffiths JM (1992) Passive tube and suction drainage after elective cholecystectomy. J R Coll Surg Edinb 37(5): 325–327
4. Fischer H (1991) Vergleichende stömungstechnische Untersuchungen unterschiedlicher Drainagen. Studienarbeit, Aerodynamisches Institut der RWTH Aachen
5. Gerngroß H, Willy C, Engeler V, Walter W (1991) Vergleichende rasterelektronenoptische und klinische Untersuchungen an PVC-, Silikon- und Polyurethan-Drainagen. In: Zumbtobel V, Schäfer K (Hrsg) Wunddrainagen in der Elektiv- und Notfallchirurgie. Pabst, Lengerich
6. Guo W, Soltesz V, Ding JW, Willen R, Liu X, Andersson R, Bengmark S (1994) Abdominal rubber drain piece aggravates intra-abdominal sepsis in the rat. Eur J Clin Invest 24(8): 540–547
7. Loh A, Jones PA (1991) Evisceration and other complications of abdominal drains. Postgrad Med J 67(789): 687–688
8. Monson JR, Guillou PJ, Keane FB, Tanner WA, Brennan TG (1991) Cholecystectomy is safer without drainage: the results of a prospective, randomized clinical trial. Surgery 109(6): 740–746
9. Sagar PM, Couse N, Kerin M, May J, MacFie J (1993) Randomized trial of drainage of colorectal anastomosis. Br J Surg 80(6): 769–771
10. Schumpelick V, Klever P, Töns CH, Zeller H (1993) Drainagen - Materialien und physikalische Grundlagen. Chirurg (1993) 64: 77–84

7.3 Problems and Future Directions of Intraperitoneal Therapy with Antineoplastic Agents

W. Schröder

During recent decades local therapy for malignant tumors, particularly those of intraabdominal origin such as gastric, colon and ovarian cancers, has attracted more interest. As ovarian cancer usually is confined to the peritoneal cavity and women die more often from the complications caused by intraabdominal tumor burden than from distant metastasis, most of the clinical investigations have been performed in patients suffering from this gynecological malignancy [1]. Moreover, ovarian carcinoma is an extraordinarily chemosensitive malignant tumor located in the peritoneal cavity [2].

The rationale of intraabdominal therapeutic procedures is based upon two major aspects of antineoplastic treatment. First, the intraperitoneal tumor is exposed directly to the cytotoxic agent, allowing a better antitumor effect of drugs whose activity against ovarian cancer is concentration dependent. This was supported by the experimental studies of Dedrick and colleagues [3] who demonstrated in a pharmacokinetic model that higher concentrations of cytotoxic drugs could be achieved by delivering the agents directly into the peritoneal cavity. A variety of chemotherapeutic agents showed pharmacokinetic advantages associated with i.p. administration, basically due to their slow clearance from the peritoneal cavity because of their macromolecular structure (Table 1). This pharmacokinetic effect also represents the basis of the second aspect of the rationale, namely the reduction of the toxic side effects of chemotherapeutic agents, particularly when applied in higher concentrations. Similar pharmacokinetic advantages and reduction of toxic side effects could be observed after administration of biological response modifiers (BRM) by the i.p. route providing additional potential applications of local antineoplastic therapy [4]. However, despite the significant pharmacokinetic advantages associated with the i.p. administration of either chemotherapeutic or immunomodulating agents, several additional factors significantly influence and limit the clinical application of this therapeutic strategy.

As cisplatin and carboplatin are currently the most effective drugs against ovarian cancer the majority of experience has been gained using these agents, both of which act directly at the DNA of the tumor cell. Penetration of both drugs into the malignancy is dependent on the concentration gradient and is therefore limited by tumor size [5]. The experimental data were confirmed by the results of the first clinical trials, showing therapeutic effects preferably in patients with minimal tumor burden [6].

Table 1. Pharmacokinetic advantage associated with intraperitoneal administration of selected cytotoxic agents [6]

Agent	Peak peritoneal cavity/plasma concentration ratio
Cisplatin	20
Carboplatin	18
Doxorubicin	474
Mitoxantrone	620
Mitomycin	71
5-Fluorouracil	298
Methotrexate	92
Taxol	1000

However, clinically noteworthy antitumor effects of directly acting cytotoxic agents applied via the i.p. route are not only dependent on tumor size but also require adequate local drug distribution for treatment of peritoneal carcinomatosis. This represents a critical weakness of intraperitoneal therapeutic procedures, as adequate distribution is potentially inhibited by massive adhesions, which, despite a considerable number of suggestions for combatting them, cannot be completely avoided because of posttraumatic induction of inflammatory reactions after intraabdominal operations [7]. In our opinion, the postoperative status per se represents no contra-indication, as small adhesions that do not involve the formation of dead spaces probably do not adversely affect the intraabdominal distribution of aqueous solutions. On the other hand, it seems more than plausible that widespread intraabdominal adhesions, particularly those described as "frozen pelvis", will not allow adequate intraperitoneal distribution of chemotherapeutic drugs. The pattern of postoperative adhesions after radical oncological operations in the abdomen is variable and has to be taken into consideration when planning an intraperitoneal therapeutic regimen.

Moreover, effective local intraabdominal therapy requires an adequate volume for satisfactory distribution. Based upon experimental studies and theoretical considerations, particularly in the Anglo-American literature, treatment volumes of 2 l and more are recommended. However, clinical application of such large volumes is often limited by intolerable abdominal pain, edema etc. [8].

Any recommendations regarding the definitive volume required for effective intraperitoneal cancer therapy also have to consider the different mechanisms of antineoplastic drug activity. As chemotherapeutics act directly on the tumor cells, immunomodulating agents are mostly effective by activating the host's local immune response. Concerning this latter issue, detection and presentation of antigens, as well as chemotactic processes, play key roles independently from strictly physical considerations of distribution. However, the question of the optimal volume for intraperitoneal drug administration remains open.

In summary, intraperitoneal therapy of ovarian or other cancers of intraabdominal origin represents an interesting approach, as not only chemotherapeutics or cytokines could be applied safely by this route. A variety of innovative antineoplastic approaches, such as antibody-guided toxins or enzyme-mediated pro-drug therapy, are based upon this route of drug administration, promising a satisfactory effect on tumor cells in the nearer future. The effectiveness of those therapeutic regimens may be reinforced by modern concepts of local adhesion prevention, i.e. by inhibition of inflammatory reactions with anti-IL-6 antibodies.

References

1. Deppe G, Malviya VK (1991) Ovarian cancer. Advances in management. Surg Clin N Am 71: 1023–1039
2. Thigpen JT, Vance RB, Kansur T (1993) Second-line chemotherapy for recurrent carcinoma of the ovary. Cancer 71: 1559–1564
3. Dedrick RL, Myers CE, Bungay PM, Devita VT Jr (1978) Pharmacokinetic rationale for peritoneal drug administration in the treatment of ovarian cancer. Cancer Treat Rep 62: 1–11
4. Schröder W, Bender HG (1992) Pharmakologische Entwicklungen zum therapeutischen Einsatz von Biological-response Modifiern. Gynakologe 25: 258–267
5. Los G, Verdegall EME, Mutsaers PHA, McVie JG (1991) Penetration of carboplatin and cisplatin into rat peritoneal tumor nodules after intraperitoneal therapy. Cancer Chemother Pharmacol 28: 159–165
6. Markman M (1993) Intraperitoneal chemotherapy. In: Markman M, Hoskins WJ (eds) Cancer of the ovary. Raven, New York, pp 317–325
7. Stangel JJ, Nisbeth JD, Settles H (1984) Formation and prevention of postoperative abdominal adhesions. J Reprod Med 29: 143–156
8. Dunnick NR, Jones RB, Doppmann JL, Speyer J, Myers CE (1979) Intraperitoneal contrast infusion for assessment of intraperitoneal fluid dynamics. Am J Roentgenol 133: 221–223

8 Pleura, Pericardium, and Peritoneal Dialysis

8.1 Indication, Technique, and Results of Therapeutic Pleurodesis: Formation of Adhesions and Parallels to Abdominal Surgery

M. Hürtgen, A. Linder, and H. Toomes

Introduction

Pleura and peritoneum both originate from the inner layer of the former coelomic cavity, which is not separated in thoracic and abdominal before the sixth week of embryological development [4]. This suggests a relationship between adhesion formation in interpleural and interperitoneal space. Understanding what happens in one cavity may shed light on problems in the other. In the present context, we focus on the formation of adhesions following different types of surgical trauma. In pneumothorax surgery, formation of adhesions is usually not looked upon as a complication, but as the goal of the procedure. In therapeutic pleurodesis, the possibility of adhesions not forming is an important factor, but the reasons for this nonformation are as yet unknown.

Indications

Common indications for pleurodesis are the following:

1. Pneumothorax
   a) Primary
   b) Secondary
2. Pleural effusion
   a) Benign
   b) Malignant
3. Chylothorax

Pneumothorax and effusions are frequent, whereas chylothorax is rare. It is desirable to select the method of pleurodesis for a given indication corresponding to the necessary extent and density of adhesions. This depends on failure of previous therapy, underlying disease, life expectancy of the patient, and the procedures usually used in the clinic concerned.

Table 1. Techniques of surgical pleurodesis

Type	Technique
Mechanical	Drainage
	Abrasion
	Pleurectomy
Foreign body	Drainage
	Talc
Thermic	Argon beam coagulation
	Electric coagulation
	Laser coagulation
	Infrared coagulation
Chemic	Tetracycline
	Glucose
	Chemotherapeutic agents
	Miscellaneous

Techniques

Various types of primary noxa to the mesothelium (Table 1) cause adhesion formation in both abdominal and thoracic surgery. The basic process responsible for adhesion formation is an inflammatory response of local tissue. The intensity and duration of inflammation are correlated to the characteristics of the trauma.

Introducing a chest drain, abrasion, and pleurectomy result in pleural defects of different extents and depths.

Thermal procedures result in third- or fourth-degree tissue burn. The depth of the burn depends on the energy source and the energy level at which the source is set and is difficult to standardize [2]. From animals trials with dogs, superficial necrosis by means of argon beam coagulation is known to produce insufficient adhesions [1]. For deeper burns with prolonged healing, more adhesions are to be expected.

The role and mechanism of pure fibrin glue pleurodesis are questionable. Without any additional trauma to reduce the fibrinolytic activity of the interpleural space, the effect of fibrin glue usually only lasts for a few days. This may not allow formation of fibrous adhesions. Fibrin glue has also been used to prevent adhesion formation in the abdomen. All this suggests that the result of fibrin glue application depends on cofactors that are difficult to define.

In chemical pleurodesis, if a chest tube is used, it is not possible to ensure that the reacting agent spreads all over the pleural surface. However, any surgical approach used for this purpose alone would be too invasive.

Foreign bodies provoke local inflammation. The extent of adhesions corresponds to the duration of the mechanical irritation. Talc leads to a lifelong local inflammation, resulting in extensive adhesions. In Germany, talc is usually only used in malignancies or in patients whose condition is very poor.

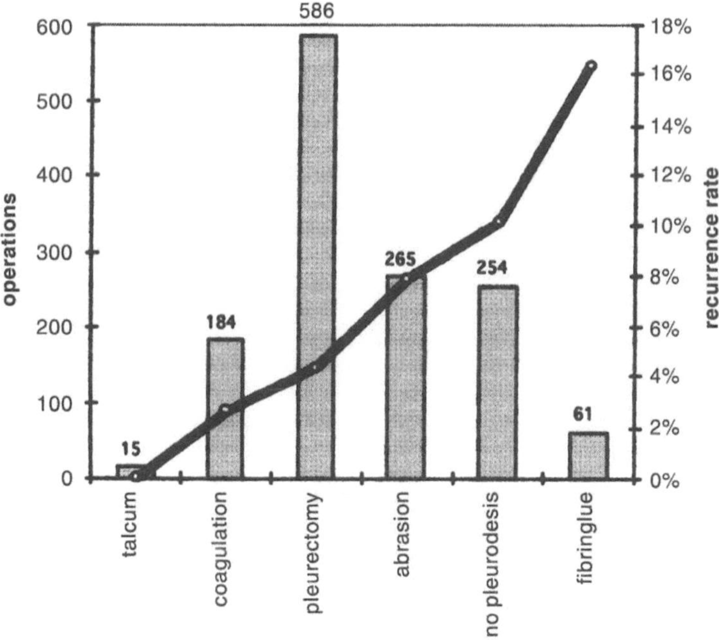

Fig. 1. Recurrence rates (*black line*) in a total of 1360 pleurodesis operations using different procedures

Survey

In a survey of 39 clinics, the Deutsche Gesellschaft für Thoraxchirurgie evaluated the current state of operative pleurodesis for spontaneous pneumothorax by video-assisted thoracoscopic surgery. Out of 20 clinics that responded, 19 of them had performed a total of 1360 operations and reported their recurrence rate (Fig. 1) and complications.

Some clinics observed contradictory results after similar procedures. This may be explained by the different extent of additional parenchymal resection. The most effective methods may be preferred for severe cases, thus probably masking differences between procedures. However, fibrin glue should be expected to work at least as well as no pleurodesis at all. Unfortunately, the recurrence rate with fibrin glue is extremely high, in some groups more than 50%. It probably even prevents adhesions, as discussed for abdominal surgery.

Grouped for duration of inflammation and time needed for wound healing, recurrence rates roughly correlate inversely with expected intensity and duration of the inflammatory response after surgery. Talc shows the best results, in spite of its restriction to difficult cases in Germany. Time is considered to be a very important factor, due to clinical observation of three kinds of adhesions (avascular "spider's webs," vascularized bridles, and dense scarring) depending on the clinical situation. In the occasional cases of reoperation, only

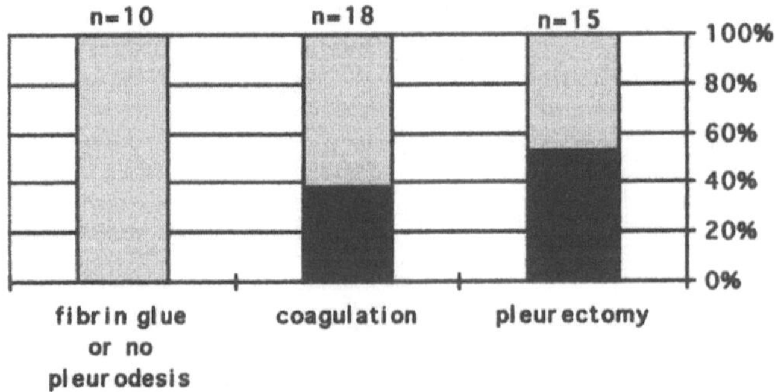

Fig. 2. Incidence of pain (*black bars*) and no pain (*shaded bars*) in different pleurodesis procedures. From [3]

limited adhesions are usually encountered, as the initial trauma only lasted for the time of normal wound healing. Blebs in recurrent pneumothorax provoke recurrent tissue response in all cases of air leak, both apparent and inapparent. Vascularized adhesions frequently originate from these blebs, as they do from sutures in the abdomen. Chronic pleuritis of any etiology may result in dense adhesions that are almost impossible to lyse.

The only complication of interest in the present context is pain, as this is also an important sequel of peritoneal adhesions. The problems of pain evaluation are well known and almost impossible to overcome in retrospective multicenter trials. For this reason, we did not even try to address this in our survey. A prospective study at the university of Giessen [3] demonstrated increasing pain with more aggressive means of pleurodesis (Fig. 2).

No conclusions for abdominal surgery should be based on this. Severe complaints after pleurodesis usually follow intraoperative damage to the intercostal nerves. There is no evidence of a similar mechanism in abdominal adhesions. Pain appears immediately after talc application and may persist for years, which can be explained by the extensive inflammatory reaction to talc.

Conclusion

Assuming a decrease in recurrence rate after pleurodesis with increasing density and extent of postoperative adhesions, interesting cross-links with adhesion formation after different types of intra-abdominal trauma are suggested. What is best in pleurodesis should be worst in the abdomen. Pleurodesis might even act as a "human model" to learn more about adhesion formation in the abdomen.

Multiple factors affect the recurrence rate as an indicator of adhesion formation. Rarely known modifiers of adhesion formation may explain strange findings such as a normal pleura on reoperation for recurrence after previous pleurectomy.

It may be presumed that it is not so important *what* is done to the pleura, but *how long* it is done for pleura.

Summary

In thoracic surgery, adhesion formation has aroused widespread interest not as a complication, but as the goal of certain procedures. In therapeutic pleurodesis, the possibility of adhesions not forming is an important factor, but the reasons for this nonformation are as yet unknown. The common origin of the pleura and peritoneum is the inner layer of the former coelomic cavity, which suggests a relationship between adhesion formation in interpleural and interperitoneal space.

The indication for therapeutic pleurodesis is usually pneumothorax or pleural effusion, and the nature of the disease determines the choice of the technique used to achieve pleurodesis. Tube thoracostomy, pleural abrasion with a sponge, and pleurectomy result in pleural defects. Thermal procedures such as argon beam, electric, laser, and infrared coagulation lead to pleural necrosis without major defects. Chemical agents (e.g., tetracyline) and foreign bodies (drainage, talc) induce pleurodesis by inflammatory response of different durations. The role of fibrin glue is difficult to determine. Interpleural adhesions may be divided into three main types: (1) avascular and easy to lyse, (2) vascularized bridles, and (3) a dense scar with almost no recognizable tissue borders.

Our conclusions concerning adhesion formation after surgery by video-assisted thoracic surgery (VATS) are based on personal experience and on 1360 operations included in a survey conducted by the Deutsche Gesellschaft für Thoraxchirurgie. Severe pain accompanies pleurectomy and talc application. Significant differences in recurrence rates after spontaneous pneumothorax as an indicator of the density of adhesions are only found after talc and fibrin glue application. The recurrence rate obviously depends on other factors such as the extent of bulla resection and modifiers of adhesion formation. The severity of trauma seems to be less important than the duration of trauma or inflammation.

References

1. Bresticker MA, Oba J, LoCicero III J, Greene R (1993) Optimal pleurodesis: a comparison study. Ann Thorac Surg 55: 364
2. Hürtgen M, Schäfer A, Lukosch Ch J, Schwemmle K (1994) Thoracoscopic treatment of pneumothorax. In: Steichen FM, Welter R (ed) Minimal invasive surgery and new technology. Quality Medical, St Louis
3. Hürtgen M, Buhr J, Kluth D, Kelm Ch, Schäfer A (1995) Thorakoskopische Operation des primären Spontanpneumothorax. Chirurg 66: 890–894
4. Langman J (1977) Medizinische Embryologie. Thieme, Stuttgart

8.2 Hazards and Prevention of Postsurgical Pericardial Adhesions

D.M. Wiseman

The Clinical Problem: Hazard and Risk

The formation of adhesions following cardiothoracic surgery places the mediastinal structures and grafts at risk of catastrophic injury [91] during a second sternotomy, making it a bloody, time-consuming, and hazardous procedure [20, 51]. Over 360 000 cardiac procedures are performed annually in the United States [37, 88] up to 10% of which are reoperations [15, 26, 41].

Approximately 4% of patients undergoing reoperation experience complications related to repeat sternal opening. If hemorrhage does occur during repeat sternotomy, there is a mortality risk of approximately 37% [20].

In addition to extrapericardial adhesions, fibrous tissue may also fill the pericardial space, obscuring the coronary vasculature. Right ventricular function may be impaired because of adhesions between the right ventricle and the chest wall [4]. Adhesion formation around ventricular assist devices makes their removal difficult [42].

Failure to close the pericardium appears to increase the risk of a hemorrhagic event during sternal reentry [16,20]; thus primary pericardial closure has been advocated [73], particularly after the pericardium has been maintained under tension during surgery to avoid graft compression [16]. Others [51] have opposed this idea, and many surgeons leave the pericardium open to avoid disturbance of extracardiac grafts and diastolic filling of the heart [61]. Other surgical methods of avoiding these problems involve the use of pericardial meshing [61] or autologous pericardial flaps [11] at the primary operation.

Accepting the inevitability of adhesion formation, innovative approaches to the heart in repeat operations have been suggested, including lateral thoracotomy [33] or pericardiotomy [79] approaches and partial removal of sternal wires, using them as a barrier between the saw and the heart during sternotomy [34].

Peritoneal and Pericardial Adhesion Formation

Since most information is known about peritoneal adhesion formation and its prevention, it is useful to compare and contrast peritoneal and pericardial adhesion formation to facilitate the design of specific approaches to pericardial adhesions.

Similarities

Adhesion formation involving pericardial tissues shares both histological [48] and biochemical characteristics with the analogous processes that occur in other tissues bounded by an internal membrane, particularly the peritoneum [7, 8, 9, 63].

Foreign materials are a well-known stimulus for adhesion formation. In cardiac surgery, pledgets used to support suture lines have been reported to act as sources for infection, scarring, adhesions, and calcification [6, 57, 99].

Fibrinolytic mechanisms have been described which have the potential to limit adhesion formation in peritoneum [78, 81] and pericardium [72, 78]. The source of this fibrinolytic activity appears to be the endothelial cells of the submesothelial vessels and the mesothelium itself. Surgical and other trauma will compromise the mesothelium and reduce its fibrinolytic activity in peritoneal and pericardial tissues [78]. Such compromise is widely accepted as a central event in the pathogenesis of adhesions [7, 24, 36, 81]. From samples obtained during cardiac surgery, Nkere et al. [74, 75] found a progressive rounding and denudation of mesothelium commensurate with the degree of inflammation and the reduction in fibrinolytic activity (mainly tissue-type plasminogen activator, t-PA) of the pericardium.

That both mesothelial damage and blood are required for adhesion formation has been shown in both pericardial [13] and peritoneal [89] tissues.

Differences

Anatomical, physiologic, and surgical factors govern the behavior of pericardial and peritoneal tissues and materials used to prevent adhesions.

Both the parietal pericardium and the subepicardium contain relatively few lymphatics compared with the peritoneum [22]. Although this would not affect the absorption of small molecules by capillaries, high molecular weight materials such as polymer degradation products would take longer to clear in the pericardium.

Both the peritoneum and pericardium are polar membranes with mesothelium on one surface. Unlike the peritoneum, the pericardium is a distinct membrane, with its antimesothelial surface unattached to surrounding tissue, except when adhesions form to the sternum. Since this epipericardial layer appears to lack a functional mesothelium, the fibrinolytic activity of submesothelial vessels and macrophages is likely to play a more prominent role in preventing adhesions than in peritoneal tissues. Furthermore, the manner in which this layer regenerates must be considered more carefully than in the equivalent layer in peritoneal tissues.

The movement of the heart imposes two requirements on barrier materials. A barrier must withstand the stresses induced by this movement, remaining both intact and in place. It must also be capable of being fixed in place by sutures or by other means.

In the days following cardiac surgery, 500–1000 ml bloody fluid is expected to drain from the chest cavity [93]. This has several implications for the design of materials for the prevention of pericardial adhesions:

1. The agent should not be flushed away through mediastinal drains, nor should it interfere with drainage and increase the risk of pericardial tamponade.
2. It must retain its integrity for the duration of this bleeding and exudation. For peritoneal tissue, it is widely held that any agent acting as an adhesion barrier must persist for at least 3 days, since this is the minimum time over which serosal (mesothelial) healing takes place [18, 80, 94]. In epicardial tissues, it may take as long as 7 days before bleeding and exudation cease.
3. Its action must not be compromised in the presence of blood. The action of some agents used in the pelvic cavity is known to be compromised if they become soaked with blood [102]. Others [104] appear to be less dependent on good hemostasis, at least at abdominal sites.

The healing of bone (sternum), coronary arterial anastomoses, and incised myocardium must not be compromised. Drugs such as t-PA can increase bleeding at any surgical site. This would be greater in cardiac surgery due to the use of heparin, which enhances the action of t-PA [2].

Even though some agents have successfully reduced pericardial adhesions and facilitated sternal reentry, they have compromised the visibility of the coronary vasculature by inducing epicardial fibrosis [5, 60]. This would hamper future revascularization procedures. We have observed that certain degradable polymers produce abrasive fragments, which may contribute to epicardial inflammation.

An important difference between cardiac and abdominal surgery is the use of cardiopulmonary bypass (CPB). Hematologic differences found when CPB is used seem to have practical implications concerning the testing of pericardial patches in animals. In sheep, pericardial xenografts performed well without CPB, but evoked severe adhesions, epicardial reactions, and in some cases graft calcification with CPB [29].

Prevention of Pericardial Adhesions

Various methods of reducing pericardial adhesions have been evaluated, mainly in animal models. Because of the difficulties in conducting second-look evaluations for efficacy, clinical studies are extremely limited.

Drugs

Although a number of drugs have been evaluated in animal models of abdominal adhesions [101], few studies have examined their effects on pericardial adhesions.

Fibrinolytic Drugs

Given the role of mesothelial compromise and fibrin deposition in the initiation of adhesion formation, it is not suprising that fibrinolytic drugs such as plasmin [46], t-PA [21, 59], streptokinase (SK) [43], and urokinase [86] have all been investigated for the reduction of adhesions, at least in abdominal models. Clinically, there is at least one report of the use of intrapericardial SK to facilitate the drainage of postoperative loculated effusion [14].

In a rabbit pericardial adhesion model, three fibrinolytic drugs were evaluated for their ability to reduce pericardial adhesions [103]. Single-dose treatment with t-PA, a t-PA analogue (Fb-Fb-CF), or SK caused reductions in the extent and tenacity of adhesion formation compared with untreated surgical controls. A modified fabric of oxidized regenerated cellulose (mTC7) used to localize the agents to the cardiac surface did little to interfere with their activity. Despite impressive reductions in adhesion formation, postoperative bruising, bleeding, and swelling were associated with treatment with t-PA and to a lesser extent with SK and Fb-Fb-CF. In studies in the abdomen, bleeding was not observed with t-PA [21, 68], suggesting a differential susceptibility of different tissues to the bleeding effects of these drugs.

Anti-inflammatory Drugs

Anti-inflammatory drugs (including nonsteroidal anti-inflammatory drugs, corticosteroids, and antihistamines) have been evaluated in a number of abdominal adhesion models with reasonable degrees of success [101]. Although these drugs are used clinically, particularly in pelvic surgery, clear demonstrations of clinical benefits of these drugs through well-conducted clinical studies have not materialized.

An early study [95] in dogs showed a reduction in pleural, but not pericardial adhesions with a combination of dexamethasone and promethazine. Methylprednisolone given for 1 week eliminated pericardial/epicardial adhesions in 14 out of 15 dogs [98], whereas dogs left untreated, as well as those treated with ibuprofen, all formed adhesions. A slight reduction in the severity of adhesions was noted in animals treated with ibuprofen. Despite these impressive results in animals, the effects of steroids on wound healing and immunosuppression remain; thus they have not achieved widespread use clinically.

Liquids

Use of Coating Solutions

Mesothelial damage may occur by tissue manipulation and desiccation. To overcome this, the periodic instillation of dilute solutions of hydrophilic polymers (e.g., carboxymethylcellulose, hyaluronic acid, polyvinylpyrrolidone) during surgery has been shown in animals to reduce adhesions when applied before, but not after, pericardial injury [23, 105]. In dogs [66], the instillation of 0.4% hyaluronic acid every 20 min over a 2-h period of peri- and epicardial desiccation and abrasion was sufficient to reduce the incidence of intrapericardial adhesions in 100% of sites examined in vehicle (phosphate-buffered saline, PBS) or surgical controls to 64%. This treatment did not compromise epicardial visibility. Although the half-life of hyaluronic acid within the pericardial space is stated as 3–4 days, i.e., beyond the onset of fibrinolysis after mesothelial injury, further studies are needed to assess the persistence and effect of hyaluronic acid in the presence of postoperative bleeding and with the use of drains over periods of several days.

Dextran 70

With mixed success and the possibility of severe adverse effects [19, 44], the use of 32% dextran 70 in gynecologic surgery has declined over the last several years. In rabbits [87] or rats [82], small volumes of dextran 70 instilled intrapericardially reduced the severity of adhesions. These effects could not be due to hydroflotation, but to lubricating or pharmacological effects. Such effects might include modulation of platelet function and enhancement of fibrinolysis [96], concentration of plasminogen activator activity at the mesothelial surface [55], and interference with lymphocyte and macrophage activity [83].

Barriers

In 1988, a minority (29%) of thoracic surgeons surveyed reported that they used pericardial substitutes [41]. When they did so, they used bovine pericardium 51.3% of the time, Silastic/silicone-based materials 17.5% of the time, and expanded polytetrafluoroethylene (ePTFE) 31.2% of the time. Less than half the respondents reported dissatisfaction with the performance of bovine pericardial xenografts or silicone-based materials stemming from anecdotal reports of dense adhesions, pericardial reactions, graft rejection, infection, and fevers attributed to the graft. Nineteen out of 22 surgeons who observed ePTFE membrane at reoperation reported their satisfaction with the result at reoperation.

The method of placement of an adhesion barrier, particularly a pericardial patch, appears to be important for a successful outcome. Revuelta et al. [84] proposed that pericardial patches be sutured on only one side of the pericardium to prevent buckling due to cardiac movement. This is because blood may accumulate in the furrows and around the margins of a loosely fastened permanent membrane and act as a nidus for adhesion formation. In models of radical pelvic surgery, adhesion formation was worse than controls when ePTFE membrane was fastened with interrupted sutures [27] and better than

Table 1. Experiences with pericardial xenografts: animal and clinical reports

Source	Positive Result	Negative Result
Bovine	Gabbay et al. [29] (S)	Gabbay et al. [29] (S)
	Bunton et al. [10] (S)	Eng et al. [25] (H)
	Mathisen et al. [54] (D)	
	Meus et al. [60] (D)	
	Opie et al. [77] (H)	Gallo et al. [32] (H)
Porcine	Gallo et al. [30] (D)	Gallo et al. [32] (H)
Equine	Mathisen et al. [54] (D)	Gallo et al. [32] (H)
	Segesser et al. [91] (H)	

Studies were conducted in humans (H), sheep (S), or dogs (D).

controls when positioned using continuous nonabsorbable sutures [69, 70]. A similar phenomenon has been described for pericardial grafts [31].

Xenografts and Heterografts

Fixed pericardial grafts of bovine, porcine, or equine origin have been used as pericardial patches for preventing pericardial adhesions with mixed results in both animal and clinical studies [40, 41] (Table 1). These materials, particularly those fixed in glutaraldehyde, may calcify [31]. Careful washing of the xenograft appears essential to success, with one suggestion that fixation in ethanol is preferable to formalin fixation [77]. Because of the problems of epicardial reaction, as well as the risk of infection potentiation, these materials should only be used with caution [32].

Human amniotic membrane has also been evaluated for adhesion prevention. Minimal extrapericardial adhesions, no epicardial adhesions, and minimal histologic reactions were found in dogs in which the pericardium was closed with glutaraldehyde-preserved human amniotic membrane [71].

Fibrin

Given the role of fibrin deposition in the pathogenesis of adhesions, the use of fibrin to prevent adhesions may seem somewhat paradoxical [35]. Several studies conducted in the abdomen of animals [17, 49, 50] indicate the contrary. Perhaps once polymerization is complete, an "adhesion barrier" is formed in situ which cannot stick to other surfaces. More fundamentally, any means of limiting bleeding [93] and uncontrolled fibrin deposition must serve to limit adhesions.

Two studies have tested this hypothesis in pericardial tissues. In the first of these [45], fibrin sealant (from human cryoprecipitate) was applied to an atriotomy incision line and to the cardiac surface before pericardial closure in four out of eight mini-pigs. Although a greater number of adhesions were found in animals in whom fibrin sealant had been used, they were less tenacious and more easily dissected than those found in control animals. Adhesions in the control group appeared to contain more fibroblasts, infiltrating leukocytes, and collagen bundles than in the treatment group. Furthermore, the density of fibroblasts and collagen bundles increased with time in the control group, but not in the treatment group.

A second study in rabbits (D.M. Wiseman, L. Kamp, and P.M. Scholz, unpublished, cited in [101]) essentially confirmed these findings and extended them to a situation in which the pericardium was not closed. Both the extent and severity of pericardial adhesions were reduced by a commercial fibrin sealant which also contained aprotinin, an inhibitor of fibrinolysis.

Nonabsorbable Adhesion Barriers

Early attempts at preventing adhesions involved materials which had a low adherence for tissue such as Silastic/silicone-based materials. With varying degrees of success [5, 47, 56, 60, 97, 100, 106], dense adhesions and epicardial reactions, they have been largely superseded by ePTFE [41].

ePTFE is commercially available for pericardial reconstruction as a thin (0.1-mm) membrane with small pore sizes (less than 1 μm), which are believed to contribute to its lack of tissue adherence.

Although not specifically indicated for the prevention of postsurgical adhesions, the commercial form is indicated for "the reconstruction or repair of passive biological membranes, specifically the pericardium or peritoneum" (Gore and Associates, Inc., Flagstaff, Arizona, USA).

ePTFE membranes have been shown in some animal models to reduce the formation of pericardial adhesions, while preserving the visibility of the epicardial vessels [40, 85]. Others have reported severe inflammatory reactions [71], and the formation of an epicardial "fibrous peel" has been observed with ePTFE [10] or other PTFE materials [60, 84, 85].

Because of the problems in making a direct assessment, few reports exist of the effects of ePTFE membrane in humans. In an uncontrolled study of 110 patients [64, 65], no complications were attributed to ePTFE membrane. In four patients in whom a reoperation was required, the chest was entered in minutes with no significant adhesions involving the patch, sternum, or epicardium and without epicardial reactions.

Four-ply ePTFE membranes were placed in an uncontrolled series of 61 children undergoing surgical repair of congenital heart defects [39]. Qualitative observations were made at resternotomy in 23 of these children. It was noted that "the retrosternal space was secured by finger dissection, and safe resternotomy was then possible." No major complications occurred, with one case of pericardial effusion and two cases of retrosternal abscess. Similar observations were made in eight of 79 patients requiring reoperation after correction of congenital cardiac defects [1]. No adhesions were noted between the chest wall and the pericardial patch, with minimal epicardial adhesions, a thin epicardial reaction, and good epicardial visibility.

Infection potentiation is at least a theoretical risk with any foreign material. With the exception of one study [39] no such effect has been reported in experiential studies with ePTFE [1, 41]. In a more specialized application for pericardial patches, there has been one report of the successful use of ePTFE membranes to reduce adhesions around ventricular assist devices in six patients [42].

Absorbable Adhesion Barriers

Interceed (TC7) Absorbable Adhesion Barrier (Johnson and Johnson Medical, Inc., Arlington, TX) is currently the only product indicated by the Food and Drug Administration (FDA) of the United States for the prevention of adhesions. Based on extensive multinational clinical studies [3, 28, 76, 92], it is used in gynecologic surgery. The action of Interceed is known to be compromised in the presence of bleeding [102]. Thus meticulous hemostasis must be obtained prior to use. However a modified form of Interceed (nTC7) appears to function even in the presence of bleeding [104] and reduces adhesions in a (Table 2) rabbit cardiac model [90].

In a canine model, a composite membrane of hyaluronic acid and carboxymethylcellulose was found to reduce the severity of intrapericardial adhesions with minimal effect on the epicardial anatomy [67]. The membrane was placed between the epicardium and the pericardium, which was then closed.

Synthetic Absorbable Polymers: A Paradigm Shift

Polylactide (PLA), polyglycolide (PGA), and their copolymers have been used for many years in medical devices, the most common of which are sutures and prosthetic meshes. Under prevailing paradigms, barriers are to be used in much the same way as dressings for cutaneous wounds: the wound (surgical site) is covered for the period of epithelialization (mesothelialization) and then removed or allowed to degrade (e.g. Interceed). The dressing (barrier) plays no active part in the process other than to protect the wound.

Table 2. Effect of a neutralized Interceed barrier (nTC7) on adhesion formation in a rabbit pericardial model

	Extent of adhesions (%)[a]	SEM	Animals (n)
Control	84	6.7	15
Interceed barrier	89	8.6	7
nTC7	41	10.3	15[*]

SEM, standard error of mean.
[a]The percentage involvement of a median strip of anterior epicardium at risk of sternal adhesions.
[*]$p < 0.01$, Student's t test, compared with controls.

According to one group of workers, the use of synthetic absorbable materials to cover the heart "appears preposterous" at first, because most of these materials can induce a strong foreign body reaction [29]. However, the findings of three groups [10, 29, 52, 53] offer an empirical case for a paradigm shift for the prevention of pericardial adhesions.

In sheep, coarse and fine PGA meshes evoked "generally favorable" epicardial reactions, and although a clear "clinical benefit" of these meshes could not be demonstrated, both meshes were replaced by a continuous collagenous membrane, with less adhesion formation and epicardial reaction found with the finer mesh [10].

Also in sheep, Gabbay et al. [29] noted that meshes of PGA (Dexon) and/or Maxon (copolymer of glycolide and trimethylene carbonate) induced strong foreign body reactions at first, which subsided after the digestion of the polymer. A thin collagenous layer then replaced the mesh which "prevented adhesion formation" and which could be peeled away easily with little epicardial reaction.

Polyhydroxybutyrate (PHB) is a polymer produced by fermentation of the bacterium Alcaligenes eutrophus. It degrades slowly to produce normal mammalian metabolites [62]. Studies in sheep with a pericardial patch made of PHB [52, 53] have confirmed and extended the findings made with PGA meshes (see above). Adhesions developed in four out of 18 animals treated with PHB patches in contrast to five out of five control animals in which the pericardium was left open. The epicardial vasculature was clearly visible in two out of 18 treated animals, but only in one out of five control animals. Histologically, as the polymer was degraded by macrophages it was replaced by a progressively thicker dense collagenous layer. At 2 months, the earliest time point observed, this patch was covered by a cell layer whose identity as mesothelial cells was confirmed by the presence of ultrastructural (scanning and transmission electron microscopy, SEM and TEM), immunohistochemical, and biochemical (prostacyclin) markers.

The notion that it is possible, at least in cardiac surgery, to view synthetic absorbable barriers as scaffolds for the formation of a neomembrane (pericardium) is not entirely without precedent at other surgical sites. In the abdomen, a polyglactin mesh used to elevate the bowel from the pelvis became replaced by fibrous tissue to form a permanent pelvic sling in patients undergoing radiotherapy [12]. In craniotomy, a composite mesh of polyglactin and collagen membrane was replaced by a neodura [58]. Finally, dermal grafts composed of fibroblasts grown on a polyglactin mesh became vascularized and replaced with a neodermal tissue as the synthetic mesh absorbed [38].

Conclusion

A unique set of anatomic and physiologic factors govern the approaches towards the prevention of pericardial adhesions. While the use of materials designed primarily for use in the abdomen is not ruled out, it may be appropriate to challenge the paradigm of a rapidly absorbable adhesion barrier as used in abdominal surgery. Studies suggesting that more slowly absorbed barriers can act as tissue scaffolds to facilitate the regeneration of a neopericardium provide encouraging support for this tissue-engineering paradigm.

Important to note here are the advances in instrumentation that are beginning to make possible endoscopic cardiac surgery without sternotomy. Such a change in surgical approach would challenge many of the assumptions made here about the design of materials for prevention of pericardial adhesions and would likely shift the emphasis to more pharmacological approaches or to approaches using rapidly absorbable barriers.

Whatever the path that surgical technology takes, agents used to prevent adhesion formation are still likely to play a role in cardiac surgery. Although animal models have replicated some of the unique features of cardiac surgery, no animal model has attempted to synthesize the complexity of cardiac surgery in testing agents for adhesion prevention. Accordingly, clinical studies remain the ultimate test of these hypotheses and paradigms. This raises the challenge of how to evaluate the efficacy of adhesion prevention treatments in humans.

Summary

Adhesion formation following cardiothoracic surgery places the mediastinal structures at risk of catastrophic injury, making a second sternotomy a time-consuming and hazardous procedure. Pericardial closure may ameliorate adhesion formation, although at some risk of fluid accumulation and pericardial tamponade. Several methods of reducing pericardial adhesions have been evaluated clinically and in animal models with mixed results. These methods include the use of pericardial xenografts, synthetic and absorbable barriers, fibrinolytic drugs, oxidized regenerated cellulose, dextran 70, fibrin glue, and hyaluronic acid derivatives.

Although the mechanism of postsurgical adhesion formation is similar throughout the body, specific anatomic and physiological factors operating at individual surgical sites will govern the choice and design of putative adhesion-prevention agents. Following cardiac surgery, extensive and prolonged bleeding is expected over the first 5 days of surgery. This means that materials must remain intact and functioning in the presence of blood. The integrity and positioning of barrier materials must not be compromised by the movement of the heart, nor should the placement of mediastinal drains interfere with their action. Some materials have been noted to evoke fibrosis of the epicardium, thus impairing the visibility of the coronary vasculature. Finally, metabolic differences associated with the use of cardiopulmonary bypass may influence the behavior of adhesion barriers.

Because of the unique anatomic and physiological considerations in cardiac surgery, it may be appropriate to challenge the paradigm of rapidly absorbable adhesion barriers as used in abdominal surgery. Recent studies suggesting that more slowly absorbed barriers can act as tissue scaffolds to facilitate the regeneration of a neopericardium provide encouraging support for a tissue-engineering paradigm, at least in cardiac surgery.

Acknowledgements. It is a pleasure to thank my colleagues and friends with whom I have collaborated in the area of pericardial adhesions: Laura Gottlick-Iarkowski, Lola Kamp, Robert Jochen, and Peter Scholz.

References

1. Amato JS, Cotroneo JV, Galdieri RJ, Alboliras E, Antillon J, Vogel RL (1989) Experience with the polytetrafluoroethylene surgical membrane for pericardial closure in operations for congenital cardiac defects. J Thorac Cardiovasc Surg 97: 929–934
2. Andrade-Gordon P, Strickland S (1986) Interaction of heparin with plasminogen activators and plasminogen: effects on the activation of plasminogen. Biochemistry 25: 4033–4040
3. Azziz R and the INTERCEED Barrier Study Group (1993) Microsurgery alone or with INTERCEED Absorbable Adhesion Barrier for pelvic sidewall adhesion re-formation. Surg Gyn Obstet 177: 135–139
4. Bailey LL, Li Z, Schulz E, Roost H, Yahiku P (1984) A cause of right ventricular dysfunction after cardiac operations. J Thorac Cardiovasc Surg 87: 539–542
5. Bonnabeau RC, Armanious AW, Tarnay TJ (1973) Partial replacement of pericardium with dura substitute. J Thorac Cardiovasc Surg 66: 196–201
6. Borst HG (1987) Dire consequences of the indiscriminate use of Teflon felt pledgets. J Thorac Cardiovasc Surg 94: 442–443
7. Buckman RF, Woods M, Sargent L, Gervin AS (1976) A unifying pathogenetic mechanism in the etiology of intraperitoneal adhesions. J Surg Res 20: 1–5
8. Buckman RF, Buckman D, Hufnagel HV, Gervin AS (1976) A physiologic basis for the adhesion-free healing of deperitonealized surfaces. J Surg Res 21: 67–76
9. Buckman RF, Hufnagel HV, Olivier G, Buckman D, Zuidema GD (1977) Some effects of Bunnell suture on otherwise uninjured tendons in subhuman primates. Surgery 82: 662–666
10. Bunton RW, Xabregas AA, Miller AP (1990) Pericardial closure after cardiac operations. J Thorac Cardiovasc Surg 100: 99–107
11. Canver CC, Marrin CAS, Plume SK, Nugent WC (1993) Autologous pericardial flap for prevention of reentry injury in cardiac reoperations. Ann Thorac Surg 55: 179–180
12. Clarke-Pearson DL, Soper JT, Creasman WT (1988) Absorbable synthetic mesh (polyglactin 910) for the formation of a pelvic "lid" after radical pelvic resection. Am J Obstet Gynecol 158: 158–161
13. Cliff WJ, Groberty J, Ryan GB (1973) Postoperative pericardial adhesions. The role of mild serosal injury and spilled blood. J Thorac Cardiovasc Surg 65: 744–750
14. Cross JH, De Giovanni JV, Silove ED (1989) Use of streptokinase to aid in the drainage of postoperative pericardial effusion. Br Heart J 62: 217–219
15. Culliford AT, Girdwood RW, Isom OW, Krauss KR, Spencer FC (1979) Angina following myocardial revascularization. J Thorac Cardiovasc Surg 77: 889–895
16. Cunningham JN, Spencer FC, Zeff R, Williams CD, Cukingnan R, Mullin M (1975) Influence of primary closure of the pericardium after open-heart surgery on the frequency of tamponade, postcardiotomy syndrome, and pulmonary complications. J Thorac Cardiovasc Surg 70: 119–125
17. de Virgilio C, Dubrow T, Sheppard BB, MacDonald WD, Nelson RJ, Lesavoy MA, Robertson JM (1990) Fibrin glue inhibits intra-abdominal adhesion formation. Arch Surg 125: 1378–1382
18. diZerega GS, Rodgers KE (1992) The peritoneum. Springer, Berlin Heidelberg, New York
19. diZerega GS (1994) Contemporary adhesion prevention. Fertil Steril 61: 219–235
20. Dobell ARC, Jain AK (1984) Catastrophic hemorrhage during redo sternotomy. Ann Thorac Surg 37: 273–278
21. Doody KJ, Dunn RC, Buttram VC (1989) Recombinant tissue plasminogen activator reduces adhesion formation in a rabbit uterine horn model. Fertil Steril 51: 509–512
22. Drinker CK, Field ME (1931) Absorption from the pericardial cavity. J Exp Med 53: 143

23. Duncan DA, Yaacobi Y, Goldberg EP, Mines M, O'Brien D, Congdon F, Carmichael MJ (1988) Prevention of postoperative pericardial adhesions with hydrophilic polymer solutions. J Surg Res 45: 44–49
24. Ellis H (1982) The causes and prevention of intestinal adhesions. Br J Surg 69: 241–243
25. Eng J, Ravichandran PS, Abbott CR, Kay PH, Murday AJ, Shreiti I (1989) Reoperation after pericardial closure with bovine pericardium. Ann Thorac Surg 48: 813–815
26. English TAH, Milstein BB (1978) Repeat open intracardiac operation. J Thorac Cardiovasc Surg 76: 56–60
27. Fowler JM, Lacey SM, Montz FJ (1991) The inability of Gore Surgical Membrane to inhibit post-radical pelvic surgery adhesions in the dog model. Gynecol Oncol 43: 141–144
28. Franklin R, Ovarian Adhesion Study Group (1995) Reduction of ovarian adhesions by the use of Interceed. Obstet Gynecol 86: 335–340
29. Gabbay S, Guindey AM, Andrews JF, Amato JJ, Seaver P, Khan MY (1989) New outlook on pericardial substitution after open heart operations. Ann Thorac Surg 48: 803–812
30. Gallo JI, Pomar JL, Artinano E, Val F, Duran CMG (1978) Heterologous pericardium for closure of the pericardial defects. Ann Thorac Surg 26: 149–154
31. Gallo JI, Artinano E, Duran CG (1982) Clinical experience with glutaraldehyde preserved heterologous pericardium for the closure of the pericardium after open heart surgery. Thorac Cardiovasc Surg 30: 306–309
32. Gallo JI, Artinano E, Duran CG (1985) Late clinical results with the use of heterologous pericardium for closure of the pericardial cavity. J Thorac Cardiovasc Surg 89: 709–712
33. Gandjbakhch I, Acar C, Cabrol C (1989) Left thoracotomy approach for coronary artery bypass grafting in patients with pericardial adhesions. Ann Thorac Surg 48: 871–873
34. Garrett HE, Matthews J (1989) Reoperative median sternotomy. Ann Thorac Surg 48: 305
35. Gauwerky JFH, Mann J, Bastert G (1990) The effect of fibrin glue and peritoneal grafts in the prevention of intraperitoneal adhesions. Arch Gynecol Obstet 247: 161–166
36. Gervin AS, Jacobs G, Hufnagel HV, Mason KG (1975) Surgical trauma and pericardial fibrinolytic activity. Am Surg 41: 225–229
37. Graves EJ (1995) National Hospital Discharge Survey: annual summary, 1993. National Center for Health Statistics. Vital Health Stat 13(121): 47
38. Hansbrough JF, Dore C, Hansbrough WB (1992) Clinical trials of living dermal tissue replacement placed beneath meshed, split-thickness skin grafts on excised burn wounds. J Burn Care Rehabil 13: 519–529
39. Harada Y, Imai Y, Kurosawa H, Hoshino S, Nakano K (1988) Long term results of the clinical use of an expanded polytetrafluoroethylene surgical membrane as a pericardial substitute. J Thorac Cardiovasc Surg 96: 811–815
40. Heydorn WH, Daniel JS, Wade CE (1987) A new look at pericardial substitutes. J Thorac Cardiovasc Surg 94: 291–296
41. Heydorn WH, Ferraris VA, Berry WR (1988) Pericardial substitutes: a survey. Ann Thorac Surg 46: 567–569
42. Holman WL, Bourge RC, Zorn GL, Brantley LH, Kirklin JK (1993) Use of expanded polytetrafluoroethylene pericardial substitute with ventricular assist devices. Ann Thorac Surg 55: 181–183
43. James DCO, Ellis H, Hugh TB (1965) The effect of streptokinase on experimental intraperitoneal adhesion formation. J Pathol Bacteriol 90: 279–287
44. Jansen RPS (1985) Failure of intraperitoneal adjuncts to improve the outcome of pelvic operations in young women. Am J Obstet Gynecol 153: 363–371
45. Joyce DH, Cichon R, Muralidharan S, Gu J, McGrath LB (1991) Alteration in pericardial adhesion formation following pretreatment with fibrin glue. J Appl Biomat 2: 269–271
46. Knightly JJ, Agostino D, Cliffton EE (1962) The effect of fibrinolysin and heparin on the formation of peritoneal adhesions. Surgery 52: 250–258
47. Laks H, Hammond G, Geha AS (1981) Use of silicone rubber as a pericardial substitute to facilitate operation in cardiac surgery. J Thorac Cardiovasc Surg 82: 88–92
48. Leak LV, Ferrans VJ, Cohen SR, Eidbo EE, Jones M (1987) Animal model of acute pericarditis and its progression to pericardial fibrosis and adhesions: ultrastructural studies. Am J Anat 180: 373–390

49. Lindenberg S, Lauritsen JG (1984) Prevention of peritoneal adhesion formation by fibrin sealant. Ann Chir Gynaecol 73: 11–13
50. Lindenberg S, Steentoft P, Sorensen SS, Olesen HP (1985) Studies on the prevention of intra-abdominal adhesion formation by fibrin sealant. Acta Chir Scand 151: 525–527
51. Loop FD (1984) Catastrophic hemorrhage during sternal reentry. Ann Thorac Surg 37: 271–272
52. Malm T, Bowald S, Bylock A, Busch C (1992) Prevention of postoperative pericardial adhesions by closure of the pericardium with absorbable polymer patches. J Thorac Cardiovasc Surg 104: 600–607
53. Malm T, Bowald S, Bylock A, Saldeen T, Busch C (1992) Regeneration of pericardial tissue on absorbable polymer patches implanted into the pericardial sac. Scand J Thorac Cardiovasc Surg 26: 15–21
54. Mathisen SR, Wu HD, Sauvage LR, Walker MW (1986) Prevention of retrosternal adhesions after pericardiotomy. J Thorac Cardiovasc Surg 92: 92–98
55. Mayer M, Yedgar S, Hurwitz A, Palti Z, Finzi Z, Milwidsky A (1988) Effect of viscous macromolecules on peritoneal plasminogen activator activity: a potential mechanism for their ability to reduce postoperative adhesion formation. Am J Obstet Gynecol 159: 957–963
56. Mazuji MK, Lett JC (1973) Siliconized Dacron as a pericardial patch. Arch Surg 87: 446–449
57. McHenry MC, Longworth DL, Rehm SJ, Keys TF, Moon HK, Cosgrove DM, Loop FD (1988) Infections of the cardiac suture line after left ventricular surgery. Am J Med 85: 292–300
58. Meddings N, Scott R, Bullock R, French DA, Hide TA, Gorham SD (1992) Collagen Vicryl – a new dural prosthesis. Acta Neurochir 117: 53–58
59. Menzies D, Ellis H (1989) Intra-abdominal adhesions and their prevention by topical tissue plasminogen activator. J R Soc Med 82: 534–535
60. Meus PJ, Wernly JA, Campbell CD, Takanishi Y, Pick RL, Zhao-Kun Q, Replogle RL (1983) Long term evaluation of pericardial substitutes. J Thorac Cardiovasc Surg 85: 54–58
61. Milgalter E, Uretzky G, Siberman S, Appelbaum Y, Shimon DV, Kopolovic J, Cohen D, Jonas H, Appelbaum A, Borman JB (1985) Pericardial meshing: an effective method for prevention of pericardial adhesions and epicardial reaction after cardiac operations. J Thorac Cardiovasc Surg 90: 281–286
62. Miller ND, Williams DF (1987) On the biodegradation of poly-B-hydroxybutyrate (PHB) homopolymer and poly-B-hydroxybutyrate-hydroxyvalerate copolymers. Biomaterials 8: 129–137
63. Milligan DW, Raftery AT (1974) Observations on the pathogenesis of peritoneal adhesions: a light and electron microscopical study. Br J Surg 274–280
64. Minale C, Hollweg G, Nikol S, Mittermayer C, Messmer BJ (1987) Closure of pericardium using expanded polytetrafluoroethylene surgical membrane (Gore-SM): clinical experience. Thorac Cardiovasc Surg 35: 312–315
65. Minale C, Nikol S, Hollweg G, Mittermayer C, Messmer BJ (1988) Clinical experience with expanded polytetrafluoroethylene Gore-Tex R surgical membrane for pericardial closure: a study of 110 cases. J Card Surg 3: 193–201
66. Mitchell JD, Lee R, Hodakowski GT, Neya K, Harringer W, Valeri R, Vlahakes GJ (1994) Prevention of postoperative pericardial adhesions with a hyaluronic acid coating solution. J Thorac Cardiovasc Surg 107: 1481–1488
67. Mitchell JD, Lee R, Neya K, Vlahakes GJ (1994) Reduction in experimental adhesions using a hyaluronic acid bioabsorbable membrane. Eur J Cardiothorac Surg 8: 149–152
68. Montz FJ, Fowler J, Wolff A, Lacy SM, Mohler M (1991) The ability of recombinant tissue plasminogen activator to inhibit post-radical pelvic surgery adhesions in the dog model. Am J Obstet Gynecol 165: 1539–1542
69. Montz FJ, Monk BJ, Lacy SM (1992) The Gore-Tex Surgical Membrane: effectiveness as a barrier to inhibit postradical pelvic surgery adhesions in a porcine model. Gynecol Oncol 45: 290–293

70. Montz FJ, Monk BJ, Lacy SM (1993) Effectiveness of two barriers at inhibiting post-radical pelvic surgery adhesions. Gynecol Oncol 48: 247–251
71. Muralidharan S, Gu J, Laub GW, Cichon R, Daloisio C, McGrath LB (1991) A new biological membrane for pericardial closure. J Biomed Mat Res 25: 1201–1209
72. Myhre-Jensen O, Larsen SB, Alstrup T (1969) Fibrinolytic activity in serosal and synovial membranes. Arch Pathol 88: 623–630
73. Nandi P, Leung JSM, Cheung KL (1976) Closure of pericardium after heart surgery. A way to prevent postoperative cardiac tamponade. Br Heart J 38: 1319–1323
74. Nkere UU, Whawell SA, Thompson EM, Thompson JN, Taylor KM (1993) Changes in pericardial morphology and fibrinolytic activity during cardiopulmonary bypass. J Thorac Cardiovasc Surg 106: 339–345
75. Nkere UU, Whawell SA, Sarraf CE, Schofield JB, Thompson JN, Taylor KM (1994) Perioperative histologic and ultrastructural changes in the pericardium and adhesions. Ann Thorac Surg 58: 437–444
76. Nordic Adhesion Prevention Study Group (1995) The efficacy of Interceed (TC7)* for prevention of reformation of postoperative adhesions on ovaries, fallopian tubes and fimbriae in microsurgical operations for fertility: a multicenter study. Fertil Steril 63: 709–714
77. Opie JC, Larrieu AJ, Cornell IS (1987) Pericardial substitutes: delayed reexploration and findings. Ann Thorac Surg 43: 383–385
78. Porter JM, Ball AP, Silver D (1971) Mesothelial fibrinolysis. J Thorac Cardiovasc Surg 62: 725–730
79. Praeger PI, Clauss RH, Reed GE (1989) Lateral pericardiotomy for a safer second operation. Surg Gyn Obstet 168: 363–364
80. Raftery AT (1973) Regeneration of parietal and visceral peritoneum. Br J Surg 60: 293–299
81. Raftery AT (1981) Effect of peritoneal trauma on peritoneal fibrinolytic activity and intraperitoneal adhesion formation. Eur Surg Res 13: 397–401
82. Reikeras O, Nordstrand K, Sorlie D (1987) Use of dextran to prevent pericardial adhesions caused by maize starch powder. Eur Surg Res 19: 62–64
83. Rein MS, Hill JA (1989) 32% Dextran 70 (Hyskon) inhibits lymphocyte and macrophage function in vitro: a potential new mechanism for adhesion prevention. Fertil Steril 52: 953–957
84. Revuelta JM, Garcia-Rinaldi R, Johnston RH, Vaughan GD (1985) Implantation of pericardial substitutes. Ann Thorac Surg 39: 190–191
85. Revuelta J, Garcia-Rinaldi R, Val F, Crego R, Duran C (1985) Expanded polytetra-fluoroethylene surgical membrane for pericardial closure. J Thorac Cardiovasc Surg 89: 451–455
86. Rivkind AI, Lieberman N, Durst AL (1985) Urokinase does not prevent abdominal adhesion formation in rats. Eur Surg Res 17: 254–258
87. Robison RJ, Brown JW, Deschner WP, Highes B, King H (1984) Prevention of pericardial adhesions with dextran 70. Ann Thorac Surg 37: 488–490
88. Rutkow IM (1989) Socioeconomics of surgery. Mosby, St Louis
89. Ryan GB, Groberty J, Majno G (1971) Postoperative peritoneal adhesions. Am J Pathol 65: 117–148
90. Saferstein L, Wolf S, Kamp L, Linsky C, Wiseman D (1992) Process for preparing a neutralized oxidized cellulose product and its method of use. United States Patent no. 5,134,229
91. Segesser L, Jornod N, Faidutti B (1987) Repeat sternotomy after reconstruction of the pericardial sac with glutaraldehyde-preserved equine pericardium. J Thorac Cardiovasc Surg 93: 616–619
92. Sekiba K and the Obstetrics and Gynecology Adhesion Prevention Committee (1992) Use of INTERCEED (TC7) Absorbable Adhesion Barrier to reduce postoperative adhesion reformation in infertility and endometriosis surgery. Obstet Gynecol 79: 518–522
93. Spotnitz WD, Dalton S, Baker JW, Nolan SP (1987) Reduction of perioperative hemor-rhage by anterior mediastinal spray application of fibrin glue during cardiac operations. Ann Thorac Surg 44: 529–531

94. Schwartz L, Diamond M (1991) Formation, reduction and treatment of adhesive disease. Semin Reprod Med 9: 89–99
95. Smith LO (1968) Prevention of surgically induced pericardial adhesions with combined dexamethasone and promethazine therapy. J Fla Med Assoc 55: 413–417
96. Tangen O, Wik KO, Almqvist IAM, Arfors AE, Hint HC (1972) Effects of dextran on the structure and plasmin-induced lysis of human fibrin. Thromb Res 1: 487–492
97. Toty L, Bakdach H, Personne C (1984) Réparation des pertes de substance de la paroi thoracique et du péricarde par un filet en matière résorbable préfabriqué. Ann Chir 38: 109–112
98. Vander Salm TJ, Okike ON, Marsicano TH, Compton C, Espinoza E (1986) Prevention of postoperative pericardial adhesions. Arch Surg 121: 462–467
99. Vincent JG, Skotnicki SH, van der Meer JJ, Kubat K (1987) Resorbable suture support for ventricular aneurysmectomy. J Thorac Cardiovasc Surg 94: 430–433
100. Weiss M, Honinger J, Belhaj M, Binet JP (1984) Etude expérimentale de quelques substituts péricardiques. Ann Chir 38: 180–187
101. Wiseman DM (1994) Polymers for the prevention of surgical adhesions. In: Domb AJ (ed) Site specific pharmacotherapy. Wiley, Chichester, pp 420–421
102. Wiseman DM, Gottlick LE, Diamond MP (1992) Effect of thrombin-induced hemostasis on the efficacy of an absorbable adhesion barrier. J Reprod Med 37: 766–770
103. Wiseman DM, Kamp L, Linsky CB, Jochen RF, Pang RHL, Scholz P (1992) Fibrinolytic drugs prevent pericardial adhesions in the rabbit. J Surg Res 53: 362–368
104. Wiseman DM, Kamp LF, Saferstein L, Linsky CB, Gottlick LE, Diamond MP (1993) Improving the efficacy of INTERCEED barrier in the presence of blood using thrombin, heparin or a blood insensitive barrier, modified INTERCEED (nTC7). In: Diamond MP, diZerega GS, Linsky CB, Reid RL (eds) Gynecologic surgery and adhesion prevention. Wiley-Liss, New York, pp 205–212
105. Yaacobi Y, Goldberg EP, Kaelin D, Bailey J, Staples M, Seeger J, Duncan DA, Carmichael MJ, Pathangey B, Normann S, Burns JW (1989) Surgical adhesions of the pericardium: prevention by hydrophilic polymer solutions in a canine model. J Invest Surg 2: 320
106. Youmans CR, White J, Derrick JR (1968) The prevention of pleural and pericardial adhesions with silastic. J Thorac Cardiovasc Surg 55: 383–388

8.3 Intra-abdominal Complications in Peritoneal Dialysis with Special Reference to Peritoneal Fibrosis

H. Schmitt, B. Hermanns, W. Boeckmann, S. Drube, and H.G. Sieberth

Introduction

Nature did not create the peritoneum as a dialysis membrane; in recent years, however, it is frequently used in this therapeutic indication. The breakthrough of peritoneal dialysis as a standard renal replacement therapy occurred with the introduction of continuous ambulatory peritoneal dialysis (CAPD)[1]. First introduced by Popovich and colleagues in 1976, this concept of equilibrium dialysis allows adequate removal of uremic toxins [1, 2]. Since that time, a rapid increase of ambulatory peritoneal dialysis has been registered worldwide. At the end of 1994, the number of patients worldwide reached 100 000, with an estimated further annual growth rate of 10%–15%. The proportion of dialysis patients maintained on chronic peritoneal dialysis shows considerable variation between different countries, ranging from 2% in Portugal to nearly 50% in the United Kingdom (Germany 9%, USA 17%, Scandinavia more than 30%).

The overall treatment success of peritoneal dialysis is quite similar to hemodialysis [3–5]. Adjusting for comorbidity as an independent risk factor, Maiorca and coworkers [5] did not find any difference in the patient survival rate when comparing peritoneal dialysis and hemodialysis in a large population. After a follow-up of 4 years, the overall technique survival rate of peritoneal dialysis, however, proved to be significantly lower (more than 20%) than on hemodialysis. This points to some specific problems of peritoneal dialysis, which seem to be related to the durability of the peritoneum as a dialysis membrane.

Four major types of intra-abdominal complications can be differentiated in peritoneal dialysis:

1. Catheter complications
2. Noninfectious complications mainly resulting from the increased intra-abdominal pressure due to the instillation of dialysate
3. Peritonitis caused by infectious microorganisms
4. Peritoneal fibrosis and sclerosing peritonitis

Catheter Complications

Catheter-related complications include exit site and tunnel infection, usually caused by *Staphylococcus aureus*, external cuff extrusion, pericatheter dialysate leakage, catheter obstruction, tip migration, peritonitis, and infusion pain [6]. In addition to the classical straight Tenckhoff catheter, some other types of double-cuff peritoneal catheters have been introduced, e.g., the Toronto Western Hospital and the swan-neck Missouri catheter, which are predominantly used with a coiled intraperitoneal segment, designed to prevent tip migration and reduce infusion pain. There is no proven difference in the overall technical survival rates of straight and coiled peritoneal catheters.

The management of catheter problems varies according to the cause and the clinical presentation [6, 7]. Tunnel infection (Fig. 1) can be easily diagnosed either clinically or by ultrasound. Early catheter removal is required in this situation. Pericatheter dialysate leaks usually occur immediately or early after starting CAPD. The best method to localize such leaks is computed tomography (CT) scan with intraperitoneal contrast application, which leads to an extravasation within the abdominal wall. A temporary discontinuation of peritoneal dialysis for 10–14 days is the appropriate management of this complication. Some other forms of catheter malfunction have been reported. Obstruction can be caused by blood or fibrin clots, kinking, adhesions, omental wrapping, and constipation or bowel loops. The treatment of these complications may be very simple, such as use of laxatives or rinsing with heparin; in some cases, however, an open surgical procedure is required (omentectomy, correction or removal of the catheter). The optimum dialysate drainage is provided with the catheter tip in the true pelvis, which is achieved with the intraperitoneal segment in a strictly craniocaudal direction. If the catheter tip translocates to the left upper abdomen (Fig. 1), the peristaltic movement of the descending colon may restore the correct position; however, a tip dislocation to the right upper abdomen usually does not return to the original position spontaneously [6]. Occasionally, a radiologically controlled reposition procedure using a guide wire may be successful. It should finally be emphasized that a malpositioned, but well-functioning catheter does not need special treatment.

Noninfectious Complications

Several noninfectious complications of peritoneal dialysis result from increased intra-abdominal pressure, which is a consequence of the instillation of dialysate into the peritoneal cavity. Up to 10% of CAPD patients may develop hernias during a 5-year follow-up [8]. Many types of hernias have been described in the literature, the most common being inguinal, umbilical, and catheter insertion (Fig. 1). These all represent sites of structural weakness, particularly under the influence of constantly elevated intra-abdominal pressure. Hernias should be repaired surgically; following operation, the patients can be managed on peritoneal dialysis with low fill volumes or may be transferred to hemodialysis for 3–4 weeks.

Major noninfectious complications other than direct hernias include genital edema and hydrothorax [8]. Recent reports suggest that up to 5% of all male CAPD patients might experience genital edema. This complication has been attributed to different pathogenetic mechanisms. First, the dialysate can flow

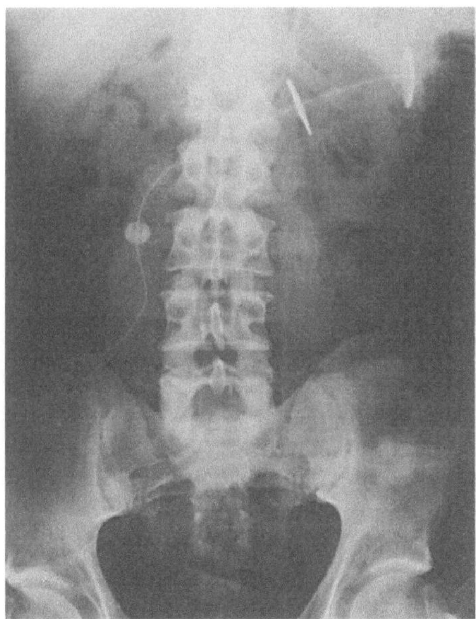

Fig. 1a–c. Complications in peritoneal dialysis related to the catheter and elevated intra-abdominal pressure. **a** Catheter dislocation. **b** Tunnel infection with cutaneous fistula. **c** Umbilical hernia

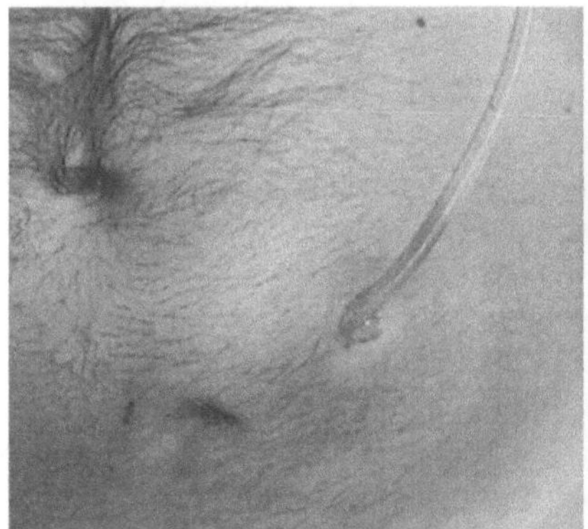

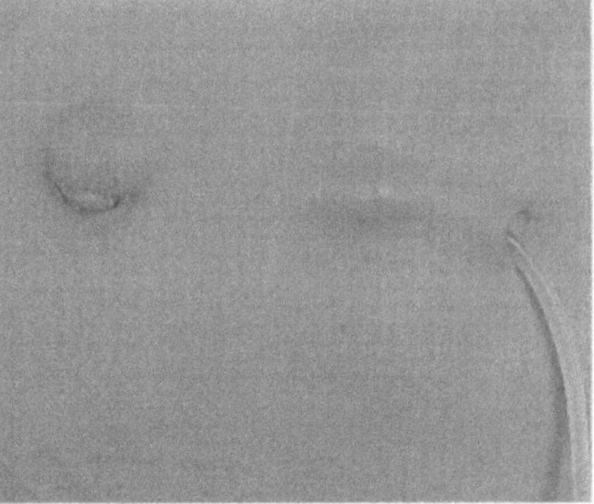

through a patent vaginal process into the scrotum, where it can penetrate into the surrounding tissue. Second, through defects of the peritoneum at the catheter incision site, the dialysis fluid may enter the anterior abdominal wall and move downwards to produce genital edema. Small leaks should be treated conservatively, applying methods to lower intra-abdominal pressure, such as small-volume dialysis in the supine position or transient discontinuation of peritoneal dialysis for several weeks. Persisting edema requires surgical correction.

The development of a large pleural effusion is an uncommon, but well-known complication of peritoneal dialysis. Its true incidence is about 1.5%, with women being predominantly affected. The pathogenesis of peritoneal dialysis related hydrothorax, which is usually located in the right pleural cavity, has not been fully elucidated. Small diaphragmatic lesions leading to a direct pleuroperitoneal communication are postulated and have been confirmed during operation and by autopsy findings in some cases. Besides a temporary or even permanent discontinuation of peritoneal dialysis, different therapeutic strategies have been recommended, such as pleurodesis with tetracycline, fibrin adhesive, or autologous blood. If recurrence is observed, surgery or even termination of peritoneal dialysis is indicated.

Peritonitis Caused by Infectious Microorganisms

The development and widespread acceptance of CAPD as a standard dialysis technique used to be affected by the high incidence of peritonitis, the most common complication of peritoneal dialysis [9, 10]. Changes in the connecting systems and the improved clinical management of peritoneal dialysis patients have significantly decreased the risk of peritonitis, which is now observed at an average rate of one episode per 24 treatment months. Typical routes of infection are transluminal or periluminal – related to the catheter – and transmural from the intestinal tract. Occasionally, other sources of endogenous infection have also been reported, such as hematogenic or ascending from the genital tract in women. A variety of microorganisms, predominantly gram-positive strains (staphylococci), were isolated in CAPD peritonitis, and numerous different treatment protocols have been established.

A standardized approach in patients presumed to have CAPD peritonitis was first published in 1987 and updated in 1993 [9]. Cloudy effluent and abdominal pain are the earliest clinical signs. The initial diagnostic evaluation should include dialysate cell count, gram stain, and culture. A gram stain is particularly helpful in the early recognition of fungal peritonitis, which frequently requires early catheter removal. The first choice of antibiotics is vancomycin with an additional cephalosporin or aminoglycoside, if clinically indicated. This combination is administered intraperitoneally and provides good protection against most causative microorganisms, since no reliable microbiological information is usually available at the start of therapy. This treatment regimen sometimes has to be modified after 24–48 h, depending on the culture results and the sensitivity testing. If *Staphylococcus aureus* has been identified and the clinical condition does not improve, rifampicin should be added. If culture reveals gram-negative or multiple organisms, including anaerobic bacteria, other sources of intra-abdominal pathology necessitating surgical exploration, e.g., diverticulitis, should be seriously considered. *Pseudomonas* or *Xanthomonas* peritonitis is extremely difficult to cure, particularly when it develops as a consequence of catheter infection. Therefore, consideration of early catheter removal is important to preserve long-term peritoneal membrane function for dialysis.

In general, clinically relevant adhesion formation is not observed following mild to moderate CAPD peritonitis. However, significant adhesion formation may occur during severe episodes of peritonitis due to *Staphylococcus aureus*, *Pseudomonas*, or other gram-negative strains, and particularly as a result of fungal infections. In this situation, peritoneal dialysis cannot be continued, because of inadequate clearance rates and loss of ultrafiltration. In addition to catheter problems, peritonitis and its sequelae, such as loss of ultrafiltration and loss of peritoneal cavity, remain the most important reasons for technical failure in CAPD [11, 12]. This is still true today, although the incidence of peritonitis has decreased significantly during the past 10 years.

Peritoneal Fibrosis and Sclerosing Peritonitis

Based on the findings from the peritoneal biopsy registry, Dobbie [13–15] contributed a great deal to our understanding of peritoneal fibrosis and developed his concept of different stages in this process as follows:

1. Opacification of the serosa
2. "Tanned" peritoneum
3. Mural fibrosis
4. Sclerosing encapsulating peritonitis

Compared to healthy individuals, the uremic peritoneum shows distinctive ultrastructural abnormalities prior to the onset of peritoneal dialysis. By transmission electron microscopy, Dobbie [13] revealed filamentous intracytoplasmic inclusions in the mesothelium, which can finally lead to a detachment of these cells from the basement membrane. In patients undergoing continuous peritoneal dialysis, additional reactive changes of the mesothelial surface have been reported [13–15], including a decrease in the number of microvilli and pinocytotic vesicles, hyperplasia of the rough endoplasmic reticulum, degenerative changes in mitochondria (mitochondrial pyknosis and intracristal swelling), alterations of the ground substance, and deposition of collagen fibers in the submesothelium. Biopsies obtained during severe episodes of peritonitis are characterized by morphological signs of acute inflammation such as fibrin exsudation, infiltration of polymorphonuclear leukocytes, and dilated capillaries. If the patient does not recover quickly, the inflammatory process may finally lead to a loss of mesothelial surface and increased collagen formation in the almost acellular submesothelial tissue. So-called diabetiform lesions such as basement membrane reduplication of the mesothelium itself and the stromal blood vessels have been observed in both diabetic and nondiabetic uremic patients on peritoneal dialysis [13, 16]. Nonenzymatic glycosylation of structural proteins is most likely the underlying pathogenetic mechanism. According to Dobbie [13], these findings are clearly associated with a history of multiple and severe episodes of peritoneal inflammation. During and shortly after peritonitis – with a transient loss of mesothelial surface – the submesothelial tissue is directly exposed to the high dialysate glucose concentrations. Based on these observations, Dobbie developed his concept that frequency and severity of peritonitis on the one hand and the nonphysiological composition of the dialysis fluid (high osmolality, low pH) on the other hand promote the process of peritoneal dialysis-related peritoneal fibrosis, which shows a wide range of morphological alterations, from opacification of the serosa, to sclerosing encapsulating peritonitis [13–15, 17].

Figures 2–4 illustrate the case of a 48-year-old man who started with peritoneal dialysis in 1991 and had not had a previous episode of peritonitis. The main dialysis problem was a slowly progressive loss of ultrafiltration. Following a few days of diarrhea, he was admitted to hospital in June 1995 with severe fungal peritonitis due to *Candida parapsilosis*, identified in the dialysate and stool culture. Despite systemic antifungal treatment (amphotericin B, flucytosine) and early catheter removal, the patient died a few days later from multiple organ failure. At autopsy "tanned" peritoneum syndrome was diagnosed.

Figure 5 depicts the X-ray findings of a 41-year-old woman who started with CAPD in 1993. Within 2 years she suffered several episodes of bacterial peritonitis (*S. aureus* and *S. epidermidis* as causative microorganisms). A gradual decrease of ultrafiltration was subsequently observed, followed by inadequate removal of uremic toxins. The peritoneal equilibration test (PET) exhibited very low rates for peritoneal transport of small solutes. A significant thickening

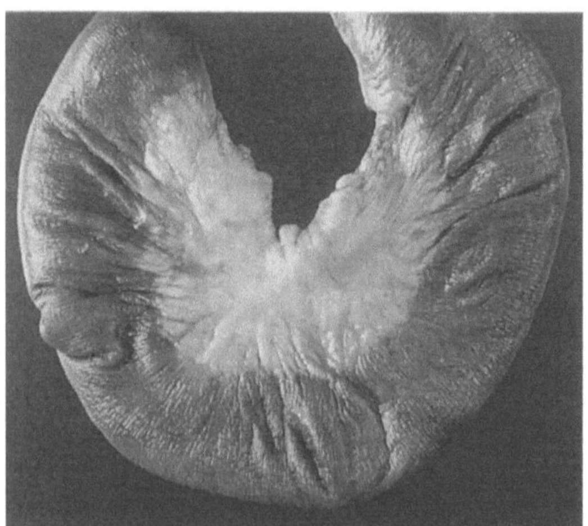

a

Fig. 2a,b. Macroscopic appearance of tanned peritoneum; leathery thickening of the peritoneal membrane which is dry, wrinkled, and light brown in colour

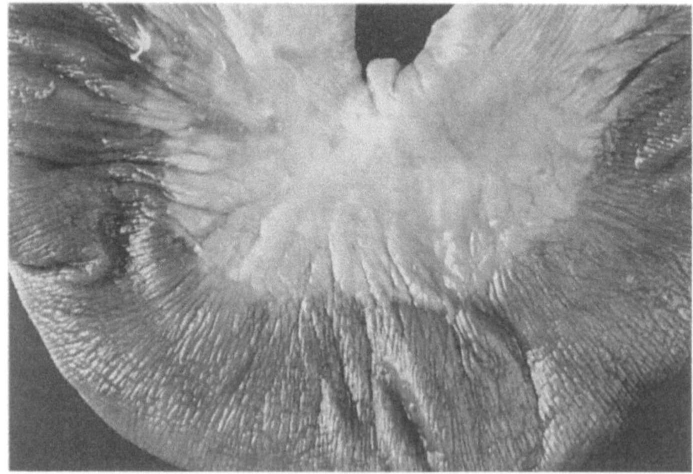

b

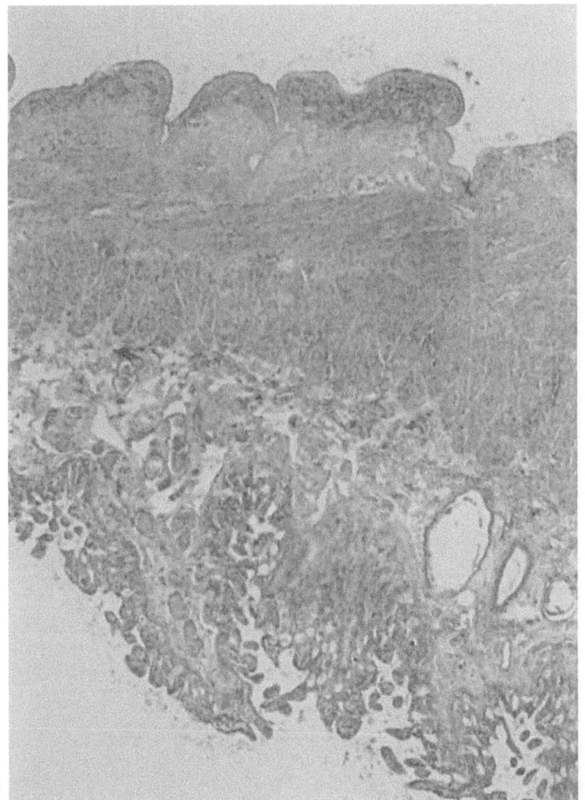
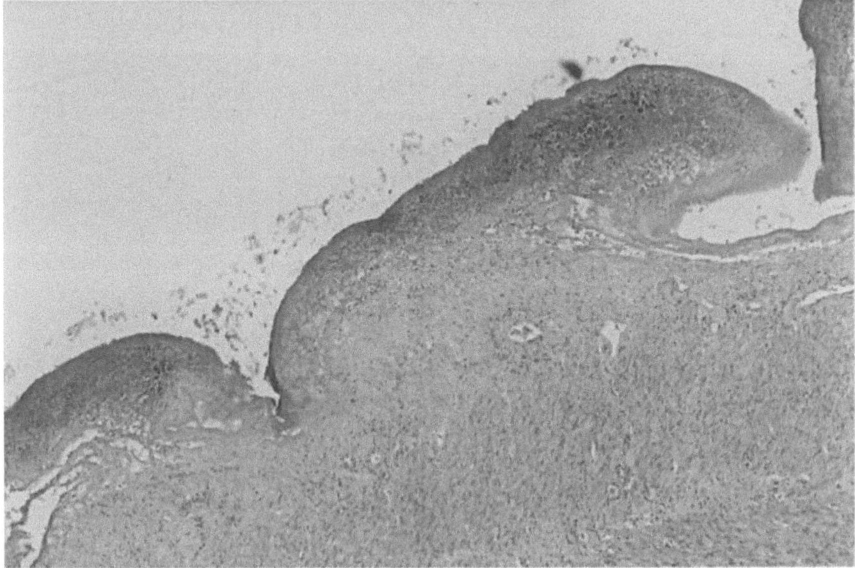

Fig. 3a,b. Light microscopy findings in tanned peritoneum; replacement of the mesothelial surface by a layer of dense fibrous connective tissue; nonspecific mononuclear infiltrate in the submesothelial area

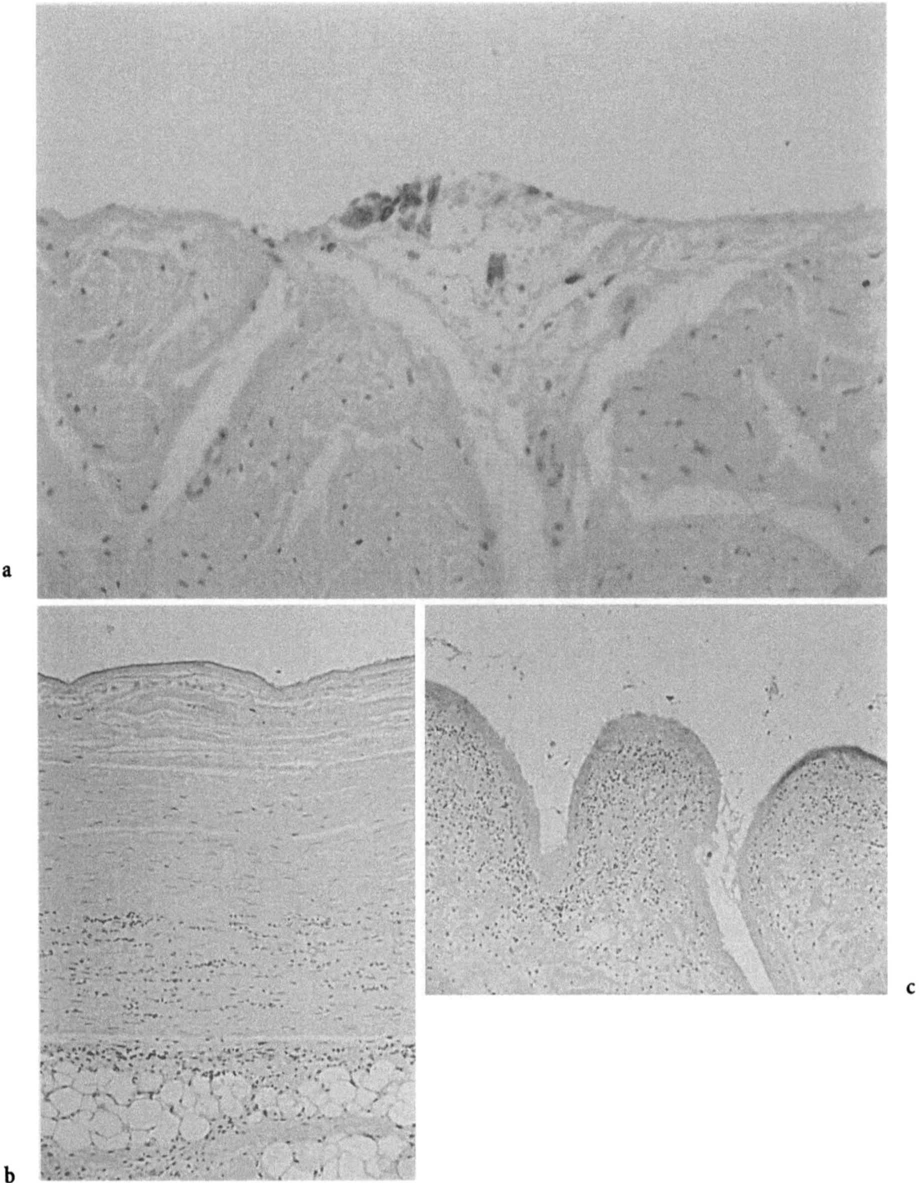

Fig. 4a–c. Immunohistochemical staining for cytokeratin in tanned peritoneum **a** Focally, a positive reaction is found in superficial cells. **b,c** The major part of the surface layer, however, remains negative, indicating the total destruction of the mesothelium

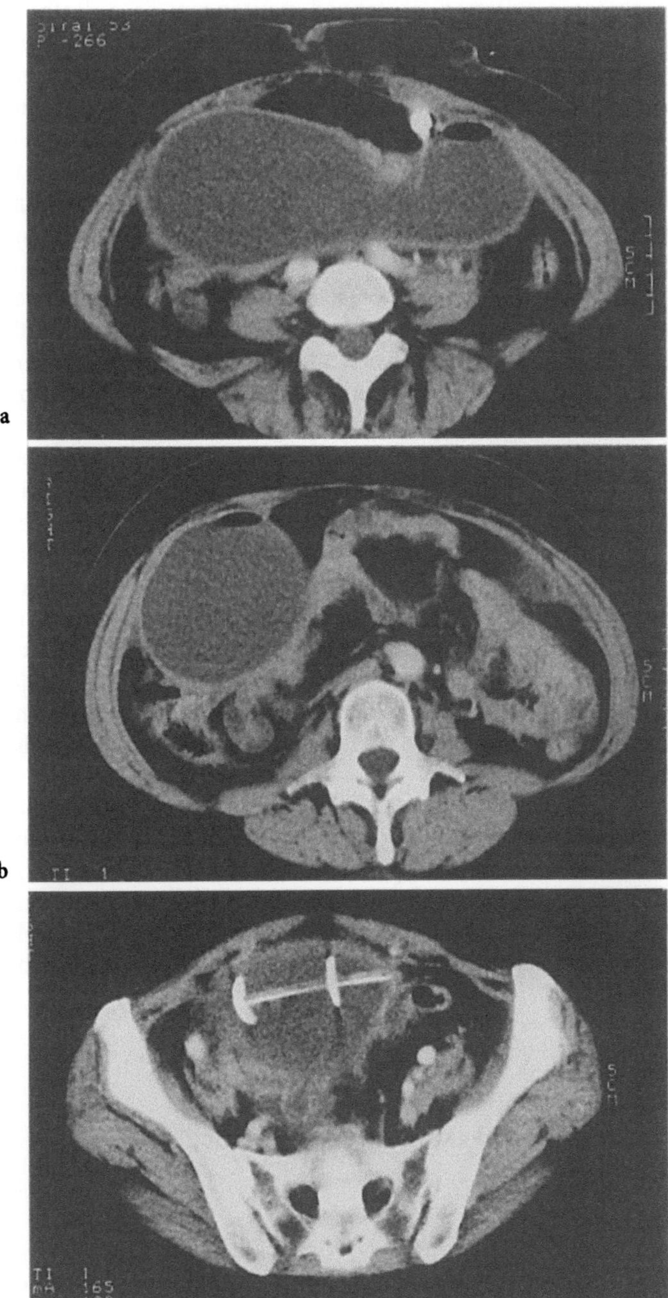

Fig. 5a–c. Abdominal computed tomography (CT) scan in severe peritoneal fibrosis, showing a significant thickening of the peritoneal membrane and formation of several compartments within the peritoneal cavity as a consequence of recurrent peritonitis

and condensation of the peritoneal membrane with concomitant reduction of the effective surface was seen on abdominal CT scan [18].

The typical macroscopic criterion of tanned peritoneum is a leathery thickening of the peritoneal membrane, which appears dry, wrinkled, and light brown in colour. On light microscopy, the mesothelium is replaced by connective tissue consisting of hyalinized collagen fibers with a striking acellularity, which was termed "cellular desert" by Dobbie [13, 14]. In addition, a nonspecific mononuclear cellular infiltrate is usually observed; calcification is another common finding in peritoneal fibrosis [19, 20]. The tanned peritoneum syndrome is predominantly seen in patients maintained on peritoneal dialysis for a considerable number of years.

Primary nonspecific inflammatory peritoneal reactions may have fatal sequelae for the long-term function of the peritoneal membrane in dialysis. With time, the dialysate itself and bacterial exo- or endotoxins may mediate a persistent damage of the peritoneum. If early healing occurs, a complete remission can be achieved. Delayed healing, however is accompanied by structural changes, which may be progressive and result in peritoneal fibrosis and new membrane formation [13, 14]. This process of fibrogenesis subsequently proceeds to an aggressive form of mural fibrosis. The term most frequently used for this disease is sclerosing encapsulating peritonitis [21–29]. Loss of ultrafiltration, vomiting, and recurrent small-bowel obstruction are the main clinical symptoms in these patients, who have a poor prognosis (mortality rate at least 50%). Surgical treatment is not recommended because of lacking efficacy and a high rate of severe postoperative complications. A recent report [30] suggesting the application of azathioprine and prednisone has not been confirmed so far. The majority of patients are transferred to hemodialysis, but the disease may nevertheless progress.

The local synthesis and secretion of interleukin-1 in the peritoneal cavity and a prolonged stimulation of mesothelial stem cells with consecutively increased collagen formation have been supposed to be important factors in the pathogenesis of peritoneal fibrosis, finally leading to sclerosing peritonitis [31, 32]. The etiology of this rare disease, however, remains unknown. Multiple causes which probably act simultaneously have been suggested and can be summarized as follows:

- Recurrent or severe peritonitis
- Acetate-containing dialysate
- Hypertonicity and low pH of the dialysate
- Contamination of the peritoneal cavity with chlorhexidine
- Plastic particles
- Beta blockers
- Formaldehyde

It seems likely that frequent episodes of peritonitis and the composition of the dialysate as well as the permanent and long-term exposure of the peritoneum to this nonphysiological solution play a key role, described by the term "bioincompatibility", and this points to the necessity for the development of alternative dialysis solutions [33, 34].

Summary

Four major types of intra-abdominal complications can be differentiated in peritoneal dialysis (PD):

1. Catheter complications include exit site and tunnel infection (usually caused by *Staphylococcus aureus*), pericatheter dialysate leakage, catheter obstruction due to kinking, fibrin clots or omental wrapping, and catheter tip migration. The management of these malfunctions varies according to the cause and the clinical presentation.

2. Several non-infectious complications of PD result form the instillation of dialysate into the peritoneal cavity: inguinal and umbilical hernias, genital edema, and hydrothorax via small defects in the diaphragm. These problems frequently require surgical repair or even termination of PD treatment.

3. In the past, the development and widespread acceptance of PD as a standard dialysis technique were affected by the high incidence of peritonitis. Changes in the connecting systems and the improved clinical management of this complication have led to a dramatic reduction in the risk of peritonitis, which nowadays occurs at an average rate of one episode per 24 treatment months. Adhesions are usually not observed following a mild to moderate PD peritonitis. However, significant adhesion formation with consecutive reduction of the effective peritoneal surface area may develop during severe episodes of peritonitis due to *Staphylococcus aureus*, pseudomonas or other Gram-negative bacteria and particularly as a result of fungal infections. In this situation PD cannot be continued because of inadequate clearance rates and loss of ultrafiltration. Faecal peritonitis due to direct perforation of the gut is a rare situation only seen during the treatment of acute renal failure using stilette catheters.

4. Peritoneal fibrosis: compared with healthy individuals the uremic peritoneum shows distinctive ultrastructural abnormalities. By transmission electron microscopy Dobbie et al. [13] revealed filamentous intracytoplasmic inclusions in the mesothelium, which can finally lead to a detachment of these cells from the basement membrane. In patients undergoing continuous PD, additional reactive changes in the mesothelial surface have been reported: e.g. decrease in the number of microvilli and pinocytotic vesicles, hyperplasia of the rough endoplasmic reticulum, alterations in the ground substance and deposition of collagen fibres in the submesothelium. Multiple and severe episodes of peritonitis are associated with morphological signs of basement membrane reduplication (diabetiform pathology), also seen in non-diabetic uremic subjects. These findings can be explained by non-enzymatic glycosylation of structural proteins in the submesothelial tissue. During and shortly after peritonitis (temporary loss of mesothelial surface), this area is exposed to the high dialysate glucose concentrations.

PD-related peritoneal fibrosis shows a wide range of morphological lesions, from opacification of the serosa to massive fibrosis. A thickened leathery appearance of the peritoneal membrane, called the "tanned" peritoneum has been described by Dobbie [14]. This syndrome is predominantly seen in patients maintained on PD for a considerable number of years. Upon light microscopy the mesothelium is replaced by collagen fibres. Subsequently, this process may proceed to an aggressive form of mural fibrosis, finally leading to signs of bowel obstruction. The clinical term most frequently used for this disease is sclerosing encapsulating peritonitis. Loss of ultrafiltration is the main symptom in these patients. A local synthesis and secretion of interleukin-1 in the peritoneal cavity and an increased production of collagen have been proposed to be important pathogenetic factors. The etiology of this rare disease, however, remains unknown. It seems obvious that the composition of the dialysate ("bioincompatibility") as well as the permanent and long-term exposition play key roles.

References

1. Popovich RP, Moncrief JW, Decherd JF, Bomar JB, Pyle WK (1976) The definition of a novel portable/wearable equilibrium dialysis technique. Trans Am Soc Artif Int Organs 5: 64
2. Popovich RP, Moncrief JW, Nolph KD, Ghods AJ, Twardowski ZJ, Pyle WK (1978) Continuous ambulatory peritoneal dialysis. Ann Int Med 88: 449–456
3. Serkes KD, Blagg CR, Nolph KD, Vonesh EF, Shapiro F (1990) Comparison of patients and technique survival in CAPD and hemodialysis: a multicenter study. Perit Dial Int 10: 15–19
4. Burton PR, Walls J (1987) Selection-adjusted comparison of life expectancy of patients on CAPD, hemodialysis, and renal transplantation. Lancet 2: 1115–1119
5. Maiorca R, Vonesh EF, Cavalli PL, De Vecchi A et al. (1991) A multicenter, selection-adjusted comparison of patient and technique survivals on CAPD and hemodialysis. Perit Dial Int 11: 118–127
6. Twardowski ZJ, Khanna R (1994) Peritoneal dialysis access and exit site care. In: Gokal R, Nolph KD (eds) The textbook of peritoneal dialysis, 1st edn. Kluwer, Dordrecht, pp 271–314
7. Gokal R, Ash SR, Helfrich GB, Holmes CJ et al. (1993) Peritoneal catheters and exit site practices: toward optimum peritoneal access. Perit Dial Int 13: 29–39
8. Bargman JM (1994) Noninfectious complications of peritoneal dialysis. In: Gokal R, Nolph KD (eds) The textbook of peritoneal dialysis, 1st edn. Kluwer, Dordrecht, pp 555–590
9. Keane WF, Everett ED, Golper TA, Gokal R et al. (1993) Peritoneal dialysis-related peritonitis treatment recommendations: 1993 update. The ad hoc advisory committee on peritonitis management. Perit Dial Int 13: 14–28
10. Piraino B, Bernardini J, Holley JL, Perlmutter JA (1993) A comparison of peritoneal dialysis related-infections in short- and long-term peritoneal dialysis patients. Perit Dial Int 13: 194–197
11. Gokal R, Jakubowski C, King J et al. (1987) Outcome in patients on CAPD and hemodialysis: 4-year analysis of a prospective multi-center study. Lancet 2: 1105–1109
12. Piraino B, Bernardini J, Sorkin M (1989) Catheter infections as a factor in the transfer of CAPD patients to hemodialysis. Am J Kidney Dis 13: 365–369
13. Dobbie JW (1994) Ultrastructure and pathology of the peritoneum in peritoneal dialysis. In: Gokal R, Nolph KD (eds) The textbook of peritoneal dialysis, 1st edn. Kluwer, Dordrecht, pp 17–44
14. Dobbie JW (1992) Pathogenesis of peritoneal fibrosing syndromes (sclerosing peritonitis) in peritoneal dialysis. Perit Dial Int 12: 14–27
15. Dobbie JW (1990) New concepts in molecular biology and ultrastructural pathology of the peritoneum: their significance for peritoneal dialysis. Am J Kidney Dis 15: 97–109
16. Di Paolo N, Sacchi G (1989) Peritoneal vascular changes in CAPD. An in vivo model for the study of diabetic microangiopathy. Perit Dial Int 9: 41–45
17. Rubin J, Herrera GA, Collins D (1991) An autopsy study of the peritoneal cavity from patients on CAPD. Am J Kidney Dis 18: 97–102

18. Korzets A, Korzets Z, Peer G et al. (1988) Sclerosing peritonitis. Possible early diagnosis by computerized tomography of the abdomen. Am J Nephrol 8: 143–146
19. Marichal JF, Faller B, Brignon P, Wagner D, Straub P (1987) Progressive calcifying peritonitis: a new complication of CAPD? Nephron 45: 229–232
20. Cox SV, Lai J, Suranyi M, Walker N (1992) Sclerosing peritonitis with gross peritoneal calcification: a case report. Am J Kidney Dis 20: 637–642
21. Clark C, Terris R (1983) Sclerosing peritonitis associated with metoprolol. Lancet 1: 937
22. Grefberg N, Nilsson P, Andreen T (1983) Sclerosing obstructive peritonitis, beta-blockers, and CAPD. Lancet 2: 733–734
23. Bradley J, McWhinnie D, Hamilton D et al. (1983) Sclerosing obstructive peritonitis after CAPD. Lancet 2: 113–114
24. Oreopoulos D, Khanna R, Wu G (1983) Sclerosing obstructive peritonitis after CAPD. Lancet 2: 409
25. Hauglustaine D, van Meerbeek J, Monballyu J, Goddeeris P et al. (1984) Sclerosing peritonitis with mural fibrosis in a patient on long-term CAPD. Clin Nephrol 22: 158–162
26. Ing T, Daugirdas J, Gandhi V (1984) Peritoneal sclerosis in peritoneal dialysis patients. Am J Nephrol 4: 173–176
27. Campbell S, Clarke P, Hawley C, Wigan M et al. (1994) Sclerosing peritonitis: identification of diagnostic, clinical, and radiological features. Am J Kidney Dis 24: 819–825
28. Krediet RT, Struijk DG, Boeschoten EW, Koomen GCM et al. (1989) The time course of peritoneal transport kinetics in CAPD patients who develop sclerosing peritonitis. Am J Kidney Dis 13: 299–307
29. Bowers VD, Ackermann JR, Richardson W, Carey LC (1994) Sclerosing peritonitis. Clin Transpl 8: 369–372
30. Junor BJ, McMillan MA (1993) Immunosuppression in sclerosing peritonitis. Adv Perit Dial 9: 187–189
31. Shaldon S, Koch KM, Quellhorst E, Dinarello CA (1984) Pathogenesis of sclerosing peritonitis in CAPD. Trans Am Soc Artif Intern Organs 30: 193–194
32. Fracasso A, Calo L, Landini S, Morachiello P et al. (1993) Peritoneal sclerosis: role of plasticizers in stimulating interleukin-1 production. Perit Dial Int 13, Suppl 2: S517–S519
33. Wieczorowska K, Khanna R, Moore HL, Nolph KD, Twardowski ZJ (1995) Rat model of peritoneal fibrosis: preliminary observations. Adv Perit Dial 11: 48–51
34. Suzuki K, Khanna R, Nolph KD, Moore HL, Twardowski ZJ (1995) Spontaneous peritonitis and peritoneal fibrosis in rats on peritoneal dialysis for 9 weeks. Adv Perit Dial 11: 52–56

9 Treatment of Peritoneal Adhesions

9.1 Indications and Therapeutic Strategy for Intestinal Obstruction Due to Intra-abdominal Adhesions

U. Schöffel, W. Sendt, R. Häring, and E.H. Farthmann

Incidence

It is commonly reported that 3%–4% of all laparotomies are performed for intestinal obstruction. It has also been suggested that an increase in inguinal hernia repair during the last few decades, leading to a decrease in obstructions secondary to hernia, along with increasing numbers of elective abdominal surgery has led to the net effect that intestinal obstruction now is primarily caused by intra-abdominal adhesions [4].

By looking at series of operations for intestinal obstruction, the actual role of intra-abdominal adhesions become apparent (Table 1). If a series combines both large- and small-bowel obstructions, about 40% are caused by intra-abdominal adhesions. If only small-bowel obstructions are evaluated, the rate increases to 70%.

In our own series of about 5000 laparotomies since 1991, 64 out of 171 cases (37.4%) operated on for intestinal obstruction were caused by adhesions. Most occurred in the group with prior abdominal operations ($n=60$), from which 11 were classified as early (within 4 weeks) and 49 as late postoperative. Within the group of 28 obstructions without prior celiotomy, only four cases resulted from adhesions. These were classified as "spontaneous."

Table 1. Intestinal obstructions secondary to adhesions

Reference	Total cases(n)	Adhesions (%)
Large and small bowel		
Nemir 1952 [12]	430	30
Bevan 1984 [1]	277	38
McEntee et al. 1987 [8]	228	32
Menzies and Ellis 1990 [9]	359	41
Füzün et al. 1991 [5]	582	44
Own series 1995	171	37
Small bowel only		
Playforth et al. 1970 [14]	111	54
Laws and Aldrete 1976 [7]	465	69
Stewardson et al. 1978 [17]	238	64
Bizer et al. 1981 [2]	405	74

Modified from [10].

Concerning bowel obstruction in cancer patients, a recent study reported on 61 patients in whom there was no relation to cancer in 28%. Obstruction was due to adhesions in only 17% [19].

With regard to the postoperative situation, repeat laparotomy rates range from 0.7% to 7.4%. These numbers include repeat laparotomies for early intestinal obstruction which become necessary after 0.2%–1.4% of all laparotomies and account for 20%–30% of all repeat laparotomies. If we presume that early postoperative adhesions are present to some degree in virtually all cases, it can be concluded that these adhesions lead to early complications in 0.2%–1.4% of cases.

Late postoperative adhesions are present in about 70%–90% of all patients as reported in a postmortem analysis [20] and in a study in surgical patients [9]. These adhesions eventually require reintervention in up to 3% of cases.

The incidence of early postoperative small-bowel obstruction certainly depends on the extent of surgical intervention. Operations involving extensive handling of the bowel generally result in higher obstruction rates. Following hepatobiliary surgery, obstruction rates of 0.1% and 0.06% have been reported. Bowel surgery led to obstructive complications in 1.8% and 2.34% of cases, respectively [21, 18]. Interestingly, in the latter series there was no difference between resections and nonresective interventions within the small-bowel group. Explorative laparotomies led to early obstruction in about 1% of cases in both studies. The overall obstruction rates were 0.8% and 0.69%, respectively.

Etiology

Intra-abdominal adhesions result from a variety of mechanisms injuring or irritating the peritoneum. Mechanical damage to the serosal lining, intra-abdominal infections, tissue necrosis, and intra-abdominal foreign material may play the initiating role. The pathophysiological mechanisms leading to adhesion formation and attempts to grade adhesions are dealt with in Chap. 4.

The term early postoperative intestinal obstruction may well be used synonymously with intra-abdominal adhesions, since other possible causes (anastomotic swelling, internal hernia, intussusception, ischemic stenosis) do not account for more than 10% of all cases. In the late postoperative period, however, obstruction is due to adhesions in about one half of the cases. In our own series of 132 late postoperative obstructions, tumors were the leading cause (n=58) followed by adhesions (n=49), inflammation (n=16), radiation injury (n=4), and hernia (n=1).

Diagnosis

Concerning the diagnosis, there is nothing pathognomonic about any intestinal obstruction (secondary to adhesions or other causes). Consequently, the diagnosis is based on very simple techniques; it requires a thorough history, physical examination, and simple imaging procedures.

Diagnostic measures should answer the following questions: Can mechanical obstruction be distinguished from an abnormality of bowel motility? Is the disorder acute or chronic? Is the obstruction partial or complete? Is differentiation possible between a noncompromised (simple) intestinal obstruction and an obstruction by strangulation with vascular compromise?

The typical history includes intermittent colicky pain, nausea, and vomiting. Obstipation is a late finding. Aggravation of pain by eating suggests a more chronic and incomplete obstruction. Persistent pain, however, is highly suggestive of intestinal compromise or an associated intra-abdominal inflammation such as intestinal necrosis.

Physical examination is more important in classifying intestinal obstruction than in making the actual diagnosis. Distension is related to the level of obstruction. High-pitched bowel sounds, often synchronous with waves of abdominal pain, are pathognomonic. A truly silent abdomen may represent an abdominal catastrophe, and signs of cough tenderness again are suggestive of an associated intra-abdominal inflammation.

Imaging techniques may be of help, but usually do not allow a definitive diagnosis. Upright chest and abdominal films are useful to rule out free intraperitoneal air and to demonstrate air–fluid interfaces proximal to the obstruction. Contrast medium administered by mouth or via a nasogastric tube and followed through the small bowel helps to differentiate between complete and partial obstruction. Ultrasound examinations usually do not increase diagnostic accuracy, but may be helpful in grading distension (complete versus partial) and bowel wall thickness (acute versus chronic) and in revealing futile peristalsis.

Regarding the preoperative findings in our own series, it is important to stress that even in the early postoperative period the typical findings of colicky pain and presence of bowel sounds are detectable in most cases (Table 2). The high prevalence of earlier intra-abdominal infections seems remarkable.

Table 2. Adhesive obstructions – preoperative findings (own series 1991–1995)

	Early postoperative[a]	Late postoperative	Without prior operation
Patients (n)	11	49	4
APACHE II Score (mean)	6.4	5.3	4.3
Colicky pain (%)	73	100	100
Earlier IAI (%)	45	43	50
Bowel sounds (%)	82	95	75
Contrast studies (%)	45	45	25

IAI, intra-abdominal infection; APACHE, Acute Physiology and Chronic Health Evaluation.
[a]Within 4 weeks.

Therapy

Nonoperative measures such as volume replacement and tube decompression are routinely applied during preparation for later surgical intervention. This may be extended as palliative therapy or may even result in definitive therapy in cases of partial obstruction. Success of nonoperative treatment in terms of relief of symptoms must always be weighed against the danger of impending vascular compromise. This normally determines the period of conservative management. Knowledge of diffuse intraperitoneal malignancy warrants prolonged attempts at intestinal intubation [19]. A short or nasogastric tube will be sufficient if there are no excessively dilated loops. Dilated small bowel may be an indication for endoscopical insertion of a long nasointestinal tube. However, it should be kept in mind that all tubes favor silent aspiration and that long tubes have inherent risks which may increase morbidity [15].

Indications for laparotomy are well defined: signs of intestinal compromise (persistent pain, cough tenderness, metabolic acidosis); failure to respond within 24 h of conservative treatment; diagnostic proof of complete obstruction; a suspected associated intra-abdominal infection.

In the postoperative setting, indications are almost the same. Our present approach to suspected postoperative obstruction is shown in Fig. 1.

Major goals of operative intervention are the prevention of intestinal ischemia and the relief of the obstruction by adhesiolysis, diversion, or bypass. Whether operative decompression is necessary and whether prevention of subsequent obstruction is feasible are matters of debate.

Elements of the operative strategy include avoiding opening the bowel and minimalizing tissue trauma. In most cases, the primary operative step is the dissection of adherent bowel from the anterior abdominal wall continuing laterally until the right and left colon are identified.

All bowel loops should be brought out of the pelvis thereby identifying the sigmoid colon and the rectum. In clarifying the relation between bowel loops, there is virtually no reason to divide any adhesions that are encountered.

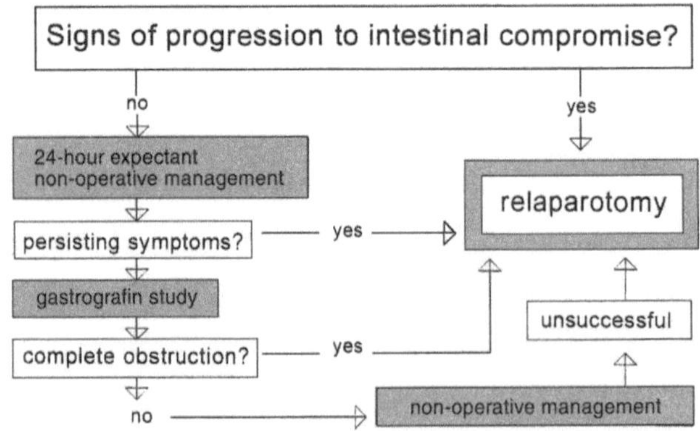

Fig. 1. Decision-making in postoperative intenstinal obstruction

Table 3. Adhesive obstructions – intraoperative findings (own series 1991–1995)

	Early post-operative (%)	Late post-operative (%)	Without prior operation (%)
Level of obstruction			
Jejunum	64	31	0
Ileum	27	53	75
Large bowel	9	14	25
Single adhesive band	36	53	50

However, examination of the small bowel from the ligament of Treitz to the ileocecal valve must be possible. Finally, compromised and obstructed segments are released; the bowel viability is checked, and it is then carefully repositioned, avoiding kinking of injured bowel or of segments with diameter changes.

In our own series, we found proximal small-bowel obstruction more often in the early postoperative period and more distal obstructions in the later course (Table 3). Single adhesive bands accounted for roughly one half of cases.

Resection was rarely necessary in the early postoperative period, but had to be performed in about one third of the cases in later events (Table 4). Long-tube stenting was applied in a considerable number of these patients. The recurrence rate (11%) and the overall mortality rate (10%) were in the expected range.

Concerning the role of laparoscopy, some skepticism seems appropriate. Laparoscopic procedures certainly merit a place in the diagnostic or therapeutic armamentarium in chronic abdominal pain. In acute, complete obstruction, however, enhanced morbidity and high conversion rates seem to limit the value of this approach [6, 16].

The prevention of recurrent obstruction is discussed in Chap. 10. Intestinal or mesenteric plication [3, 13] with its inherent risks of fistulization, intestinal infarction, and bleeding appears to be of historical interest. Intraluminal tube stenting to prevent acute angulation seems an appealing concept. However,

Table 4. Adhesive obstructions – operative procedures (own series 1991–1995)

	Early postoperative	Late postoperative	Without prior operation
Patients (*n*)	11	49	4
Adhesiolysis (%)	91	92	75
Resection (%)	9	33	25
Diversion (%)	0	0	0
Long-tube stenting (%)	64	22	25
Recurrence (%)[a]	0	12	25
Mortality (%)	9	10	0

[a]Requiring reoperation.

there is no proof that the development of "favorable" adhesions, if achievable at all, outweighs the risks of long-time stenting [15].

Chemical prophylaxis concentrates on anti-inflammatory measures, emulsifying effects, locally enhanced fibrinolysis, or the enhancement of gut motility.

From the abdominal surgeon's point of view, some questions remain: How should intraoperative decompression be performed? Closed by manual squeezing, open via an enterotomy, or by the application of a long tube? What is the best way to place a long tube? Nasointestinal, as has been recommended previously [11, 17]? Or via a gastrostomy or jejunostomy, as reported recently [15]? What additional measures should be taken? When and how should chemical prophylaxis be performed? What is the role of translocation of bacteria and bacterial products in intestinal obstruction? Further studies will be necessary to clarify these questions.

Summary

Intra-abdominal adhesions will eventually require operative intervention in up to 3% of cases. Three to 4% of all laparotomies and 20% to 30% of all repeat laparotomies are for intestinal obstruction. About 40% of intestinal obstructions are caused by intra-abdominal adhesions which may result from a variety of peritoneum-injuring or -irritating mechanisms.

In the clinical situation, it is of utmost importance to differentiate between mechanical obstruction and abnormalities of bowel motility; between acute and chronic disorders; between partial and complete obstruction; and between simple obstruction and obstruction by strangulation with vascular compromise.

General indications for laparotomy for intestinal obstruction are signs of vascular compromise, failure to respond within 24 h of conservative treatment, the diagnosis of complete obstruction, and the suspicion of associated intra-abdominal infection. The best way of performing intra-operative decompression and indications for prophylaxis of subsequent obstruction are still under discussion.

Reference

1. Bevan PG (1984) Adhesive obstruction. Ann R Coll Surg Engl 66: 164–169
2. Bizer LS, Liebling RW, Delaney HM, Gliedman HL (1981) Small bowel obstruction. The role of non-operative treatment in simple intestinal obstruction and predictive criteria for strangulation obstruction. Surgery 89: 407–413
3. Childs WA, Phillips RB (1960) Experience with intestinal plication and a proposed modification. Ann Surg 152: 258–265
4. Fabri PJ, Rosemurgy A (1991) Reoperation for small intestinal obstruction. Surg Clin North Am 71: 131–146
5. Füzün M, Kaymak E, Harmancioglu Ö, Astarcioglu K (1991) Principal causes of mechanical bowel obstruction in surgically treated adults in western Turkey. Br J Surg 78: 202–203

6. Hallfeldt KKJ, Kantelhardt T, Waldner H, Schweiberer L (1995) Die laparoskopische Adhäsiolyse in der Therapie chronischer Abdominalschmerzen. Zentralbl Chir 120: 387–391
7. Laws HL, Aldrete JS (1976) Small bowel obstruction: a review of 465 cases. South Med J 69: 733–734
8. McEntee G, Pender D, Mulvin D, McCullough M, Naedeer S, Farah S, Badurdeen MS, Ferraro V, Cham C, Gillham N, Matthews P (1987) Current spectrum of intestinal obstruction. Br J Surg 74: 976–980
9. Menzies D, Ellis H (1990) Intestinal obstruction from adhesions – how big is the problem? Ann R Coll Surg Engl 72: 60–63
10. Menzies D (1993) Postoperative adhesions: their treatment and relevance in clinical practice. Ann R Coll Surg Engl 75: 147–153
11. Nelson RL, Nyhus LM (1979) A new long intestinal tube. Surg Gynecol Obstet 149: 581–582
12. Nemir P (1952) Intestinal obstruction: ten year statistical survey at the Hospital of the University of Pennsylvania. Ann Surg 135: 367–375
13. Noble TB (1937) Plication of the small intestine as prophylaxis against adhesions. Am J Surg 35: 41–44
14. Playforth RH, Holloway JB, Griffin WO Jr (1970) Mechanical small bowel obstruction: a plea for earlier surgical intervention. Ann Surg 171: 783–788
15. Rodriguez-Ruesga R, Meagher AP, Wolff BG (1995) Twelve-year experience with the long intestinal tube. World J Surg 19: 627–631
16. Schrenk P, Woisetschläger R, Wayand U, Rieger R, Sulzbacher H (1994) Diagnostic laparoscopy: a survey of 92 patients. Am J Surg 168: 348–351
17. Stewardson RH, Bombeck CT, Nyhus LM (1978) Critical operative management of small bowel obstruction. Ann Surg 187: 189–193
18. Stewart RM, Page CP, Brender J, Schwesinger W, Eisenhut D (1987) The incidence and risk of early postoperative small bowel obstruction. Am J Surg 154: 643–647
19. Tang E, Davis J, Silberman H (1995) Bowel obstruction in cancer patients. Arch Surg 130: 832–836
20. Weibel MA, Majno G (1973) Peritoneal adhesions and their relation to abdominal surgery. Am J Surg 126: 345–353
21. Zer M, Dux S, Dintsman M (1980) The timing of relaparotomy and its influence on prognosis. Am J Surg 139: 338–343

9.2 CO$_2$ Laser Adhesiolysis

B. Lehman

Introduction

In the course of his/her profession each surgeon has met patients suffering from adhesions who have gone through a series of operations and hospital stays. These patients often chronically need analgestics or another form of pain therapy, e.g., a morphine pump. It has to be taken into account that these patients being permanently under medication suffer from a large loss of quality of life and, despite therapy, are often not without pain.

The CO$_2$ laser offers the possibility of a tissue-saving and thus promising reoperation for patients for whom other surgical procedures either no longer guarantee success or can no longer be applied, e.g. in case of extended intestinal adhesions. Although with CO$_2$ laser there is also no guarantee of success, the results achieved so far justify a certain optimism.

Method of CO$_2$ Laser adhesiolysis

Physical Prerequisites

The CO$_2$ laser is a cutting laser with a relatively low coagulation effect. It works at a wavelength range of 10 600 nm and is thus not visible to the human eye. When using CO$_2$ laser, a pilot ray is required, usually consisting of a helium-neon laser.

Due to its properties, which are determined by the wavelength, the CO$_2$ laser has to be passed on by an optical system of lenses and mirrors (in contrast to the neodym-YAG-laser which is passed on via a fiber) such that the *non-touch process* has to be applied.

A second consequence of the CO$_2$ laser wavelength is the fact that it loses its effect very rapidly when emerged in liquids, i.e., blood, rinsing liquid or cell water; thus its penetration depth remains limited.

Depending on the power setting (Watt value and the reaction time), there is a very differentiated treatment, depending on cell layer depth. In its property as light ray, the CO$_2$ laser offers the possibility to work in the focussed ray path, the cutting effect being then prevalent, and also the possibility of defocussing, resulting in a stronger coagulation effect.

Clinical Implementation of the Physical Prerequisites

In the field of operative adhesiolysis therapy, the above mentioned physical properties offer optimum conditions for the operative use of the CO$_2$ laser.

Non-touch Process

By using the non-touch process, sensitive tissue is saved, i.e., the tissue layers to be separated will not be touched. As a cutting laser with a low coagulation effect, the laser separates the tissue layers, e.g., intestine from peritoneum, by vaporizing, i.e., evaporating the cells that are hit. Depending on the power setting (Watt value) this is where the effect of the CO$_2$ laser stops.

Focussed and Defocussed Ray Path

When applied in a focussed ray path, the CO$_2$ laser has a lower coagulation effect, such that small vessels, normally found in adhesions, are immediately closed. Thus the laser adhesiolysis results in no or only very little bleeding. Only larger vessels (diameter > 1 cm) cannot be vaporized, even in the defocussed ray path, and electrical coagulation may have to be used. Just as with light, CO$_2$ laser has a focus point behind which the laser beam is again defocussed, such that damage to the tissue behind an adhesion is very small, depending, of course, on power and reaction time.

The tissue behind adhesions may be protected by lavage solutions or wet swabs, as these absorb the laser.

Tissue Stimulation

Another biological effect of the CO$_2$ laser is the stimulating effect on organic tissue. If there are no other irritations leading to tissue damage, e.g., microtraumata by abdominal towels, swabs, or suture material, even the worst adhesions may result in a restitutio ad integrum.

Laparoscopy vs Laparotomy

Laparoscopy is, of course, always superior to laparotomy. Nevertheless there are some cases in which laparoscopy is not possible, such that laser adhesiolysis via laparotomy may still offer, given the necessary microsurgical precautions, the possibility of a permanent improvement of the patient's condition.

Table 1. Adhesion causes ($n=70$ patients)

Cause	Percentage
Inflammations	43
Endometriosis	
Total	49
Stage I-II AFS	29
Stage III-IV	20
Pre-operations	
Total	63
1-2 pre-operations	51.5
3-10 pre-operations	11.5

Clinical Study

This study is based on a clinical course observation I was able to perform, from 1989 to 1991, with 70 female patients. Due to an increasing work load, I was not able to follow these patients; however, I was able to laparoscopy them again and thus get an objective view of the results.

Patient Selection and Adhesion Causes

The female patients had been selected by chance. They had been admitted into the hospital with chronic relapsing pain, existing for years or decades. The pain was described by 71% of the patients as severe, strongly impairing quality of life. In many cases, pain therapy had been administered and/or pre-operations because of adhesions had been performed.

The causes for the adhesions detected intra-operatively can be subdivided into three groups, as shown in Table 1.

Operative Procedure

Preferably, a laparoscopy was performed; however, a relaparotomy became necessary in 34% of the patients. In 11% of the patients this was the fourth to eleventh laparotomy. (Table 2).

Table 2. Operative procedure

Procedure	Percentage
Laparoscopies	66
Relaparotomies	34
1-2 preoperations	51.5
3-10 preoperations	11.5

Table 3. Pre-operative vs postoperative complaints

	None	Slight	Severe
Pre-operative	0%	29%	71%
6 months post-operative	60%	33%	2 patients
12 months post-operative	51%	34%	2 patients

Method of Data Collection

The initial interview was performed upon hospitalization, and after 6 and 12 months the patients were asked to judge their current condition. Due to the personal nature of the relationship between the female patients and the female surgeon, a response rate of 85% resulted after half a year and 75% after 1 year. The results may be judged as significant in combination with the objective findings acquired in the meantime by re-laparoscopy for other reasons with regard to CO$_2$ laser adhesiolysis.

Study Result

Table 3 shows a comparison of the pre- and postoperative conditions of the patient.

It should be noted that the two patients who stated that their conditions had not improved were in stationary psychotherapeutic and/or psychiatric treatment.

Summarizing it may be said that the patients had a significant increase in quality of life, after many of them had lived for up to 15 years with continuous pain.

Discussion

The problem in performing this study was the extensive follow-up that was required but which, due to time constraints, could not be carried out. For ethical reasons, no control laparoscopies were done. Nevertheless, in the subsequent years, there were repeated possibilities to confirm the results described by the patients.

Problems and Possible Complications of Laser Adhesiolysis

The CO$_2$ laser offers both a cutting and a coagulation device, and thus makes special demands on the surgeon. In general, laser adhesiolysis requires a high degree of patience, operative skill and experience, more than required in conventional surgical procedures.

Surgical Preparations

In general, patients to be treated with laser adhesiolysis will have been operated on several times before and most of them will have endured and suffered extensive pain. Of course, the patients are afraid of a new operation; therefore an essential part of the surgical preparation is an extensive discussion between the surgeon and the patient. This offers the patients the opportunity to talk about their fears and to ask questions, thus reassuring the patient.

Intraoperative Difficulties

Danger of Intestinal Lesions

It is in the nature of an abdominal operation that it includes an increased danger of intestinal lesions. In order to reduce this risk to a minimum, an exact localization of the problem should be performed by the surgeon prior to the operation, such that the Verres needle and the trocar can be introduced in a direction that is presumably free from adhesions.

Cicatrization of the Abdominal Wall

Due to frequent prior operations, the abdominal wall is sometimes cicatrized to such an extent that introduction of the Verres needle is impossible. In some cases an open laparoscopy is required or a re-laparotomy has to be performed. This has to be discussed with the patient in advance.

Extraperitoneal position of the Verres Needle

When introducing the Verres needle, a not definitive intraperitoneal position may result. Visual examination or open laparoscopy is then the method of choice. In case of lack of success, here too a relaparotomy has to be performed.

Relaparotomy

Even in case of a relaparotomy there may be considerable problems caused by fixation of the intestine at the abdominal wall; here too, the gentle non-touch process of CO_2 laser adhesiolysis permits spontaneous separation of the tissue layers.

Postoperative Complications

These include the following:

1. Inflammation reaction: Due to the heat effect during extensive laser adhesiolysis, there will always be a certain inflammation reaction, possibly with fibrin exudation, requiring an adequate prophylaxis (see below).

2. Intestinal violation: In the course of adhesiolyses near the intestine, unnoticed violations of the intestinal wall may happen due to the remote effect of the laser in the defocussed ray path. Normally this complication arises after several days, requiring regular post-operative follow-up of the patients.

3. Adhesion relapses: Renewed adhesion creation will be increased by a too early strain on the patients. Of course, there may be other reasons for the creation of renewed adhesions.

Follow-up Treatment After Laser Adhesiolysis

To prevent inflammation, we perform post-operative prophylaxis with Solu-Decortin for 3 days at a dosage of 100 mg, 75 mg, 50 mg. In addition, we use physical measures such as moor baths and shortwave or stimulation current treatments starting on the fifth post-operative day. This therapy will be continued at home and is reported by the patients to be very soothing. Normal saline solution or Ringer's solution at body temperature is always be used during laparoscopy and a little rinsing liquid is left in situ. Also, we recommend physical rest for about 2 weeks.

Summary

Looking at the results of the study and the findings collected in the re-operations, the CO$_2$ laser adhesiolysis is an excellent method to surgically treat adhesion-related pains. It is important to consider the procedure not as a new surgical method, but rather in the context of pre- and post-operative patient care.

9.3 Laparoscopic Treatment of Peritoneal Adhesions: A Clinical Study of 53 Patients

M. Schnabel, W. Dietz, U. Malewski, and H. Feist

Introduction

Peritoneal adhesions are a common complication after intraabdominal surgical procedures and inflammatory diseases [5]. The pathomorphological process which leads to the formation of adhesions was described by Milligan and Raferty [7]. The starting point is a fibrin matrix which is replaced by vascularized granulation tissue containing macrophages, fibroblasts and giant cells. The interaction of fibroblasts and collagen allows the adhesion to mature into a fibrous band [7]. The pathophysiological mechanism is the dysbalance between fibrinogenesis and fibrinolysis caused by multiple factors after damage to the peritoneum [11]. In 65% of patients with prior abdominal surgery adhesions were found, and for 3%–6% of these cases further surgery is necessary [4]. The economical implication of adhesions is demonstrated clearly by the cost. In the United States, in 1988, nearly 1.2 million dollars were needed for the treatment of lower abdominal adhesions, not considering outpatient treatment and work loss [8]. Apart from severe complications (e.g., ileus), pain is the main reason why patients consult a doctor. Other clinical symptoms are various and mostly nonspecific. The final diagnosis of adhesions must first exclude many other possible diagnoses. Most patients consult many doctors and undergo time-consuming diagnostic and therapeutic procedures before they reach the surgeon and request assistance. To verify the diagnosis of adhesions, the peritoneal cavity must be inspected; however, such procedures may themselves induce adhesions. Adhesiolysis should thus be performed at the same time, with as little surgical trauma as possible. These demands appear to be satisfied by laparoscopic surgical techniques. Since the main indication for such operations is pain, the technique should improve the patient's quality of life, assessed especially by pain reduction. In this study the influence and potential benefit of laparoscopic adhesiolysis on the quality of life was investigated.

Patients and Methods

Patients

The study involved prospective clinical observations without a comparative control group. Between January 1992 and December 1994, 62 patients with abdominal pain were treated for possible peritoneal adhesions at the surgical

Table 1. Prior surgical interventions in the patient group (n=53)[a]

Prior surgery	Number
Appendectomy	44
Hysterectomy	12
Abdominal wall hernia	7
Adnexectomy	5
Ileus	4
Meckel's diverticulum	3
Cholecystectomy	3
Adhesiolysis	3
Laparoscopic sterilization	2
No prior surgery	1

[a]Patients may appear more than once.

clinic of Delmenhorst. All patients with acute and inflammatory diseases were excluded from the study. Patients with severe complications of adhesions like ileus were also not included in this selected group. Patients ages at presentation ranged from 14 to 65 years (median 34.1 years). The sex distribution was unbalanced with 95% female and 5% male patients. Previous operations are listed in Table 1.

Clinical Examinations

Prior to laparoscopy, to verify the suspected adhesions, acute, inflammatory and infectious as well as gynecological, urological and other nonsurgical diseases were excluded by laboratory, clinical, ultrasonographic, endoscopic, and, in some cases, radiologic examinations. All patients with preoperative pathological findings were excluded from the treatment group. Standardized questionnaires were employed to evaluate the clinical history of the patients. All clinical, laboratory and ultrasonographic examinations were also standardized.

Operative Treatment

The laparoscopic operation methods were standardized. Before proceeding, powder was washed from the gloves to prevent foreign body granuloma formation and adhesions. The approach for the optical trocar was infra- or supraumbilical, depending on the suspected adhesions. The open approach was obligatory. A second 5 mm trocar was visually placed in the left lower abdomen. A third trocar was sometimes necessary for difficult preparation procedures. The whole abdomen was then systematically examined. Enteroenteral adhesions were excluded by exploration of the bowel. Adhesions were classified according to Luciano [5, 6]. Bowel adhesions to the peritoneum were cut either by diathermy or with scissors depending on the vascularization. Enteroenteral adhesions were treated by open surgery. Before ending, a thorough lavage was performed. Removal of the 5 mm trocars was visually followed. The fascia at the umbilical incision was closed by a surture to prevent hernia.

Postoperative Examinations

Postoperatively, convalescence was monitored, and, in particular, all complications during the hospital stay were noted. The development of clinical complaints was registered daily using the visual analog pain scale (VAPS), which ranged from zero (no pain) up to 100 (unbearable pain) [2].

Follow-Up

A follow-up was performed 6–24 months postoperatively in 34 (56%) patients by clinical and ultrasonographic examination. Additionally, a questionnaire was completed by the patient. Using our laparoscopic adhesiolysis treatment score (LATS), the questionnaire provided an assessment of the success of the laparoscopic treatment.

Scoring System

The patients scored their discomfort concerning daily life, work, eating, digestion, fear, pain and sleep with 0–3 points. The number of medical consultations and hospitalisations was also transferred into points (Table 2). The patients were scored twice. By adding the points, as shown in Table 2, a comparison between the preoperative value and the result after the operations was possible. The overall assessment is shown in Table 3.

Table 2. Laparoscopic adhesiolysis treatment score (LATS): for patient 21[a]

Preoperative				Patient's ID	Postoperative			
0	1	2	3*	Work	3	2	1	0*
0	1	2	3*	Private/sport	3	2	1	0*
0	1	2*	3	Eating	3	2	1	0*
0*	1	2	3	Digestion	3	2	1	0*
0	1*	2	3	Sleep	3	2	1	0*
0	1*	2	3	Fear	3	2	1	0*
0	1	2*	3	Pain	3	2	1	0*
0	1*	2	3	Medical consultations	3	2	1	0*
0	1*	2	3	Hospitalisations	3	2	1	0*
14				Sum	0			

Items work, private/sport, eating, digestion and sleep: 0, no; 1, little; 2, considerable; 3, severe influence. Items fear and pain: 0* no. 1* little; 2* considerably; 3* severe. Item medical consultations: 0, no; 1, some; 2, each month; 3 each week. Item hospitalisations: 0, no; 1, 1; 2, 2-3; 3, more than 3. The selected values are indicated by an asterisk. [a]The patient was a 24 year old female.

Table 3. Overall assessment of the differences between the preoperative and the follow-up by LATS scoring

Assesment	Difference
Excellent	A total of 0 points in the follow-up
Good	Reduction > 50% and no increase in any category
Equal	A difference of ± 1 point compared to preoperative score and all cases not equal to "good"
Poor	Decrease of > 2 points

[a]Points preoperative minus points scored in the follow-up.

Results

In 62 patients a diagnostic laparoscopy for suspected adhesions was performed; intraabdominal adhesions were found in 57 cases. Twice there were no pathological findings. Unexpected gynecological diseases were found in three patients (adnexitis, ovarial cyst, endometriosis). The preoperative ultrasound examinations were without significant predictive value for adhesions. Laparoscopic adhesiolysis was performed in 53 cases. Preoperatively the patients were assigned to an ASA (American Society of Anesthesiologists) risk group [1]. A total of 38 were classified as ASA I, 12 as ASA II and three as ASA III. The duration of the complaints was less than 24 h in 19 cases, between 1 day and 1 week in 12, between 1 and 4 weeks in 10 and more than 4 weeks in 11 patients. Open treatment was necessary in four patients because the position of the adhesions were associated with a high risk of complications by injuring, e.g. the small bowel. The conversion rate from laparoscopic to open treatment was 7%. According to the classification of Luciano, three patients had first grade, 10 had second grade and 40 had third grade adhesions. The median duration of the operation was 51 min (range 14–121 min) (Fig. 1). The operation time

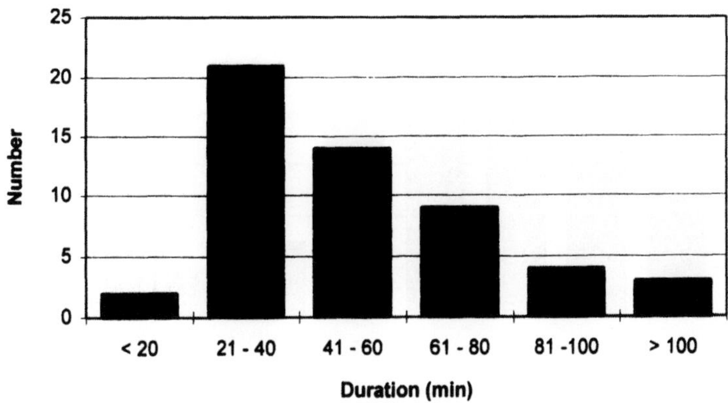

Fig. 1. Duration of surgical procedure

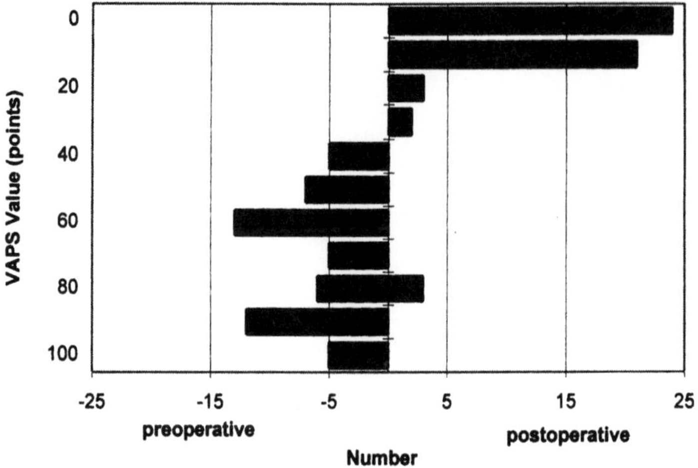

Fig. 2. Value on the visual analog pain scale (VAPS) preoperatively and 3 days postoperatively

decreased during the period of observation with increasing degree of experience. Intraoperative bleeding occurred only twice and was controlled easily with a Röder loop. Postoperatively, three patients had a periumbilical infection. In a female patient with marked obesity this umbilical infection had to be treated by opening the wound. All patient with infections were ASA II. Hematomas were found in three patients at the cutaneous wound site without signs of infection. Patients perception of pain (pre- and postoperative) is illustrated in Fig. 2. Preoperatively, the median value was 72 VAPS points; it was reduced to only 11 points 3 days postoperatively. In the three cases with a high postoperative VAPS value a significant decrease was noted over the following days. Most patients left the hospital within a week (Fig. 3). Patients who left the clinic within 3 days postoperatively judged the duration of hospitalisation as adequate.

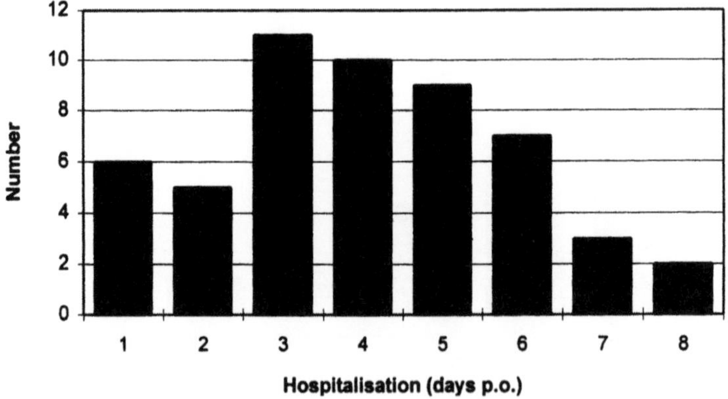

Fig. 3. Postoperative hospitalisation

In the follow-up, 36 patients (68%) were scored by LATS, half were free of complaints. A significant reduction in the LATS score was noted in 13 patients, with no change in four cases. One patient had a higher postoperative than preoperative LATS score. The laparoscopic surgery technique was classified by all patients, regardless of success, as careful and less traumatizing as open surgery, which all but one patient had previously undergone. Severe incidents in this group which would have led to further operations did not occur.

Discussion

Peritoneal adhesions are a common problem after surgical procedures and inflammatory diseases [5]. Adhesions are a complication not a disease entity themselves. Thus adhesiolysis is not a curative treatment and excellent results are unlikely. Pain is a main symptom in patients with adhesions. Also, gastrointestinal discomfort with various symptoms and severe consequences, e.g. ileus, occur. The surgical decision-making process, whether to operate in cases of pain or not, is complex. A main problem is the fact that any diagnostic interventions by laparoscopy might in themselves cause adhesions [3]. For cases of laparotomy and laparoscopy without pathological findings, post-operative adhesions are a disaster. Severe complications of adhesions such as ileus are not predictable. Moreover the conclusion that the presence of adhesions is equal to complaints is wrong. In many patients, adhesions without clinical symptoms were diagnosed during various laparoscopic procedures. Thus the surgeon must consider each patient and his or her complaints individually, although the lack of objective clinical parameters makes this difficult. The indication whether to operate or not depends on various subjective features which represent a multidimensional construct, i.e. patient's quality of life. Quality of life is defined by the WHO as the assembled reflection of physical, psychological and social well-being as well as the symptoms of disease and therapy [10]. Nevertheless quality of life is an individual perception. Disease could be reflected as a learning process with changes in the individual's assessment of the quality of life [9]. The main question assessing the results of any treatment is, "Did the therapy reduce or remove the patient's complaints and is there any improvement in his or her estimation of quality of life?" This question is unanswerable by objective clinical parameters, but can be answered by a score which is predominately based on subjective parameters. Our further demands on the score were that it was simple, understandable, user-friendly and less time-consuming. Highly sophisticated scores are of high scientific value but not practicable for several reasons during our daily work. Therefore we developed the laparoscopic adhesiolysis treatment score (LATS) to evaluate the advantage of the laparoscopic treatment of peritoneal adhesions in patients with the main symptom of pain and without severe functional disturbance. The score considers mainly subjective and only a few objective parameters. The chosen characteristics for the LATS represent those complaints which were mentioned by the patients as having considerable influence on their quality of life. In the follow-up, the patients were also asked to grade the quality of life benefit with the ratings excellent, good, equal or poor. In all cases, the overall assessment by the patient was similar to our scoring by the LATS. This indicates that the LATS in an instrument to estimate the individual's quality of life. The changes in the various areas of daily life and the individual perception of organic function could be differentiated in the follow-up by using the LATS.

Conclusion

Laparoscopic adhesiolysis is a careful method to verify intraabdominal adhesions or locate other intraabdominal diseases which can not be diagnosed by other examinations. In cases of adhesions, simultaneous treatment is possible. The method is well accepted by the patients and classified by them as less traumatizing than open surgery. Further investigation is necessary to assess the long-term results. Our laparoscopic adhesiolysis treatment score is a simple instrument for use in our daily work to estimate the benefit of the treatment to the patient's quality of life.

Acknowledgement. The authors gratefully acknowledge Dr. Madeleine Ennis, University of Belfast, for helping to prepare the manuscript for publication.

References

1. Ahnefeld FW, Dölp R, Kilian J (eds) (1984) Anästhesie. Kohlhammer, Stuttgart, pp 13–14
2. Castiglione M (1990) Meßbarkeit und Beurteilung der Lebensqualität. In: Aulbert E, Neiderle N (eds) Die Lebensqualität des chronisch Krebskranken. Thieme, Stuttgart, pp 15–26
3. diZerega GS (1994) Zeitgemäße Adhäsionsverhütung. Fertil Steril 61: 1–16
4. Hamelmann H, Dohrmann P (1990) Chirugische Maßnahmen zur Verhinderung abdomineller Verwachsungen. Langenbecks Arch Chir Suppl 2: 1023
5. Klaiber C, Metzger A (eds) (1992) Manual der laparoskopischen Chirurgie. Hans Huber, Bern, pp 185–206
6. Luciano AA, Maier DB, Koch EI, Nulsen JC, Whitman GF (1989) A comparative study of postoperative adhesions following laser surgery by laparoscopy versus laparotomy in the rabbit model. Obstet Gynecol 74: 220–224
7. Milligan DW, Raferty AT (1974). Observations on the pathogenesis of peritoneal adhesions: alight and electron microscopical study. Br J Surg 61: 274–280
8. Ray NF, Larsen JW, Stillman RJ, Jacobs RJ (1993) Economic impact of hospitalisations for lower abdominal adhesiolysis in the United States in 1988. Surg Gynecol Obstet 176: 271–276
9. Schara J (1990) Was bedeutet Lebensqualität bei Krebs? In: Aulbert E, Niederle N (eds) Die Lebensqualität des chronisch Krebskranken. Thieme, Stuttgart, pp 1–14
10. World Health Organizations (1958) The first ten years of the World Health Organizations. Geneva
11. Zühlke HV, Lorenz EMP, Straub EM, Savvas V (1990) Pathophysiologie und Klassifikation von Adhäsionen. Langenbecks Arch Chir Suppl 2: 1009

9.4 Efficiency of Laparoscopy in Treatment of Acute Small Bowel Obstruction Caused by Adhesions

G. Federmann, J. Walenzyk, A. Schneider, C. Scheele,
and G. Bauermeister

Introduction

Adhesions and bands are amongst the most frequent causes of acute small bowel obstruction. They often result from previous operations or inflammation. In many cases ileus is caused by single bands, leading to obstruction and strangulation. This can be treated by simple cutting with scissors or scalpel. In these cases conventional laparotomy itself can result in further bands or adhesions and furthermore seems to be a complicated approach to solve a simple problem.

Laparoscopy is, meanwhile, a widely used diagnostic and therapeutic procedure. As a minimally invasive approach to the abdomen, it should cause fewer adhesions or bands than with open laparoscopy [4]. Laparoscopic adhesiolysis is an established procedure in treatment of chronic adhesions causing recurrent abdominal pain or obstruction. Mainly the small bowel is treated by this approach. We therefore investigated laparoscopy in treatment of acute small bowel obstruction caused – as an acute complication – by bands or adhesions.

Preoperative Diagnostics

In order to preoperatively distinguish between different ileus situations, we admitted all patients showing ileus to a diagnostic program consisting of: (1) clinical anamnesis and investigation; (2) blood chemistry; (3) ultrasonography; (4) X-ray investigation.

All steps of investigation were aimed at determining whether acute small bowel obstruction, adhesions, tumor or other causes of ileus were present.

As contraindications to a laparoscopic approach we defined: colon ileus, small bowel ileus caused by tumor (or after tumor operation), gallstones, recurrent ileus, prolonged ileus, and incarcerated preabdominal hernias, as well as general contraindications to laparoscopy, e.g., liver cirrhosis or cardiopulmonary insufficiency.

Ultrasonography revealed very important findings (Table 1), clearly detecting small bowel obstruction. This was defined as having diameters of more than 2.5–3 cm, mostly with collapsed terminal ileum. Prolonged obstruction

Table 1. Sonographic findings in examination of the ileus

Small bowel ileus: diameter >2.5 cm and <3.5 cm
Location of ileus gut and normal gut
Exclusion of other ileus origins, e.g., tumors, gallstones, diverticulitis
Exclusion of general contraindications e.g., liver cirrhosis
Determination of laparoscopic approach (first trocar placement) using
inspirative movement of the gut under the abdominal wall

---

was more than 3.5 cm in diameter and was excluded, as a very small intraabdominal operation "tent" was to be expected. Ultrasonography also could
detect many contraindications, but furthermore could show probable adhesion-free areas of the abdominal wall [4, 10], thus locating placement, of the
first trocar.

As indication for laparoscopic adhesiolysis we defined small bowel obstruction most likely caused by adhesions or bands.

Preoperative criteria for a laparoscopic ileus approach were:

1. Small bowel ileus
2. Gut diameter < 2.5 cm–>3.5 cm
3. Adhesions highly probable
4. Absence of broad adhesions between gut and abdominal wall
5. Absence of major accompanying diseases
6. Presence of an experienced surgical team

The following conversion criteria we defined and observed were instru-
mental problems ($n=0$); complications/injuries ($n=2$); and laparoscopical
problems including insufficient procedure ($n=1$).

Surgical Technique

Usually, the first optic trocar was placed in the left upper bowel. The location
was determined by ultrasonography according to the presumed location of
obstruction and sonographically adhesion-free abdominal wall. Two further
trocars (5 mm) were visually placed and the abdomen was investigated.
Usually, the revision of the small bowel started at the terminal ileus and led to
the obstruction. In a few cases, the obstruction was identified first, and after
adhesiolysis the complete small bowel was revised. Bands and adhesions were
cut by scissors; the small bowel was moved by an atraumatic forceps.

Results

Between April 1, 1992 and December 31, 1994, 109 patients with ileus were
treated in our clinic and recruited to our trial according to the described
selection. There were 25 patients who showed colon ileus; 84 patients suffered
from different kinds of small bowel ileus. After selection according to the above

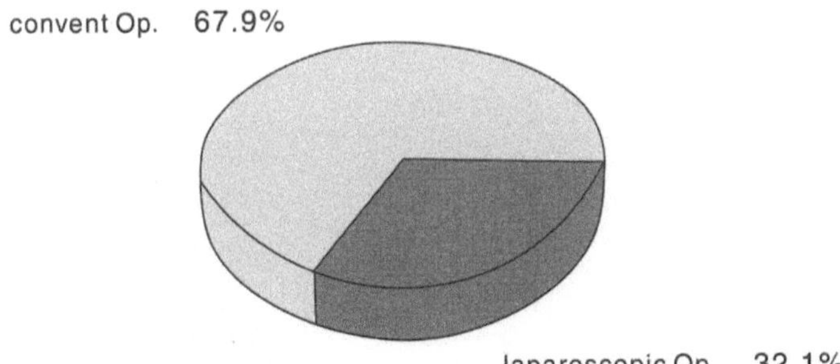

Fig. 1. Different treatments of small bowl ileus

Table 2. Causes of obstruction in conventionally operated on small bowel ileus (n=57)

Cause	n
Adhesions	26[a]
Ileus after extensive earlier operations and tumors	18
Gallstones	2
Recurrent ileus	8
Mesenterial infarction	2
Crohn's disease	1

[a]Six might have been treated by laparoscopy.

detailed criteria, 27 patients were treated by laparoscopy primarily and 57 were operated on conventionally (Fig. 1, Table 2).

Regarding those 57 patients who had contraindications to laparoscopic approach 24 were expected to have severe adhesions or prolonged ileus and two could not be treated laparoscopically because of absence of an experienced surgical team. Of these 26 patients, six might have been treated by laparoscopy according to the surgeon's reports (6/84 pts with small bowel ileus 7.4%). The other 31 patients had defined exclusion criteria to laparoscopy.

A total of 27 patients were primarily treated by laparoscopy (Fig 2, Table 3): 17 patients were treated by laparoscopic adhesiolysis. After localization the bands or adhesions were cut as described above. Five patients were diagnosed laparoscopically but operated on conventionally due to severe adhesion (n=3) and acute appendicitis or mesenterial infarction (n=2). Three patients had to be converted after laparoscopic start because of injuries (leakages) of the gut (n=2) or surgical problems (conversion rate 11.1%). Two patients had non-obstructive ileus and only underwent diagnostic laparoscopy.

Figure 3 summarizes the overall treatment of our patients with small bowel ileus: 20.2% were treated successfully by laparoscopy; approximately 10% might have been treated by laparoscopy (including 6% converted patients vs. 7% conventionally performed operations which might have been done by laparoscopy).

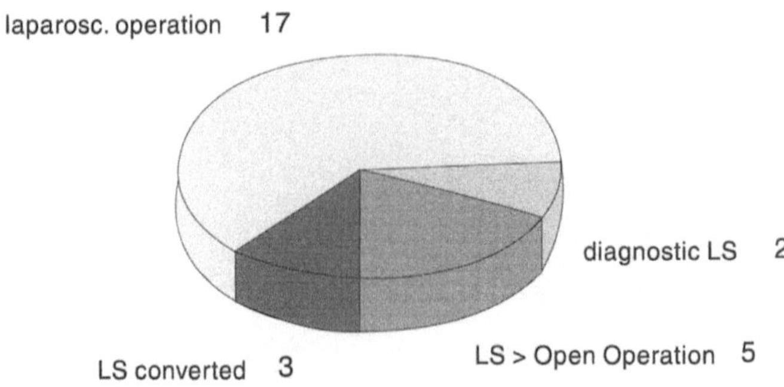

Fig. 2. Distribution of laparoscopic procedures (n=27)

Table 3. Laparoscopic procedures in small bowel ileus (n=27)

Procedure	n
Laparoscopic operation	17
Adhesions	15
Incarcerated internal hernias	2
Laparoscopic converted operation	3
Diagnostic laparoscopy, open surgery	5
Extensive adhesions	3
Mesenterial infarction /appendicitis	2
Diagnostic laparoscopy	2

Small bowel obstruction due to adhesions or bands shows a different distribution (Fig. 4): 33.3% of patients were treated sufficiently by laparoscopy, 9.8% had to be operated on conventionally, 5.9% had to be converted, and 51% were treated conventionally.

There were no major complications: in three patients we saw injuries of the gut, two of them were converted and one was sewed laparoscopically. All patients recovered without any problems.

Peristaltic movement of the gut could be seen in every laparoscopically treated patient before the end of the operation. The postoperative course was

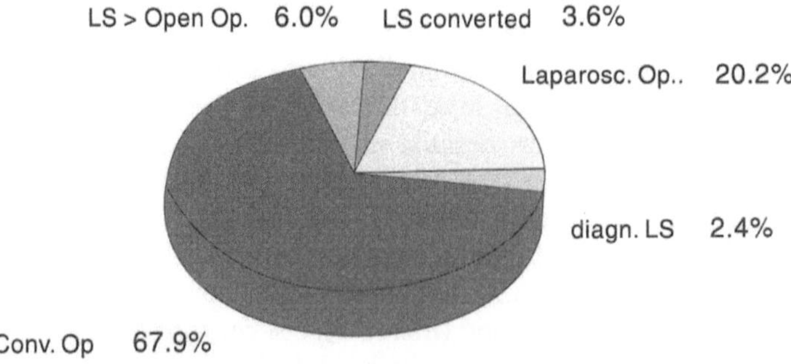

Fig. 3. Distribution of treatment in small bowel ileus (n=84)

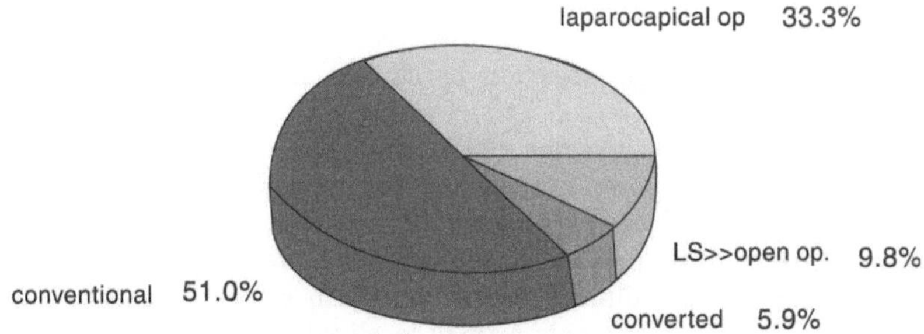

Fig. 4. Distribution of treatment in small bowel obstruction caused by adhesions (n=57)

unremarkable and normal nutrition could be reached within 3–5 days. The hospital stay ranged between 5 and 8 days and could be shortened with increasing experience. Due to our selection, a comparison with open operated patients was not possible.

Operation time ranged from 45 to 150 min and showed a typical learning curve.

No recurrent ileus could be seen among the laparoscopically treated patients (postoperative time 9–40 months).

Discussion

Adhesion-caused pain and obstructive symptoms can very often be seen following previous abdominal operations or inflammation. Mainly these symptoms are chronic and can be treated by adhesiolysis, which can be performed laparoscopically [6]. Acute small bowel obstruction due to adhesions or bands demonstrate the acute complication of adhesions and usually are treated by conventional surgery [5.7]. In dealing with laparoscopic adhesiolysis in chronic adhesions, we investigated the ability of the laparoscopic approach to treat such acute ileus.

The main preoperative problem was in distinguishing acute small bowel obstruction caused by bands or adhesions from those caused by other reasons. We did this mainly by clinical and sonographic investigation [5, 8, 11] and thus could select those patients fulfilling preoperative criteria for laparoscopic treatment. Based on this we could treat laparoscopically one third of all patients with small bowel obstruction due to adhesions or bands. Another 10% can be expected to be treated this way (those who were treated conventionally or in part those who were converted). All together about 40% of our patients with small bowel obstruction due to adhesions or bands might be treated by laparoscopical adhesiolysis.

These results differ from those demonstrated by other groups. Eypasch et al. [3] found only a few cases which could be treated laparoscopically, Levard et al. [9] investigated 25 patients with small bowel ileus, but had to convert to an open approach in about 50%. These authors discussed an inefficient preoperative patient selection. Further reports [1, 2, 7, 12] showed the ability of a laparoscopic procedure in some cases. Obviously, in our investigation there was an efficient preoperative selection by clinical and sonographic means which led to our results.

Laparoscopy seems to have some major advantages compared to conventional treatment of small bowel obstruction. The minimal invasive approach itself reduces the risk of new adhesions. Laparoscopic ileus diagnosis can surgically disqualify those patients suffering from acute ileus caused by enteritis, which can be very difficult to distinguish in some patients[2, 3, 7]. Diagnostic laparoscopy causes only a small localized incision, in contrast to treatment of the obstruction by open surgery, and laparoscopic adhesiolysis can solve the problem in many cases. It permits revision of the whole small bowel and observation of peristaltic movement before the end of the operation. Due to pneumoperitoneum even in prolonged surgery the small bowel does not show edema as occurs in prolonged conventional ileus surgery. The intraabdominal gas pressure seems to prevent this and might hinder this aspect of ileus disease. All these – in part hypothetic – features support a laparoscopic approach to adhesion-caused small bowel ileus.

As mentioned above, a careful selection should be provided for. And, of course, there must be a well-trained surgical team. Our results indicate that, based on these considerations, efficient laparoscopic treatment of acute small bowel obstruction caused by adhesions or bands can be done successfully.

References

1. Adams S, Wilson T, Brown AR (1993) Laparoscopic management of acute small bowel obstruction. Aust N Z J Surg 63: 39–41
2. Duh QH (1993) Laparoscopic procedures for small bowel disease. Baillieres Clin Gastroenterol 7: 833–850
3. Eypasch E, Mennigen R, Spangenberger W, Troidl H (1993) Laparoskopie beim akuten Abdomen. Langenbecks Arch Chir (Suppl): 134–141
4. Gai H, Thiele H (1992) Sonographische Selektionskriterien für die laparoskopische Cholecystektomie Chirurg 63: 426–431
5. Hentschel M (1982) Akuter Darmverschluß In: Häring RH(ed) Dringliche Bauchchirurgie Thieme, Stuttgart, pp 222–319
6. Keese-Röhrs T, Röhn D (1993) Die diagnostische Laparoskopie Ein Konzept zur topographischen und histopathologischen Klassifikation von Verwachsungen. Minim Invasive Chir 2: 121–129
7. Kraas E, Raude H, Löhde E (1995) Laparoskopie beim Ileus. In: Boekl O, Waclawiczek HW (eds) Standards in der Chirurgie. Zuckschwerdt, München, pp 252–255
8. Klotter H-J, Zielke A, Nies C, Sitter H, Rothmund M (1992) Sonographie beim akuten abdominellen Notfall. Chirurg 63: 597
9. Levard H, Mouro J, Schiffino L, Karayel M, Berthelot G, Dubois F (1993) Celioscopic treatment of acute obstruction of the small intestine. Immediate results in 25 patients. Ann Chir 47: 497–501
10. Martin G, Bergama S, Miola E, Caldironi MW, Dagnini G (1987) Prelaparoscopic echography used to detect abdominal adhesions. Endoscopy 19: 147–149
11. Meiser G, Meissner K (1985) Zum Stellenwert der sonographischen Ileusdiagnostik. Chirurg 56: 46–49
12. Silva PD, Cogbill TH (1991) Laparoscopic treatment of recurrent small bowel obstruction. Wis Med J 90: 169–170

9.5 A New Probe Optimizes Closed Decompression and Temporary Intestinal Splinting in Small Intestine Ileus

J. Ermisch

Introduction

All types of ileus share intestinal distension as a common pathologic feature and the starting point of several pathophysiologic processes. The elimination of intestinal distension and bacterial-toxic intestinal secretion can therefore be compared to the removal of a septic focus.

Long intestinal probes allow this treatment to be performed postoperatively by temporary intraluminal intestinal drainage. Probe systems can also be used to give local antibiotics or agents exciting peristalsis.

In all types of ileus, the operative procedure is basically determined by three important goals: (1) to combat intestinal distension; (2) to eliminate the cause of ileus; and (3) to avoid ileus relapses.

In order to eliminate intestinal distension two basic approaches are possible: (1) open decompression and (2) closed decompression.

The great number of complications occurring after enterotomy in patients with ileus caused Wangensteen and Leonhard [10] to look for new transoral intubation techniques. The development of ileus probes has mainly been based on balloon sound systems. The low delivery rate and the sophisticated and time-consuming handling of nasogastric balloon sounds that are required brings about problems which were very impressively described by Nissen and Maurer [6] already in 1965: "Any attempt to push a Miller-Abbott's tube, which has been left in the stomach, into the small intestine often remains wishful thinking unless you use rough force which should be abhorred and rejected in ileus condition."

Despite the advantages of the closed decompression procedure, the unsatisfactory transoral technique prompted us to develop a new absorbable guiding system for ileus probes [2, 3, 4].

Material, Patients and Methods

An ileus decompression probe has been designed as an alternative to the balloon sound system. Its advantages include:

1. A single lumen probe of optimum delivery
2. Easy probing based uncomplicated operative procedure

3. A guide which dissolves entirely after completion of decompression and splinting (time of function >60 min)
4. Use of a probe material of high biological acceptance

Gelatin was chosen as the basic material for the protein guiding probe (PGP) because it is pharmacologically harmless [5]. The microbiologic cleanliness of the gelatin capsule complies with the guidelines stipulated in DAB 10/VIII for the manufacture of pharmaceutics.

The new probe system (Figs. 1,2) has been used in 48 patients for intraoperative closed transoral decompression and intestinal splinting and in four patients for transanal decompression and intestinal splinting ($\male$=21/ $\female$=31). The patients were between 14 and 95 years of age (average age 63.3 years).

Indications for closed decompression and intestinal splinting included (Table 1):

1. Postoperative early and late ileuses with extensive adhesions
2. Mixed ileus with peritonitis
3. Advanced primary ileus
4. Paralytic ileus found intraoperatively

Probing Procedure

The anesthetist positions the probe with the aid of the mandrin (Figs. 1, 2) in the stomach, where it is received by the operating surgeon (Fig. 3). After removal of the mandrin, the highly flexible PGP can easily be pushed forward

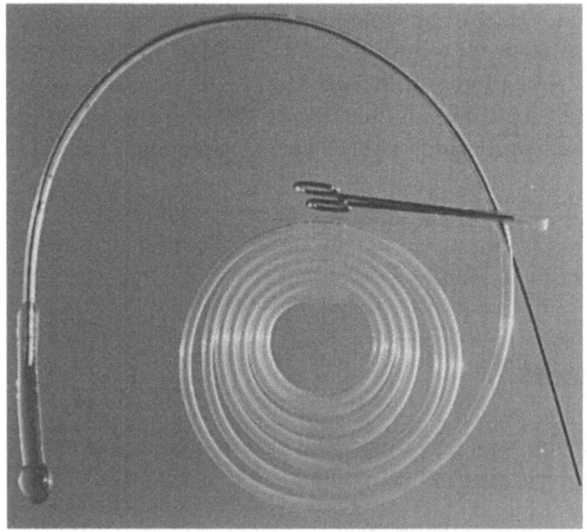

Fig. 1. Protein guiding probe (patented) with glass fiber mandrin and retention clamp

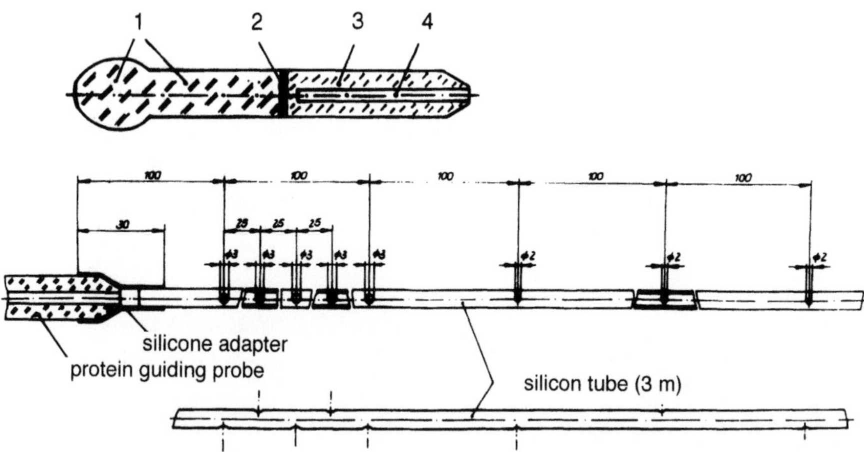

Fig. 2. Longitudinal section of protein guiding probe and hole geometry of silicone tube (Silkomed-Rüsch, outer diameter 6 mm, inner diameter 4 mm). *1*, flexible probe head (soft gelatin); *2*, boundary layer between soft and hard gelatin; *3*, rigid portion of probe shaft (hard gelatin); *4*, probe channel to accommodate mandrin.

Table 1. Types of ileus in 52 patients treated with complete or partial small intestinel splints (1987–1993)

Types of ileus	n
Paralytic	6
Advanced primary	15
Early postoperative	15
Late postoperative	16

into the small intestine. After splinting has been completed, the ileus probe, located orally, is connected with a tube which has been introduced through the nose and is retrogradely led out. A stomach tube is inserted in addition to the intestinal splint. The average retention time of the splint was 7 days. A radiologic check of the location is made on the second and fifth postoperative days using peritrastoral (Fig. 4).

Results

After a certain routine had been acquired in working with the anesthetist, the probing time into the jejunum was about 10 min. The small intestine could not be reached transorally in three patients with benign esophageal stenosis and extensive epigastric adhesions.

Postoperative complications caused by probing did not occur in 51 patients (0.5%). The probe could not be removed from one female patient due to a twisting of the bowels. As a result, a relaparotomy had to be performed. The total mortality of ileus patients with splinted small intestines was 25% (13/52).

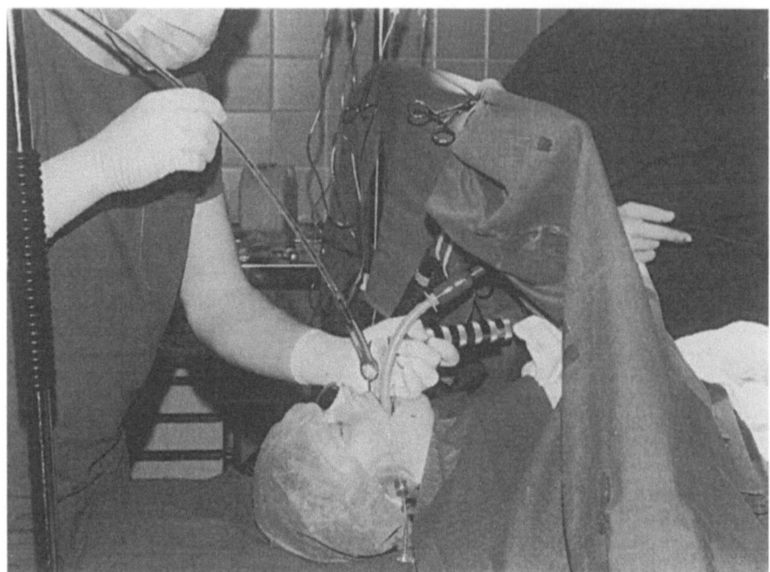

Fig. 3. Transoral probing procedure

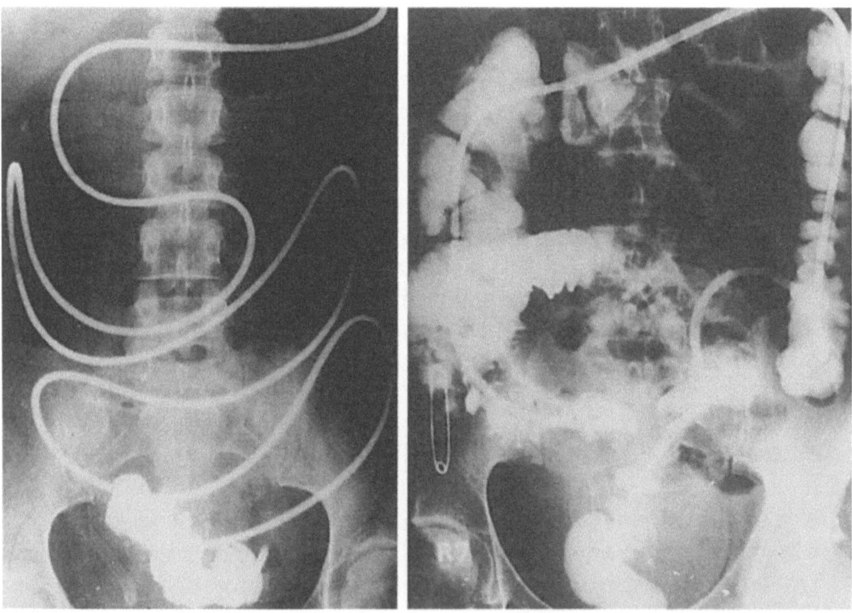

Fig. 4. *Left*, orthograde transoral small intestine splinting; *right*, retrograde transanal intestinal splinting

The 46.7% (7/15) mortality of patients with mixed ileus with peritonitis was considerably higher than the 5.5% (1/18) mortality of adhesion ileus patients.

Early ileus relapses did not occur after intestinal splinting. However, manual decompression according to Korn caused relapsing ileuses in four patients with early ileus. The complicated ileus conditions could be mastered after intestinal splinting.

Transanal decompression and splinting could be performed without difficulties [3] in two patients with postoperative early ileus after extended colon resection with a predisposition towards ileosigmoidostomy, cecum volvulus and adhesion ileus after gynecologic operations.

Summary

The efficiency of closed transoral decompression in small intestinal ileus is undisputed. According to Wangensteen [10], its status will be significantly enhanced if an improved probing procedure can be demonstrated. Indications of intestinal splinting are differently assessed in the literature, with the complicated procedure involved in nasogastric balloon sounds and the risk of iatrogenic perforation being cited decisive counterarguments.

In light of the probe-specific complications described in the literature and considering our own experience, it is always important to weigh the splinting risks against the risk of ileus relapses [1, 8, 9]. Reifferscheid and Pip specify that the relapse rate of splinted compared to nonsplinted small intestine ileus is 3.9% to 11%; that is, the relapse rate of intestinal splinting is significantly lower [7].

The capabilities of the new probe system were clearly shown when it was used in a 95-year-old female patient, whose advanced small intestinal bridle ileus (1500 ml of ileus fluid) could be operated on successfully. Taking into account the generally advanced average age of ileus patients, the operative procedure, in particular the quick elimination of the highly toxic ileus fluid and intestinal gas, plays a decisive role in the prognosis, despite modern intensive care. It is the practical aim of the new probe system to replace decompression and splinting methods using balloon sounds by a more efficient technique which provides fast and safe access by probes to each portion of the intestine.

References

1. Diettrich H, Herrmann U, Hildebrandt J (1990) Zur Problematik der Dünndarmschienung beim Adhäsionsileus. Z Klin Med 45: 481–483
2. Ermisch J, Schneider H (1988) Führungssonde zur Dünndarmschienung. Patentschrift P 3820213.1, München, pp 1–6
3. Ermisch J, Schauer K (1991) Transanales Dekompressionsverfahren bei akuter Pseudoobstruktion des Kolons. Zentralbl Chir 116: 575–579

4. Ermisch J, Schneider H (1995) Neue Sonde zur Optimierung der geschlossenen Dekompression und temporären Darmschienung beim Dünndarmileus. Chirurg 66: 235–238
5. Hüttenrauch R, Fricke S (1984) Der Einfluß des Glyzerols auf die helikale Konformation der Gelatine. Pharmazie 39: 500–501
6. Nissen R, Maurer W (1965) Zur Pathogenese und Behandlung des Darmverschlusses. Zentralbl Chir 90: 1533–1535
7. Reifferscheid M, Pip M (1984) Indikation und Risiko der inneren Darmschienung. Chirurg 55: 395–399
8. Roscher R, Beger HG(1985) Neue Vorstellungen zur Pathophysiologie des mechanischen Dünndarmileus. In: Häring R(Hrsg) Ileus-Chirurgische und gastroenterologische Praxis. de Gruyter, Berlin, pp 15–19
9. Waclawiczek HW, Henkel M, Rieger R (1987) Die innere Sondenschienung des Dünndarmes zur Ileusprophylaxe bei Peritonitis und rezidivierenden Adhäsionen. Zentralbl Chir 112: 1222–1227
10. Wangensteen OH (1969) Historical aspects of the management acute intestinal obstruction. Surgery 65: 363–383

9.6 Benefit and Risk of Long Intestinal Tubes in Intestinal Obstruction

J. Faß, S. Müller, M. Jansen, G. Ages, K.-H. Treutner, S. Truong, and V. Schumpelick

Introduction

Postoperative adhesions are the most common cause of intestinal obstruction and have a prevalence of 20%–48% [13]. Nearly 1% of all abdominal operations performed are due to this condition [9]. Many attempts have been made to prevent the postoperative formation of adhesions, but the value of the different procedures is questionable. Long intestinal tubes are used in the surgical therapy of small intestinal obstruction for two different indications. First, endoscopically placed long intestinal tubes have the capability to decompress a distended bowel and break through the pathophysiologic cascade of ileus (Fig. 1). Second, long intestinal tubes can be used for intraluminal stenting after adhesiolysis to prevent recurrent obstruction.

There is an ongoing discussion about the value of long intestinal tubes in the treatment of ileus. While one group of researchers saw a benefit in this kind of therapy [1, 4, 6, 11, 12, 15], another did not find fewer obstructions after tube therapy but observed more complications and a higher mortality correlated with the tube therapy itself and the therapeutic delay due to preoperative decompression [2, 3, 14, 16]. However, serious complications such as wound infections, peritonitis, and generalized sepsis seem to result from the trans-abdominal approach to the intestinal lumen via the stomach, small bowel or cecum and can be prohibited by transnasal insertion of the tube [6, 8, 10]. There are no data from larger studies using modern endoscopic methods as a part of the surgical concept that have assessed therapy with long intestinal tubes.

In the period from 1985 to 1995 we used long intestinal tubes in a total of 464 patients with small intestinal obstruction (Table 1). Decompression by an endoscopically placed tube was the indication in 319 patients, whereas 145 patients had their long intestinal tube placed intraoperatively for the indication of intraluminal stenting. A follow-up could be achieved in 179 patients with decompression and 84 patients with intraluminal stenting and adhesions. The patients with advanced malignancy were not included in the study, as their postoperative cause was mainly influenced by progression of the tumor and not by adhesions. Thus, there were 260 patients in our retrospective study. In all patients a Dennis tube [6] was used with a length of 270 cm and three channels for irrigation, suction and balloon blocking.

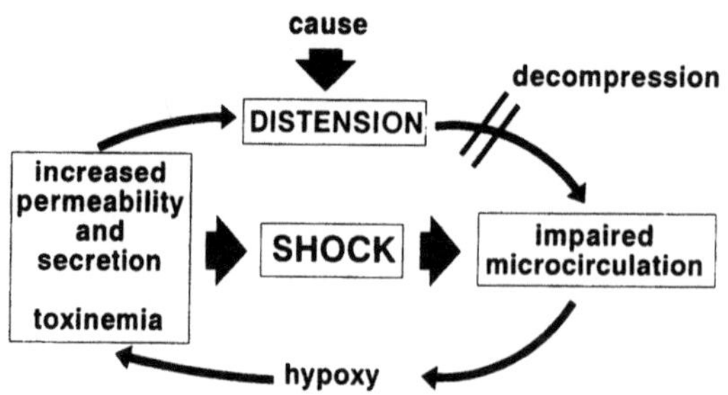

Fig. 1. Pathophysiologic basis of therapy using long intestinal tubes in small bowel obstruction

Table 1. Characteristics of 464 patients treated with long intestinal tubes (1985–1995)

Decompression		Intraluminal stenting		Total
		Adhesion	Malignancy	
Total	319	98	47	464
Follow-up	179	84		263

Here, we describe our results using long intestinal tube therapy for decompression and intraluminal stenting of obstructed small intestines.

Decompression

Indications

The pathophysiological aims of decompression of obstructed small intestine using long intestinal tubes are to relieve the distension, overcome disturbed microcirculation, end bacterial translocation and endotoxemia, and allow equilibration of fluid and electrolytes. The clinical aims are prevention of unnecessary operations and improvement of the patient's condition before necessary surgery. The main indications are paralytic ileus and incomplete mechanical ileus of different causes (Table 2). A complete mechanical ileus of any cause; the suspicion of strangulation, incarceration or ischemia; peritonitis; a history of upper GI-hemorrhage due to esophagitis; or portal hypotension are contraindications for tube decompression.

Technique

Generally, the long intestinal tube is placed endoscopically. For this purpose the patient is brought into an upright position to prevent vomiting and aspiration during the endoscopic maneuver. The tube is introduced transnasally and extracted through the mouth to be connected with the gastroscope. Then the tube is brought down to the stomach together with the endoscope and placed transpylorically with the help of a biopsy forceps (Fig. 2). After this

Table 2. Indications and contraindications for therapy using long intestinal tubes

Indications	Contraindications
Paralytic ileus	Complete mechanical ileus of *any* cause
Intoxications	Suspicion of strangulation, incarceration, or ischemia
Motility disorders	Peritonitis
Retroperitoneal trauma	History of GI hemorrhage or esophagitis (>2nd degree)
Metabolic disturbances	
Incomplete mechanical ileus	
Crohn's disease[a]	
Recurrent obstruction (adhesions)[a]	
Early postoperative stage	
Intraabdominal tumor dissemination	

[a]Without strangulation.

maneuver, the balloon is blocked and the endoscope is extracted. After the procedure an X-ray of the abdomen is made to document correct positioning of the tube. The balloon is then blocked with 15 ml of water to allow transport of the tube with the help of intestinal peristalsis. The block volume of the balloon should not be extended to prevent intestinal obstruction, and a second tube should be inserted into the stomach to drain the gastric succus and avoid

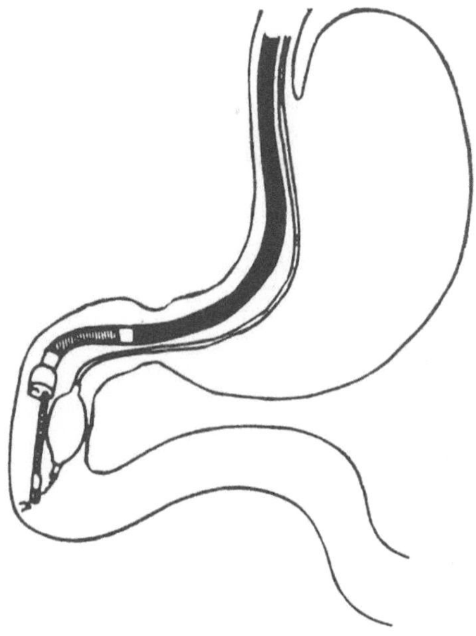

Fig. 2. Endoscopic placing of long intestinal tubes

distention. Then the tube is moved forward 5 cm every 2 h under intermittent suction. Until continuous equilibration is maintained the patient is followed up thoroughly under daily clinical and radiological controls to document the ongoing transport of the tube. When the small bowel is decompressed and the patient has regular defecations, a barium contrast enema is added to clarify the cause of obstruction and to help determining the proper surgical procedure. If there are no bowel movements after 5 days and the tube does not show any further transport, an explorative laparotomy is performed.

Results

In the 179 patients in whom a follow-up was possible, endoscopic placing of a long intestinal tube was successful in 174 patients (97.2%). The medium time needed for the procedure was 28 min (16–72 min). The causes of endoscopic failure in the five remaining patients were stenosis of the nasopharynx in two patients, one esophagitis, one gastric outlet obstruction and one broncho-spasm. The medium age of the 174 patients was 64.8 years.

In 157 patients, previous operations were the cause of the intra-abdominal adhesions and subsequent obstruction. The most common previous operations were appendectomy (21%) and gynecologic operations (19%). Some 18% of the patients presented with a recurrent intestinal obstruction due to an adhesive disease (Table 3). Complications of the tube therapy were rare: 8% of the patients complained of mild esophagitis, which disappeared immediately after removing the tube. Three patients showed minor gastrointestinal bleeding and one patient had a perforation of the upper jejunum that had to be operated upon. The rate of complications was similar to that reported in the literature (Table 4).

There were 75 patients (43.1%) who had to be operated on for intestinal obstruction after long intestinal tube decompression. In 60 of these patients, surgery was elective, while 15 patients (20%) had to be operated on under urgent conditions. In 99 patients (56.9%) an operation could be avoided by long intestinal tube decompression. Most of these cases involved early post-operative obstruction and paralytic ileus (Fig. 3). While most of the patients with malignancy and recurrent obstruction had to be operated on, only 60% of patients with Crohn's disease needed surgical intervention. We observed 15

Table 3. Indications for small bowel decompression with long intestinal tubes (n= 202)

Indication	n	Percent
Appendectomy	43	21
Gynecological operations	39	19
Obstruction	36	18
Colonic resection	22	11
Gastric resection	8	4
Bile duct operations	49	24

Table 4. Complications of small bowel decompression following treatment with long intestinal tubes: comparison with data from the literature

Reference (n)	Invagination (%)	Bleeding (%)	Perforation (%)	Fistula (%)	Esophagitis (%)
Kapral 1984 [7] (160)	1.3, 1.1	–	0.6	–	–
Weigelt et al. 1980 [16] (154)	0.6	–	–	3.2	–
Eckert et al. 1977 [5] (98)	1.0	2.0	1.0	–	–
Aachen 1995 (174)	–	1.7	0.6	–	8.0

deaths (8.6%), all of which were correlated with the patient's underlying disease and not with long intestinal tube decompression. In this situation, mortality was highest in patients with intra-abdominal disseminated malignancy.

Intraluminal Stenting

Indications

A national survey in Germany [13] showed that intraluminal stenting for the prevention of intestinal obstruction after adhesiolysis is used in 40% of all surgical clinics, without regard to frequency of abdominal operations. Since the value of this therapy is still unclear we performed a retrospective study in our

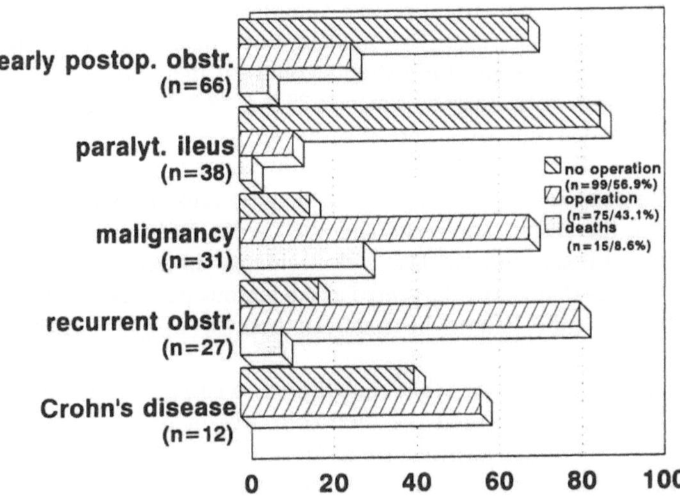

Fig. 3. Outcome of 174 patients with small bowel decompression treated with long intestinal tubes

own patient collective, evaluating intraluminal stenting by long intestinal tubes. Indications were the combination of obstruction and extended adhesiolysis, small bowel resections, or peritoneal carcinosis. The pathophysiological aims of this procedure were intra-abdominal decompression of obstructed bowel and/or administration of an intraluminal placeholder for the period when the adhesions became organized. The clinical aims were the prevention of recurrent obstruction, early restoration of postoperative motility and protection of anastomoses in preoperatively obstructed small bowel.

Technique

The technique used in our clinic was the endoscopically or manually performed transnasal introduction of a Dennis tube. After complete adhesiolysis the balloon of the tube was guided manually through the small bowel under suction to achieve a decompression of the obstructed bowel. At the same time, we could demonstrate complete restoration of the passage. Finally, the balloon was introduced into the ascendic colon. On the first postoperative day, the balloon was unblocked and the tube was left for at least 10 days without suction.

Results

Patients with intraabdominal malignancy and intraluminal stenting were not included into the study, because in these cases the results mostly depend on the underlying disease rather than on long intestinal tube therapy. Of the 98 patients who underwent intraluminal stenting because of adhesive disease, 84 had a complete follow-up. Of these, 63 patients (75%) were operated on for obstruction caused by primary adhesions, while 21 patients (25%) had a recurrent adhesive ileus. There were no intraoperative complications. The duration of tube therapy was 10.0 ± 4.3 days. The median time until the first bowel movement was 4.6 ± 2.9 days and the patients could eat their first solid food after 13.4 ± 3.4 days. The total hospital stay was 25.7 ± 18.2 days; for 7.1 ± 4.9 days the patients needed intensive care. Of the 84 patients, 37 (44%) had mostly minor complications correlated with long intestinal tube therapy. Most common were lipasemia ($n=26$) and a mild esophagitis caused by mechanical mucosal erosion of the distal esophagus and the cardia. Only five of the 26 patients with elevated lipase and amylase measurements showed morphologic changes of the pancreas that were interpreted as edematous pancreatitis. In two patients the intestinal tube had to be removed because of gastrointestinal bleeding (Fig. 4).

To further evaluate those factors that contributed to complications of long intestinal tube therapy, we analyzed the total collective of patients with decompression and intraluminal stenting ($n=263$). The most important factor that correlated with the development of complications was the duration of long intestinal tube therapy (Fig. 5). Only patients with a therapy of more than 10 days showed a relevant number of complications.

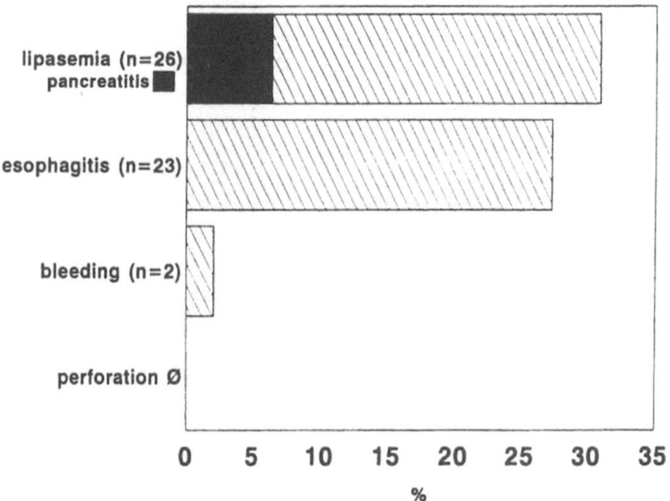

Fig. 4. Complications due to intraluminal stenting with long intestinal tubes in patients with small bowel obstruction caused by adhesions

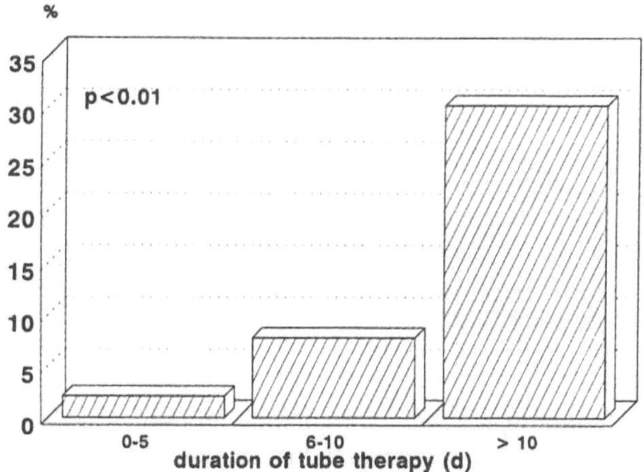

Fig. 5. Complications in all patients with small bowel decompression and intraluminal stenting with a complete follow-up (n=263), correlated with the duration of tube therapy

The median follow-up time of patients who received intraluminal stenting was 62.3 ± 27.8 (3–114) months. In this period 13 (15.5%) out of 84 patients had to be operated on for a recurrent intestinal obstruction caused by intra-abdominal adhesions. All recurrencies occurred within the first 4 years after the primary operation (Fig. 6). In the group of 13 patients with reoperations,

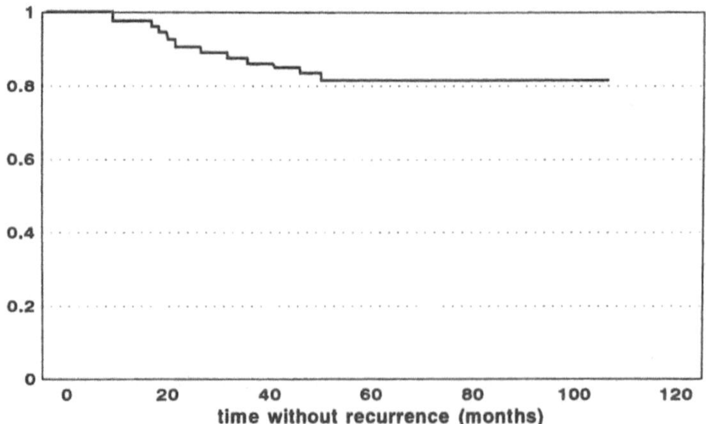

Fig. 6. Probability of being reoperated on for small bowel obstruction after intraluminal stenting with long intestinal tubes ($n=84$)

eight belonged to the initial group with recurrent adhesions, while only five patients had primary adhesions at the first operation. So the relative risk of patients with recurrent adhesions to experience another recurrency was much higher (8/21, 38.1%) than that of patients with an obstruction caused by primary adhesions (5/63, 7.9%).

Conclusions

The decompression of obstructed small bowel by endoscopic placing of a long intestinal tube is possible in 97% of patients. In about 10% of these, minor complications occur that disappear when the tube is removed. In more than half of the patients, surgery can be prevented by tube therapy. In patients who absolutely require surgery to treat their obstruction after long intestinal tube decompression, 80% can be operated on electively.

After intraluminal stenting with long intestinal tubes for small bowel obstruction caused by intra-abdominal adhesions, mostly minor complications occur in 44% of patients. Lipasemia and amylasemia, without morphologic changes of the pancreas, and a mechanically induced mild esophagitis of the distal esophagus and cardia region are the most common complications. Most of the complications occur after a tube therapy of more than 10 days.

Some 15% of our patients with intraluminal stenting had to be reoperated on for recurrent obstruction. All recurrencies occured within the first 4 years. Most of the patients with recurrent obstructions had re-reobstruction. Thus, there is probably a distinct group of patients who have a high risk for re-obstruction; however, the factors that contribute to this predisposition are still unknown.

References

1. Baker JW (1959) A long jejunostomy tube for decompressing intestinal obstruction. Surg Gynecol Obstet 109: 519–520
2. Brightwell NL, McFee AS, Aust JB (1977) Bowel obstruction and the long tube stent. Arch Surg 112: 505–511
3. Brolin RE (1983) The role of gastrointestinal tube decompression in the treatment of mechanical intestinal obstruction. Am Surg 49: 131–137
4. Close MB, Christensen NM (1979) Transmesenteric small bowel plication or intraluminal tube stenting – indications and contraindications. Am J Surg 138: 89–96
5. Eckert P, Eichfuß HP, Kippner A (1977) Die innere Schienung des Dünndarms. Aktuelle Chir 12: 20–28
6. Dennis C (1969) The gastrointestinal sump tube. Surgery 66: 309–312
7. Kapral W (1984) Die Schienung des Dünndarmes mit der Miller-Abbott-Sonde – eine kritische Analyse von 160 Fällen. Chirurg 55: 391
8. McMillin RD, Bivins BA, Griffen WO (1981) Intraluminal stenting in the management of recurrent intestinal obstruction. Am Surg 47: 74–77
9. Menzies D, Ellis H (1990) Intestinal obstruction from adhesions – how big is the problem? Ann R Coll Surg Engl 72: 60
10. Nelson RL, Nyhus LM (1979) A new long intestinal tube. Surg Gynecol Obstet 149: 581–582
11. Rodriguez-Ruesga R, Meagher AP, Wolff BG (1995) Twelve-year experience with the long intestinal tube. World J Surg 19: 627–631
12. Sanderson ER (1971) Decompression of the small intestine by retrograde intubation. Surg Gynecol Obstet 132: 1073–1075
13. Treutner K-H, Bertram P, Löser S, Winkeltau G, Schumpelick V (1995) Prophylaxe und Therapie intraabdomineller Adhäsionen – Eine Umfrage an 1200 Kliniken in Deutschland. Chirurg 66: 398–403
14. Turner DM, Croom RD (1983) Acute adhesive obstruction of the small intestine. Am Surg 49: 126–130
15. Wangensteen OH, Rea CE, Smith BA (1939) Experience with employment of suction in the treatment of acute intestinal obstruction. Surg Gynecol Obstet 68: 851–868
16. Weigelt JA, Snyder WH, Norman JL (1980) Complications and results of 160 baker tube plications. Am J Surg 140: 810–815

10 Prevention and Control of Adhesion Formation

10.1 The Management of Adhesive Disease

C.L. Kowalczyk and M.P. Diamond

Introduction

It is well known that pelvic adhesions play a major role in female infertility; adhesions may interfere with ovum pick-up by the fallopian tube, may create a spatial interference between the ovary and tube, cause fixation of one or both organs in the pelvis, or the tube/ovary may be encapsulated by the adhesions [1, 2, 3]. Adhesions may also be associated with other conditions such as acute and chronic pelvic pain, and small bowel obstruction. Predisposing factors for the development of pelvic adhesions include pelvic inflammatory disease or other pelvic infections, appendicitis, previous ectopic or reproductive surgery and hemorrhage; the most common factor being prior surgery [4]. Such predisposing factors and complications of adhesive disease prompt the appropriate use of meticulous surgical technique as well as effective barriers to adhesion formation. This chapter will review the importance of meticulous surgical technique in adhesion prevention. Then, various adjuvant therapies/barriers that have been developed to prevent adhesions will be discussed.

Surgical Techniques

The mainstay of adhesion prevention is excellent surgical and microsurgical technique. There should be minimal tissue handling as excess disruption of tissue may lead to tissue trauma. Tissue trauma in turn decreases plasminogen activator activity, suppresses fibrinolytic activity and allows fibrin to persist intraperitoneally. This is followed by an infiltration and organization of the coagulum by fibroblasts, followed by vascular and cellular ingrowth. The result is permanent fibrous adhesion formation [5]. Talc on surgical gloves and lint from the surgical drapes may elicit a foreign body reaction and tissue trauma that will subsequently lead to adhesions. Woven material used as an intraabdominal packing may cause abrasions if the organ surfaces are dry, subsequently leading to adhesions. Constant irrigation/moistening of the tissues with Ringer's lactate solution is important as such measures will prevent drying and subsequent abrasion of tissues [6]. Meticulous hemostasis is necessary as persistent blood in the peritoneal cavity and over denuded surfaces will be a nidus for fibrin deposition and adhesion formation.

The size of the suture and the tension applied in closing a defect is also important. The choice of suture material should be fine and of low reactivity as this can act as a foreign body. Suture that causes tissue ischemia as opposed to reapproximation will lead to subsequent adhesion formation secondary to inadequate blood flow and disruption of the fibrinolytic process.

The surgeon should take great care in implementing meticulous surgical technique to decrease any possible iatrogenic predisposing factors that would lead to the formation of adhesions.

The type of instrumentation at the time of surgery does not seem to alter the degree of adhesion formation. In a review by Corfman et al., scalpel, cautery, and CO_2 laser were compared for their benefit in treating/preventing adhesions [7]. At high power densities, electrocautery was noted to be comparable to both the scalpel and high power density laser in terms of adhesion formation and histology. Cautery was superior to the scalpel in terms of hemostasis with minimal adverse tissue healing effects. Although the CO_2 laser allowed for more precise incisions, minimal tissue handling, a more bloodless field, and minimal operative time, it did not result in consistent reductions in adhesions as seen at second-look laparoscopy.

Adjuvant Therapy

The equivocal results obtained with various surgical techniques and instrumentation also led to the development of a variety of instillates and barriers to prevent adhesions (Table 1). Adjuvants may act by decreasing vascular permeability, histamine release or leukocyte migration. They may alternatively have immunosuppressive effects, initiate fibrinolysis, or provide a mechanical separation through hydroflotation or third spacing. Some of the various adjuvants and their associated mechanisms are presented in Table 2. Some of these adjuvants and barriers will be discussed in this chapter.

Fibrinolytic Agents

Fibrinolytic agents act to prevent adhesion formation directly by reducing the fibrinous mass and indirectly by stimulating plasminogen activator activity [9]. Plasminogen activator is a serine protease that converts plasminogen to plasmin at the level of the fibrin clot. When plasminogen activator was topically applied as a gel to abraded rabbit uterine horns, there was a significant reduction of adhesion formation. Also, after adhesiolysis, when the gel was applied there was a decrease in adhesions. Use of fibrinolytic agents at high doses, however, may have associated hemorrhagic complications. The development and use of fibrinolytic agents remains to be investigated in human studies.

Table 1. Classes of adjuvants used in an attempt to minimize the occurrence of postoperative adhesions

---

Fibrinolytic agents
  Fibrinolysin
  Papain
  Streptokinase
  Urokinase
  Hyaluronidase
  Chymotrypsin
  Trypsin
  Pepsin
  Plasminogen activator
  Calcium channel blockers
Anticoagulants
  Heparin
  Citrates
  Oxalates
Antiinflammatory agents
  Corticosteroid
  Ibuprofen
  Antihistamines
Antibiotics
  Tetracyclines
  Cephalosporins
Mechanical separation
  Intraabdominal instillates
    Dextran
    Mineral Oil
    Silicone
    Povidine
    Vaseline
    Crystalloid solutions
    Carboxymethylcellulose
Barriers
  Endogenous tissue
    Omental grafts
    Peritoneal grafts
    Bladder strips
    Fetal membranes
  Exogenous material
    Oxidized cellulose
    Oxidized regenerated cellulose (Interceed TC7)
    Gelatin
    Rubber sheets
    Metal foils
    Plastic hood
    Photopolymerizable gels/Flowgel
    Goretex surgical membrane

Modified from Diamond and DeCherney [4].

Table 2. Proposed mechanisms of adhesion prevention by class of adjuvants

Class of adjuvant	Proposed mechanism
Antiinflammatory	Reduce vascular permeability, reduce histamine release and stabilize lysosomes
Progestins	Immunosuppression: decreased antibody production, inhibition of human mixed lymphocytic culture and leukocyte migration, decreased vascular permeability
Fibrinolytic enzymes	Fibrinolysis; stimulation of plasminogen activator
Antibiotics	Prevent infection
Mechanical separation	Surface separation, hydroflotation, siliconization

Reproduced with permission from Diamond [8].

Anticoagulants

Anticoagulants, specifically heparin, have been studied in preventing adhesions via the mechanism of decreasing fibrin deposition. Heparin in irrigating solution has not been shown to be beneficial in adhesion prevention. And, although high dose heparin given intraperitoneally or systemically did show a decrease in adhesion formation, there were significant complications noted, especially with regard to hemorrhage and wound disruption [4]. However, in rabbits low dose heparin in conjunction with local delivery (in this case Interceed TC7) showed a significant decrease in adhesion formation and reformation (see below).

Antiinflammatory Agents

Antiinflammatory agents are used to reduce vascular permeability, reduce histamine release and stabilize lysozymes. This includes such diverse agents as corticosteroids, nonsteroidal agents, progestins, antihistamines, and calcium channel blockers. Corticosteroids act in reducing the inflammatory response by the general principles mentioned above. In small animal studies, they have been shown to be effective, but only in large doses [10]. Associated with such large doses of corticosteroids is the risk of immunosuppression, infection and would dehiscence. Nonsteroidals act by inhibiting prostaglandin synthesis and plasmin inhibitors. In animal models, oxyphenbutazone and indomethacin showed a decrease in adhesion formation [10]. Ibuprofen, which also inhibits platelet aggregation and leukocyte activity, failed to show an efficacy in adhesion reduction in several animal studies [4]. Antihistamines, such as promethazine, inhibit the inflammatory response, stabilize lysosomal membranes and inhibit fibroblast proliferation. The use of antihistamines to prevent adhesions has been administered in conjunction with glucocorticoids and has not been shown to be effective in human studies [4]. Progesterone has both antiinflammatory activity via a decrease in vascular permeability and leukocyte migration as well as immunosuppressive activity via decreased antibody production. Results of adhesion formation in animal studies have been conflicting.

In a guinea pig model, aqueous progesterone given intraperitoneally resulted in a decrease in adhesion formation, while depo Provera in a rat model increased adhesion formation [10]. There are currently no human studies to support progestin as an adjuvant therapy. Calcium channel blockers (nifedipine) act by a variety of potential mechanisms including limiting tissue ischemia, as well as by limiting the release of prostaglandins E and F. Adenosine triphosphate, which induces platelet aggregation, is also limited and fibroblast migration is inhibited. Calcium channel blockers conversely induce vasodilation via the stimulation of prostacyclin I-2 [11]. Studies so far have been limited to animal studies; Steinleitmer et al. showed a reduction in pelvic adhesions along with the absence of side effects in hamsters [12, 13]. However, we were unable to confirm those observations (Diamond et al., unpubl observations).

Antibiotic Therapy

The theory behind the use of antibiotic therapy is the prevention of infection thereby decreasing the inflammatory response that would predispose to adhesion formation. The two most commonly used antibiotics to date have been tetracycline and cephalosporins. There has been, however, no significant data in animal or human studies supporting these therapies in the prevention of adhesion formation (perhaps because the incidence of intraabdominal postoperative infections following elective surgery is so low).

Hyskon

Although only approved by the FDA for uterine distension during hysteroscopy, one of the more common adjuvants that has been used is Hyskon (32 dextran 70), which is a high viscosity instillate. The premise of this adjuvant therapy involves the separation of raw surfaces after surgery by producing a siliconizing effect on the tissues, thus preventing the formation of early fibrin adhesions. Hyskon has also been shown to stimulate plasminogen activator activity, thus enhancing fibrinolysis and preventing adhesion formation. Approximately 100–200 ml of Hyskon is instilled into the cul de sac and subsequently, thrd spacing of fluid occurs into the abdominal cavity creating an intraperitoneal flotation bath. In prospective randomized blinded multicenter trials, Hyskon was shown to significantly decrease adhesion formation as observed at second-look laparoscopy [4]. Alternatively, in a study by Diamond et al. comparing the effectiveness of Hyskon vs carboxymethylcellulose (CMC) in reducing adhesion formation, utilization of 50 ml of 32% Dextran 70 did not reduce adhesions compared with control rabbits [14]. Although Hyskon in some respects may be effective in reducing adhesion formation, side effects have been noted. The side effects that have been associated with Hyskon use include fever, anaphylaxis, wound separation, shock, ARDS (Adult respiratory distress syndrome), serum sickness, DIC, labial edema, allergy peritonitis, hypokalemia, pleural effusion, and pseudopulmonary embolus [10].

Carboxymethylcellulose

Another potential adjuvant is carboxymethylcellulose (CMC). This adjuvant is produced by reacting sodium monochloride with cellulose. Its proposed mechanism is also that of hydroflotation allowing third spacing of fluid into the abdominal cavity to occur. In addition, it has a siliconization effect whereby CMC is able to coat intraperitoneal surfaces, thus preventing their direct apposition [15]. In studies by Diamond et al. using the rabbit uterine horn model, intraperitoneal instillation of CMC significantly reduced postoperative adhesion formation as well as reformation [14, 16].

Hyaluronic Acid

Hyaluronic acid is a glycosaminoglycan that under aqueous conditions forms a viscous solution. One mechanism by which adhesions are prevented is by coating of the injured surfaces with hylauronic acid. It is beneficial, however, when the surfaces are coated with this substance before injury takes place to minimize injury. In rat studies, instillation of hyaluronic acid before cecal abrasion reduced adhesion formation [17], while coating serosal surfaces after tissue injury was ineffective [18]. In a study by Grainger, using a rabbit model, hyaluronic acid was used at three different viscous concentrations and as a polymer slab of the substance. None of the hyaluronic acid solutions resulted in a reduction of ovarian adhesions; only the polymer slab significantly reduced adhesions when applied as a barrier [19]. In other studies, preformed sheets of hyaluronic acid and CMC have been shown to reduce adhesion reformation [20].

Poloxamer

Poloxamers are groups of surfactant compounds that have the ability to convert from a liquid state (at room temperature) to a gel form (T>25 °C). Once recooled, the polymer returns to its liquid form and the cycle can be repeated. In previous studies, poloxamers provided the means to deliver drugs over localized regions including dexamethasone to chemical burns and pilocarpine to reduce intraocular pressure [21].

Poloxamer 407 of Flowgel is derived from a 4000 kDa hydrophobe and is composed of 70% polyoxythylene hydrophile. Studies have been performed with this poloxamer to determine if it can reduce adhesion formation. In a study by Rice et al. [22] 0.5–1.5 ml poloxamer solution was used to cover uterine and sidewall defects in rabbit models. There was noted to be a significant reduction in primary postsurgical adhesions; 95% of the control side had adhesions compared to 40% of the treated side. This observation has been confirmed in other studies.

Interceed

Several studies are available with respect to the effectiveness of Interceed TC7 alone or in combination with adjuvants in preventing adhesions in animals. Interceed TC7 absorbable adhesion barrier (Johnson and Johnson Medical, Inc.) is a knitted fabric of oxidized regenerated cellulose. It can be considered an altered form of Surgicel and differs with respect to several characteristics including its degree of oxidation, weave, and smaller pore size. Several animal studies have shown a beneficial effect of Interceed on adhesion formation and reformation [23]. The Adhesion Barrier Study Group II in 1993 presented data from 13 centers comparing microsurgery alone to microsurgery in combination with Interceed for pelvic adhesion reformation. A total of 134 patients, all with bilateral pelvic sidewall adhesions, undergoing adhesiolysis via microsurgery at laparotomy were included. After adhesiolysis, one sidewall in each patient served as her own control while the other sidewall was covered with Interceed. Microsurgery alone showed a 55.6% reduction in the area of adherent peritoneum and a 60% and 39% reduction in filmy and severe adhesions, respectively, at second-look laparoscopy. The use of Interceed significantly further reduced the area of adherent peritoneum with a 72% and 61% reduction in filmy and severe adhesion reformation, respectively. In this study, in those patients with a differential outcome, 90% of those patients benefited from the use of Interceed barrier as assessed by greater reduction on the treated side [24].

The use of Interceed requires a very hemostatic field. Failure to achieve hemostasis prior to applying Interceed will result in the material "blackening," rendering it ineffective. Though desirable, meticulous hemostasis is not always achievable. Therefore, the use of Interceed with other adjuvants has been studied in animal models. Diamond et al. [23] incorporated the rabbit uterine horn model to evaluate the synergistic effects of Interceed plus various adjuvants in reducing adhesion formation. In comparing a variety of adjuvants in combination with Interceed (including indomethacin, promethazine, dexamethasone, progesterone, and heparin), heparin plus Interceed significantly reduced adhesion formation. Heparin delivery alone via intraperitoneal lavage, intravenous injection or intraabdominal instillation failed to prevent adhesions. Additionally, heparin in combination with other barriers including carboxymethylcellulose or Hyskon failed to demonstrate efficiency. Interceed, therefore, may be utilized as a carrier for heparin to traumatized tissues and the combination in turn may be more effective in preventing adhesions [25]. Interceed in combination with heparin has also been shown to prevent adhesion reformation as shown in the same rabbit uterine horn model [26]. However, clinical studies have failed to demonstrate any significant improvement compared to Interceed alone [27]. Additional human studies are now needed to further evaluate these findings.

Interceed in combination with thrombin has recently been investigated. Using a modified rabbit uterine horn model, "oozing" and "bleeding" sites were created. The use of thrombin alone, Interceed alone, or achieving hemostasis with thrombin then applying Interceed were compared. Although thrombin or Interceed alone did not reduce adhesions at bleeding sites, a significant reduction in adhesions was achieved with the application of thrombin first to provide hemostasis followed by the application of Interceed. Efficiency was further improved when the Interceed was moistened with heparin, rather than saline, after placement on the sidewall [28].

A modified version of Interceed nTC7 that is blood insensitive has also proved efficacious in reducing adhesions formation and reformation in animal studies [29]. The results using the nTC7 Interceed are comparable to those obtained with Interceed in combination with heparin. Further animal studies and human studies are needed, but the results thus far appear quite promising.

Goretex Surgical Membrane

Another barrier that has shown promise has been a polytetrafluoroethylene (PTFE) or Goretex surgical membrane. Goretex has been successfully used in cardiovascular and thoracic surgery for many years as a membrane for pericardial or vascular grafts [30–32]. In contrast to the material used for vascular grafts that is 1 mm in pore size and is designed to encourage adhesion/cell proliferation, the Goretex surgical membrane used in pelvic surgery is $< 1\ \mu m$ in pore size, thus inhibiting tissue attachment. It is also nontoxic, nonreactive, and antithrombogenic; it is not absorbed and is unaffected by tissue enzymes [30–32]. It is therefore a permanent membrane unless it is surgically removed at a later time point. The results of animal studies using this membrane are promising. In a study by Boyer et al. [33], Goretex was used in a model of New Zealand rabbits to cover ischemic defects in the pelvic sidewall peritoneum. The extent of adhesion formation between the rabbit uterine horn/pelvic sidewall model with and without the Goretex surgical membrane was determined. The mean adhesion score for the surgical membrane covered lesions was significantly lower than that of controls ($p < 0.001$). Histologically, none of the Goretex covered lesions had adhesions to the membrane itself, while 79% of the control lesions showed dense adhesions at the injury site [33]. This suggests that the Goretex surgical membrane as a barrier is quite effective in preventing adhesions. In a study by March et al., 18 patients with extensive pelvic adhesions and 10 undergoing myomectomy had Goretex placed over the myomectomy or adhesiolysis sites. At second-look laparoscopy, the membranes were removed easily and there were minimal adhesions noted [34]. Further human studies are necessary to continue to investigate the effectiveness of the Goretex membrane.

Conclusions

Excellent surgical technique with minimal tissue handling, frequent irrigation to maintain moist tissue surfaces, adequate tissue approximation and meticulous hemostasis remain of utmost importance in minimizing pelvic adhesions. In addition, the various adjuvant therapies discussed have been developed to aid in the prevention of adhesion formation. Despite all of these interventions, however, the battle over pelvic adhesion development has yet to be won. Incorporating the measures mentioned above may help to decrease the formation/reformation of pelvic adhesions. Advances in the field of molecular biology may prove useful in the investigation of adhesion formation; modifications of current and developments of new adjuvant/barrier therapies continues and are required to provide better adhesion prevention. By incorporating new technologies, techniques, and adjuvants in combination with meticulous surgical technique, the prevention of adhesion formation may possibly be achieved, but for now the battle continues.

References

1. Bronson RA, Wallach EE (1977) Lysis of periadnexal adhesions for correction of infertility. Fertil Steril 28: 613
2. Caspi E, Halpern Y, Bukovsky I (1979) The importance of peritoneal adhesions in tubal reconstructive surgery for infertility. Fertil Steril 31: 296
3. Gomel V (1983) Salpingoovariolysis by laparoscopy in infertility. Fertil Steril 40: 607
4. Diamond MP, DeCherney AH (1987) Pathogenesis of adhesion formation/reformation: application to reproductive pelvic surgery. Microsurgery 8: 103–108
5. Gervin AS, Puckett CL, Silver D (1973) Serosal hypofibrinolysis: a cause of postoperative adhesions. Am J Surg 125: 80–88
6. Montz FJ, Shimanuki T, Dizerega GS (1987) Postsurgical mesothelial reepithelialization. In: DeCherney AH, Polan ML (eds) Reproductive surgery. Yearbook Medical Publishers, Chicago, pp 31–48
7. Corfman RS, Diamond MP, Laser, cautery or scalpel: which is best? Lasers in Gynecology, WB Saunders, Philadelphia, pp 309–319
8. Diamond MP, Hershlag A (1990) Adhesion formation/reformation. Treatment of postsurgical adhesions, pp 23–33
9. Doody KJ, Dunn RC, Buttram VC (1989) Recombinant tissue plasminogen activator reduces adhesion formation in a rabbit uterine horn model. Fertil Steril 51: 509–512
10. Holtz G (1984) Prevention and management of peritoneal adhesions. Fertil Steril 41: 497–507
11. Mehta J, Mehta P, Ostrowski N (1986) Calcium channel blocker diltiazem inhibits platelet activation and stimulates vascular prostacyclin synthesis. Am J Med Sci 20: 291
12. Steinleitner A, Lambert H, Montoro L et al. (1988) Use of diltiazem for preventing postoperative adhesions. J Reprod Med 33: 891
13. Steinleitner A, Lambert H, Montoro L et al. (1988) The use of calcium channel blockade for the prevention of postoperative adhesion formation. Fertil Steril 50: 818
14. Diamond MP, DeCherney AH (1988) Assessment of carboxymethylcellulose and 32% Dextran 70 for the prevention of adhesions in a rabbit uterine horn model. Int J Fertil 33(4): 278–282
15. Elkins TE, Bury RJ, Ritter JL et al. (1984) Adhesion Prevention by solutions of sodium carboxymethylcellulose in the rat I. Fertil Steril 41: 926
16. Diamond MP, DeCherney AH et al. (1988) Adhesion reformation in the rabbit uterine horn model: 1 Reduction with carboxymethylcellulose. Int J Fertil 33(5): 372–375
17. Yaacobi Y, Goldberg EP, Patahaangey B et al. (1989) Prevention of postoperative abdominal adhesions in a rat cecal abrasion model. J Invest Surg 2: 320
18. Urman B, Gomel V, Jetha N (1991) Effect of hyaluronic acid of postoperative intraperitoneal adhesion formation in the rat model. Fertil Steril 56: 563
19. Grainger DA, Meyer WR, DeCherney AH, Diamond MP (1991) The use of hyaluronic acid polymers to reduce postoperative adhesions. J Gynecol Surg 7: 97–101

20. Skinner KC et al. (1992) The evaluation of HAL-F bioresorbable membrane for the prevention of postsurgical adhesion formation in two animal models. 2nd Int Symp on Gynecologic Surgery and Adhesion Prevention, Palm Beach
21. Henry RL, Schmolka IR (1989) Burn wound coverings and the use of poloxymer preparations. Clin Rev Biocompatibil 5: 207–220
22. Rice VM, Shanti A, Moghissi K et al. (1993) A comparative evaluation of Poloxymer 407 and oxidized regenerated cellulose (Interceed TC7) to reduce postoperative adhesion formation in the rat uterine horn model. Fertil Steril 59: 901–906
23. Diamond MP, Cunningham T, Linsky CB et al. (1990) Interceed (TC7) as an adjuvant for adhesion reduction: animal studies. Treatment of post surgical adhesions. Wiley Leis, New York, pp 131–143
24. Azziz R, Adhesion Barrier Study Group II (1993) Microsurgery alone or with Interceed absorbable adhesion barrier for pelvic sidewall adhesion reformation. Surg Gynecol Obstet 177: 135–139
25. Diamond MP, Linsky CB, Cunningham T et al. (1991) Synergistic effects of Interceed TC7 and heparin in reducing adhesion formation in the rabbit uterine horn model. Fertil Steril 55: 389–394
26. Diamond MP, Linsky CB, Cunningham T et al. (1991) Adhesion Reformation: reduction by the use of Interceed TC7 plus heparin. J Gynecol Surg 7: 1
27. Reid RL, Lie K, Spence JE, Tulandi T, Yuzpe A (1993) Clinical evaluation of the efficacy of heparin-saturated Interceed for prevention of adhesion reformation in the pelvic sidewall of the human. Gynecologic Surgery and Adhesion Prevention, Wiley-Liss, New York, pp 261–264
28. Wiseman DM, Gottlick LE, Diamond MP (1992) Effect of thrombin-induced hemostasis on the efficacy of an absorbable adhesion barrier. J Reprod Med 37: 766–770
29. Wiseman DM, Kamp LF, Saferstein L et al. (1993) Improving the efficacy of Interceed barrier in the presence of blood using thrombin, heparin or a blood insensitive barrier, modified Interceed (nTC7). Gyn Surg and Adhesion Prevention, Wiley-Leiss, New York, pp 205–212
30. Rvuelta JM, Garcia-Rinaldi R, Val F, Crego R, Duran CMG (1985) Expanded PTFE surgical membrane for pericardial closure. J Thorac Cardiovasc Surg 89: 451
31. Matsumoto H, Hasegawa T, Fuse K, Yamamoto M, Saigusa M (1973) A new vascular prosthesis for a small caliber artery. Surgery 74: 519
32. Fujiwara Y, Cohn LH, Adams D, Collins JJ Jr (1974) Use of Goretex grafts for replacement of the superior and inferior venae cavae. J Thorac Cardiovasc Surg 67: 774
33. Boyers S, Diamond MP, DeCherney AH et al. (1988) Reduction of postoperative pelvic adhesions in the rabbit with Goretex surgical membrane. Fertil Steril 49: 1066
34. March CM, Boyers S, Franklin R et al. (1993) Prevention of adhesion formation/reformation with the Goretex Surgical Membrane. Prog Clin Biol Res 381: 253–259

10.2 Adhesion Prophylaxis in Gynecology

M. Korell

Introduction

The formation of adhesions is very common following every type of intra-abdominal surgery. It represents one of the major complications, especially of reproductive surgery, which may lead to sterility and abdominal symptoms going as far as ileus [8, 9]. In order to prevent the extent of postoperative adhesions several methods have been investigated but without significant clinical success [3, 4]. Only the covering of the damaged peritoneal surface has promised a substantial reduction of adhesion formation. Two commercially available barriers are in use in clinical practice: Interceed TC7 (Johnson & Johnson Medical GmbH, Norderstedt Germany) and Goretex SM (W.L. Gore, Flagstaff/Arizona USA). Both methods have been proven effective both experimentally and clinically [1, 5, 7, 10]. We have compared several different methods for prevention of adhesions, peritoneal flaps, Interceed TC7 and Goretex surgical membrane (SM).

Methods

In 118 patients, we performed tubal reconstructive surgery or removal of ovarian cysts, endometrial implants esp. uterine fibroids. The approach to the abdomen was laparotomy (n=67) or laparoscopy (n=51). To reduce the risk of adhesions Goretex SM or Interceed TC7 were used and the serosal defects and wound area, respectively, were covered with the barriers. The location of the membranes was mainly the uterus (n=76), followed by the fallopian tube (n=48), the ovary (n=29), the pelvic sidewall (n=18) and the small bowel (n=1). In Fig. 1, the indications for Interceed TC7 and Goretex SM are listed. Interceed TC7 was moistened with Ringer's solution and Goretex SM was secured in place by interrupted suturing with 4–0 Nylon sutures. Figure 2 shows the operative situs after removal of a fibroid. The suture area is covered with Interceed TC7.

In 45 patients, a second-look laparoscopy was performed to evaluate the incidence and extent of postoperative adhesions.

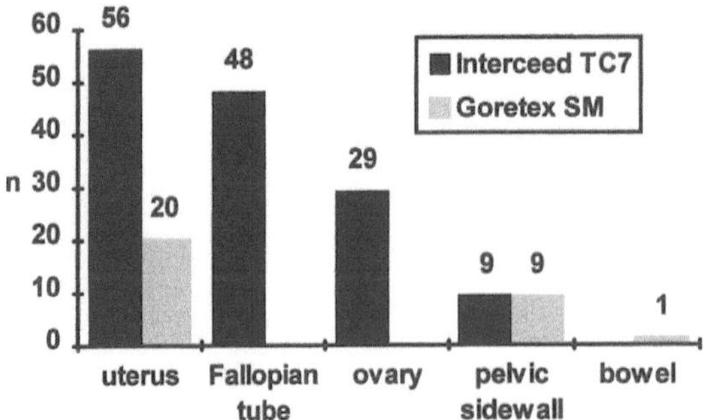

Fig. 1. Indications for barrier methods (Interceed TC7 and Goretex SM) in gynecology

Results

After removal of uterine fibroids, we found an absence of adhesions with Goretex SM or Interceed TC7 in 56.3% and 54.5%, compared to only 21.4% in the uncovered control group. Accordingly, there was a reduction of severe adhesions from 64.3% to 18.7% or, respectively, 13.6% with the barrier methods. Figure 3 shows the results as distributed based on free of adhesions, moderate adhesions and severe adhesions.

Additionally, we found good results using Goretex SM in cases of extensive surgery for endometriosis (Fig. 4).

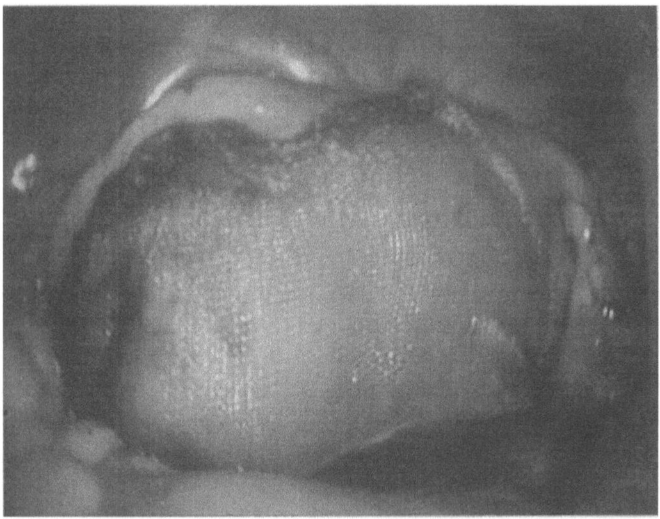

Fig. 2. Situs following removal of uterine fibroids. Covering of the suture area with Interceed TC7

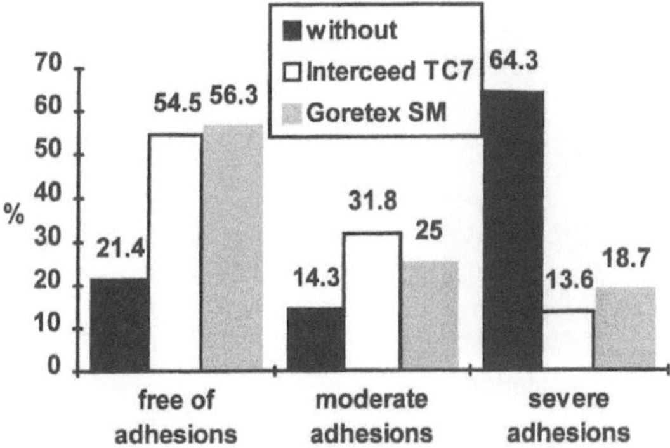

Fig. 3. Influence of Interceed TC7 and Goretex surgical membrane on adhesions after myomectomy

Discussion

The problem of postoperative adhesions is still unsolved. Especially in gynecologic surgery, the incidence can reach up to 96% following reconstructive tubal surgery [2], but even after myomectomy there is a risk of adhesions in up to 93.7% of patients (Fig. 5; [11]). Several agents were tested but without significant success. Only the barrier methods Interceed TC7 and Goretex SM seem to offer a chance of adhesion reduction [5, 10].

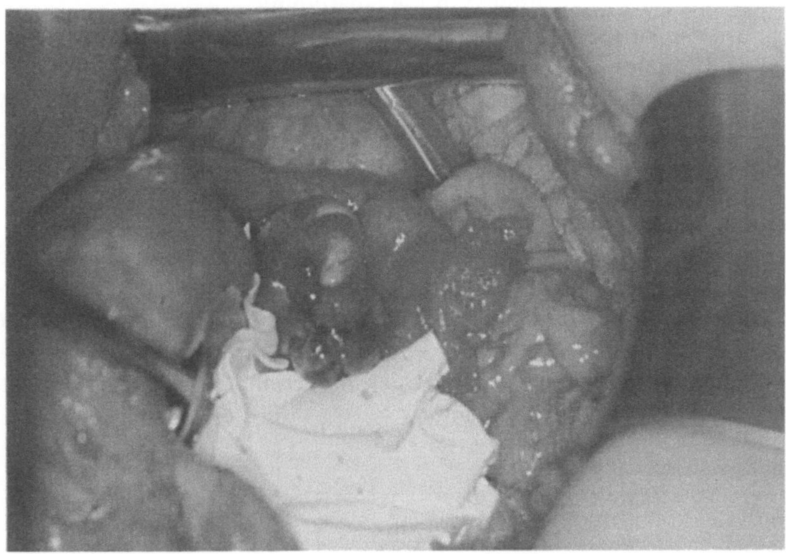

Fig. 4. Situs after extensive surgery for endometriosis. Covering of the pouch of Douglas and both pelvic sidewalls with Goretex surgical membrane

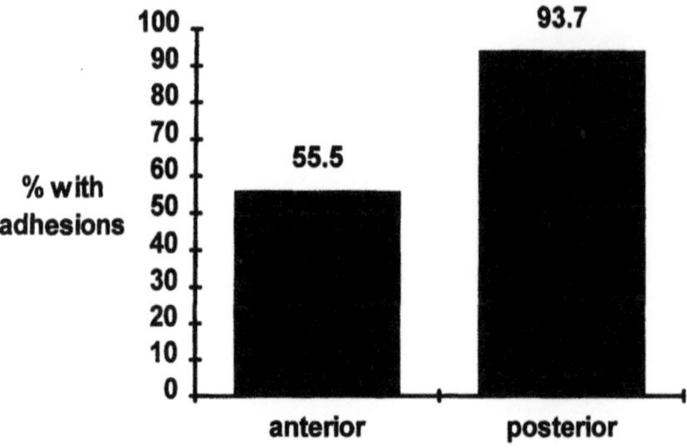

Fig. 5. Incidence of adhesions following myomectomy – influence of the site of fibroid (anterior versus posterior). (From [11])

Of decisive importance in adhesion prophylaxis is firstly, critical assessment of indications and careful performance of the operation, with observance of the principles of microsurgical interventions. This applies equally to so-called keyhole surgery (MIS), which is affected by adhesions to the same degree. Despite this, a high incidence of postoperative adhesions has to be expected particularly after interventions involving the fallopian tube, ovary or uterus. Serosal defects in the visceral peritoneum have to be covered, otherwise the formation of adhesions is practically unavoidable.

In microsurgical tubal reconstruction, we have used peritoneal transplants to cover the serosal defects with good clinical and experimental success [6]. Peritoneal flaps combine effective adhesion prophylaxis and avoidance of foreign material. But the mobilization and preparation of the grafts is time-consuming and their use is limited to the laparotomy.

In endoscopic surgery, the commercially available barrier methods Interceed TC7 and Goretex SM serve as particularly good alternatives. According to our clinical experience, both barriers can be used easily and effectively thereby significantly reducing high incidence of postoperative adhesions following removal of uterine fibroids (Fig. 3). Even in the presence of blood, Interceed TC7 and Goretex SM were equieffective. Tables 1–3 show the different characteristics of peritoneal flap, Interceed TC7 and Goretex SM.

The avoidance of peritoneal trauma by careful preparation for surgery and atraumatic operative techniques are the first steps in the prevention of adhesion. This seems to be sufficient in cases of nonreconstructive surgery. The removal of organs, e.g., ovary or uterus, and a caesarean section can be classified as "low-risk" with respect to adhesion induction (Table 4). By contrast,

Table 1. Characteristics of peritoneal flap

Advantage	Disadvantage
Natural material	Donor side
Unlimited availability	Time consuming/only in laparotomy

Table 2. Characteristics of Interceed TC7

Advantage	Disadvantage
Resorbable	Not in the presence of blood
No suture necessary	No ascites

Table 3. Characteristics of Goretex SM

Advantage	Disadvantage
Less tissue reaction	Suture necessary
In the presence of blood	Not resorbable (removal ?)

Table 4. Incidence of adhesions in gynecology

Low risk	High risk
Parietal peritoneum	Ovary
Adnexectomy	Fallopian tube
Hysterectomy	Uterus
Caesarean section	Bowel

defects of the visceral peritoneum following surgery on the ovary, fallopian tube or bowel often lead to postoperative adhesions which may influence the success rate in terms of pregnancies or complications like ileus or pain. These are "high-risk" cases according to our classification in Table 4. Here, the use of barrier methods is absolutely recommended; nonetheless, severe adhesions occur in some cases. Figure 6 shows a second-look laparoscopy following removal of uterine fibroids. One can see a shrinking of the membrane and severe adhesions to omentum and bowel. Fixation of the membrane and a wide overlap seem to be very important when using Goretex SM. By contrast, Interceed TC7 must only be moistened without suturing. Additionally the cellulose matrix is resorbable and provokes no feeling of a foreign body.

Conclusion

The barrier methods should be used to cover defects since their efficacy in adhesion prophylaxis has been demonstrated both experimentally and clinically. Peritoneal flap transplantation is used only in laparotomy; it requires much more time to perform, but is practically always available. As a non-absorbable membrane, Goretex SM induces only slight tissue reactions but has to be fixed with sutures and, if necessary, has to be removed in a second operation. Interceed TC7 is an absorbable cellulose reticulum that is suitable

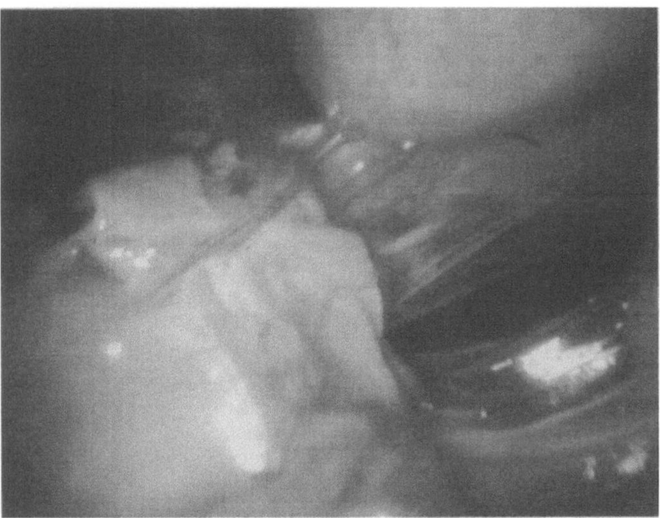

Fig. 6. Severe adhesions following myomectomy in spite of Goretex surgical membrane

for the fallopian tube, ovary and uterus. Fixation with sutures and a second operation for removal are unnecessary. It is thus particularly appropriate for endoscopic operations such as myoma enucleation, ovarian cyst extirpation and reconstructive fallopian tube surgery.

References

1. Boyers S, Diamond M, DeCherney A (1988) Reduction of postoperative pelvic adhesions in the rabbit with Gore-Tex Surgical Membrane. Fertil Steril 49: 1066–1070
2. diZerega G, Rodgers KE (1992) The Peritoneum. Springer, Berlin Heidelberg New York
3. diZerega G (1994) Contemporary adhesion prevention. Fertil Steril 61: 219–235
4. Holtz G (1984) Prevention and management of peritoneal adhesions. Fertil Steril 41: 497–511
5. Interceed Adhesion Barrier Study Group (1989) Prevention of postsurgical adhesions by Interceed (TC7), an absorbable adhesion barrier: A prospective, randomized study. Fertil Steril 51: 933–938
6. Korell M, Scheidel P, Hepp H (1994) Experimental animal model for readhesion formation study. J Invest Surg 7: 409–415
7. Linsky C, Diamond M, Cunningham T et al. (1987) Adhesion reduction in the rabbit uterine horn model using an resorbable barrier, TC7. J Reprod Med 32: 17–20
8. Monk B, Berman M, Montz F (1994) Adhesions after extensive gynecologic surgery: clinical significance etiology and prevention. Am J Obstet Gynecol 170: 1396–1403
9. Stone K (1993) Adhesions in gynecologic surgery. Curr Opin Obstet Gynecol 5: 322–327
10. Surgical membrane study group (1992) Prophylaxis of pelvic sidewall adhesions with Gore-Tex surgical membrane: a multicenter clinical investigation. Fertil Steril 57: 921–923
11. Tulandi T, Murray C, Guralnick M (1993) Adhesion formation and reproductive outcome after myomectomy and second look laparoscopy. Obstet Gynecol 82: 213–215

10.3 Prevention of Postoperative Formation and Reformation of Pelvic Adhesions

B. Larsson

The most effective way of preventing postoperative reformation of adhesions and formation of de novo adhesions is to avoid any trauma to the abdominal serosa. Even a slight trauma to the serosa, observed as petechiae, indicates a risk of adhesion formation. The previously described, less traumatic microsurgical technique in operations for fertility includes a number of specific advantages [3].

During the past decade, I have evaluated in experimental studies in rats and pigs and in clinical series the significance of the particular advantages of the less traumatic and bloodless technique in operations for fertility.

In separate studies, we have registered the benefits of keeping the serosa constantly irrigated [6], of removing adhesions by use of microelectrodes and of avoiding trauma to the serosa by use of non-woven operating towels [7], of avoiding necrotic residues by use of adequate suturing technique and of keeping the number and size of the sutures at a minimum. In experimental studies we have shown that blood and fibrinogen per se do not induce any adhesions [2], while, fibrin, by contrast, induces adhesion formation [7]. Reconstructive surgery even of huge sactosalpinges has proved to result in a promising number of intrauterine pregnancies when the gentle microsurgical technique combined with high doses of cortisone was used [3, 4]. According to my clinical experience, there is much to gain by microsurgical reconstructive tubal surgery, even in huge sactosalpinges, at least when the tubal persistaltic activity (registered during the operation by use of Millar microtransducers in the tubal lumen) is normal (unpubl. data; [4]).

The aim of the operation for fertility is to make it possible for the patient to get pregnant. The results of the treatment could consequently be given in numbers of full-term pregnancies. However, such an evaluation includes in addition a number of other factors in the fertilization procedure to be taken into consideration. Thus, the results of tubo-ovarian microsurgery might preferably be given in reduction of adhesion scores, when considering specifically the effect of preventing reformation of adhesions and formation of de novo adhesions.

By use of the microsurgical technique per se we have observed a reduction in the adhesion scores by at least 50 % in tubo-ovarian reconstructive surgery [8]. It is, however, not possible in all cases to completely avoid any trauma to the serosa when performing adhesiolysis, and in these cases adjuvant therapy is mandatory. A number of substances have been used and I would like to report on some of them.

Over the years, working together with a group of gynecologists from the Scandinavian countries and Finland, we have performed prospective, randomized, multicenter clinical studies on agents reported to reduce postoperative adhesion formation. All surgeons were well experienced in the less traumatic microsurgical technique and the scoring system was used throughout all our multicenter studies.

In two separate series, headed by me, we concluded that Solu-Medrone (Upjohn, Göteborg, Sweden) (unpubl. data) and Dextran (Pharmacia, Uppsala, Sweden) [5] did not significantly reduce the reformation of pelvic adhesions, when randomly applied to the abdominal cavity at the end of microsurgical laparotomy. Saline was administered in the control patients. When de novo adhesions were considered separately, there was, however, a significant reduction of adhesions on the oviducts in the cortisone-treated group compared to the control group. In conclusion, our experiences do not support the use of either Dextran or corticosteroids (Fig. 1) for prevention of postoperative adhesions.

On the contrary, in another multicenter study, also headed by me, the adjuvant effect of a locally applied Interceed barrier proved to significantly prevent reformation of abdominal adhesions in reconstructive, less traumatic, tubo-ovarian surgery [8] (Fig. 2). This series included 66 patients suffering from infertility due at least in part to bilateral tubal disease with bilateral adhesions attached to ovaries, fallopian tubes and fimbriae. Adnexa, randomly covered with Interceed, had significantly lower adhesion scores than the control adnexa, which means an improvement of 39% compared with micro-

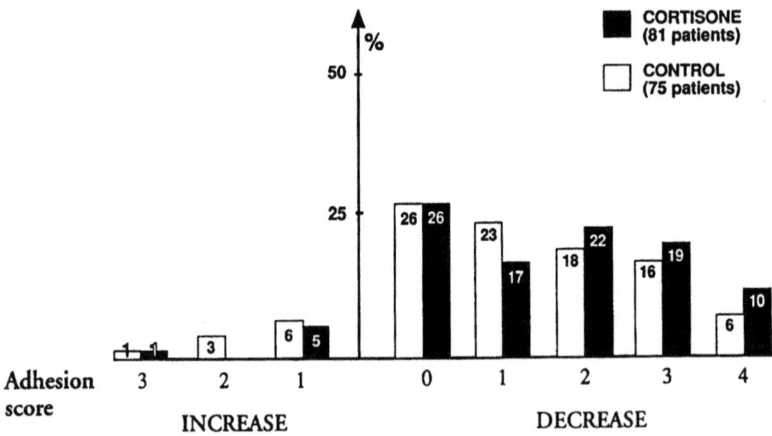

Fig. 1. The distribution in percent decrease and increase, based on 1–4 score units, of adhesions observed at control laparoscopy in comparison to those at laparotomy. *0*, no difference in adhesion scores between the laparotomy and the control laparoscopy. Observations were made on the ovary, and figures are given for the cortisone-treated group and the control group

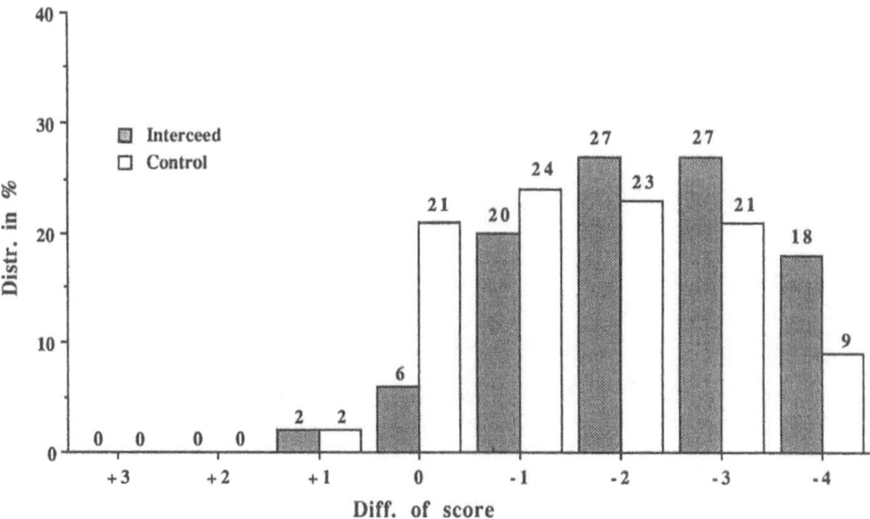

Fig. 2. The distribution in percent decrease and increase, based on 1–4 score units, of adhesions observed at control laparoscopy in comparison to those at laparotomy. *0,* no difference in adhesion scores between laparotomy and control laparoscopy. Observations were made on the ovary, and figures are given for adnexae treated with Interceed and nontreated controls

surgery alone in reducing adhesion reformation scores. When combined with microsurgical techniques, Interceed reduced adhesion reformation scores by 70%. The number of ovaries, fallopian tubes, and fimbriae without any adhesions at the time of second-look laparoscopy was significantly increased by approximately two-fold when organs were covered with Interceed.

The beneficially preventive effect on the ovaries was also shown in an international multicenter study [9]. Fifty-five patients with bilateral ovarian disease (adhesions, cysts, and/or endometriosis) were treated at initial laparotomy. At the end of the operation, one ovary was randomly assigned to be wrapped with Interceed; the other ovary was left uncovered as a control. Second-look laparoscopy was performed 10–98 days later to evaluate the incidence, extent, and severity of adhesions. Treatment with Interceed eliminated the incidence of adhesions in nearly twice as many ovaries compared to the ovaries left uncovered. This means an 86% improvement over the control in preventing adhesion development. Moreover, the differential score in the severity of adhesions showed that the ovaries treated with Interceed had a significantly larger reduction in the severity of adhesions compared to controls.

Some patients suffer from infertility because of fibroids. In an on-going clinical study, my preliminary data indicate a beneficial effect of Interceed. The barrier is placed over the area of enucleation. Especially after removal of large myomata, significant tension may exist between the two edges of the myometrial incision. This makes it almost impossible to approximate the edges by use of the otherwise generally advocated (for fertility operations) very thin sutures, as they most often incise the myometrium. Our current routine procedure includes 3:0 sutures in the uterine wall after enucleation and Interceed to cover the sutured region. This procedure has been used in ten cases, so far, and at control laparoscopy about 10 weeks later no postoperative adhesions have been observed.

Interceed is very easy to apply to any region of the abdominal cavity, not only at laparotomies but also in laparoscopic surgery.

References

1. Swolin K, Bends A, Larsson B, Tronstad SE, Bengtsson R, Hamberger L, Svanberg S (1974) Traumatization of the abdominal serosa. A comparison between non-woven and cotton abdominal swabs. Acta Chir Scand 140: 203–204
2. Nisell H, Larsson B (1978) Role of blood and fibrinogen in development of intraperitoneal adhesions in rats. Fertil Steril 30: 470–473
3. Larsson B (1982) Late results of salpingostomy combined with salpingolysis and ovariolysis by electromicrosurgery in 54 women. Fertil Steril 37: 156–161
4. Rosenborg L, Tronstad SE, Sponland G, Larsson B (1982) Results of electromicrosurgery in 78 women for correction of infertility. A two-center comparative study. Infertility 5: 35–41
5. Larsson B, Lalos O, Marsk L, Tronstad SE, Pehrson S, Bygdeman M, Joelsson I (1985) Effect of intraperitoneal instillation of 32% Dextran 70 on postoperative adhesion formation after tubal surgery. Acta Obstet Gynecol Scand 64: 437–441
6. Larsson B, Perbeck L (1986) The possible advantage of the uterine and intestinal serosa irrigated with saline in operations for fertility - An experimental study in rats. Acta Chir Scand Suppl 530: 15–18
7. Fianu S, Larsson B, Jonasson A, Hedström CG, Thorgirsson T (1986) Mechanism of action of a fibrin sealant in transabdominal urethrocystopexy: experimental study in monkeys. In: Schlaug G (ed) Fibrin sealant in operative med gynecology and obstetrics-urology, vol 3. Springer, Berlin Heidelberg New York
8. Nordic Adhesion Prevention Study Group (1995) The efficacy of Interceed (TC7) for prevention of reformation of postoperative adhesions on ovaries, fallopian tubes, and fimbriae in microsurgical operations for fertility: a multicenter study. Fertil Steril 63: 709–714
9. Franklin R, Malinak L, Larsson B, Jansen R, Rosenberg S, Webster B, Diamond M (1995) Reduction of ovarian adhesions by the use of Interceed. Obstet Gynecol 86: 335–340

10.4 Immunomodulation of the Acute Postinjury Phase of Mesothelial Repair

A. Steinleitner

Introduction

Inflammatory adhesion formation and postsurgical adhesion reformation have been the bane of generations of surgeons. Despite intense efforts of researchers since the 1960s and the clinical application of anti-inflammatory drugs and the new generation of barrier materials, adhesion reformation remains the rule rather than the exception. Although we have made progress in increasing the efficiency of adhesion prevention, we have yet to reach our objective of zero adhesion reformation.

What predisposes the body to oppose the surgeon's efforts to improve organ function with reconstructive surgery? Perhaps this question is best approached from a teleologic perspective. Mechanisms for wound homeostasis and repair have evolved to achieve a primitive objective: survival. The wounded animal's goal is to live to fight another day.

To this end, cascades of interlocking systems act to maintain corporal integrity. Inflammatory cells serve as a network of sensors and effectors, gathering information concerning the twin threats of traumatic tissue injury and infection. Macrophages and neutrophils are dispatched to remove necrotic tissue and fight sepsis. Concurrently, platelet activation and fibrin deposition act to staunch bleeding and prevent death from exsanguination. To err on the side of caution, the body employs an "all out" response. After all, there may be no second chances for the wounded animal in the bush.

Unfortunately, in its maximal response to invasive trauma, otherwise undamaged tissues may be sacrificed in the maelstrom of the acute inflammatory response. Furthermore, healing with precise restoration of anatomic relationships may be an unaffordable luxury for the injured animal. Anticipating that it may be called again to fight sooner rather than later, the body forms dense collagenous adhesions to reinforce the wound.

The problem facing reconstructive microsurgeons is the simple fact that the body cannot distinguish a finely honed scalpel from a filthy spear. The organism isn't "smart" enough to recognize the surgeon's benevolent intent. Instead, the surgical wound is regarded as a major threat to existence. Thus, the surgeon is greeted with same all out response that served so well in the wild. Adhesion formation occurs as a result of the survival instinct.

Conceptually, the role of the surgeon is to cajole, placate, and sometimes fool the body into believing that the surgical incision may be treated with less than a maximal homeostatic response. In this review we will examine the use of "immunomodulatory agents" – medications which have not been classically regarded as possessing anti-inflammatory properties – as a means of intervening in the acute post-injury phase of healing.

Acute Postinjury Events and the Course of Mesothelial Repair

The process of mesothelial wound repair occurs in three phases. The initial 6–24 h constitute the acute postinjury phase. The objective of this phase is to stabilize the wound and re-establish homeostasis. After the wound has been stabilized a phase of fibrinolysis is initiated with the secretion of tissue plasminogen activator (tPA) by intact mesothelial cells and macrophages. Macrophage-directed reperitonealization occurs over the ensuing 4–6 days, culminating in the restoration of mesothelial continuity.

The severity of the inflammatory response during the postinjury phase of healing exerts a profound impact on the ultimate course of peritoneal repair. Inflammatory tissue injury and the pattern of growth factor production weigh heavily on the balance between aberrant healing and normal repair. In many instances the extent of adhesion formation is determined within an hour of the surgical incision. Consequently, interventions which ameliorate postinjury phase inflammation may have value as anti-adhesion therapies.

The influence of postinjury phase inflammation events on mesothelial repair may be both obvious and subtle. Marked surgical trauma, poor hemostasis, and dehydration of mesothelial surfaces are gross insults that are well known to cause adhesion formation and reformation. For over two decades careful surgical technique has stood as the basis for adhesion prevention regimens. Contemporary surgeons strive to minimize mesothelial trauma by employing microsurgical incisions and closures, and meticulous hemostasis wherever possible. Tissue dehydration leading to injury of previously undamaged tissue surfaces and subsequent reduction in mesothelial tPA production is minimized by employing endoscopic techniques where possible and by carefully moistening tissues in patients having open procedures.

New avenues for developing adhesion prevention strategies may be found by manipulating the subtle inflammatory events of wound homeostasis during the acute postinjury phase of repair. These acute postinjury phase events are summarized below.

Inflammatory Cell-Mediated Tissue Injury

A clean precise surgical incision ordinarily elicits a minimal degree of tissue injury. The impact of this injury may, however, be amplified by excessive production of inflammatory mediators (leukotriene B_4, complement factor C5a, formyl methionyl peptides, collagen and fibrinonectin fragments) for granulocytes and macrophages. The activation of granulocytes (principally polymorphonuclear leukocytes, PMNs) is a critical determinate of postsurgical tissue injury. Granulocytes serve as the effector cell for macrophage-directed bacteriostasis and tissue phagocytosis during the acute post-injury phase of healing. PMNs constitute the predominate inflammatory cell type during the initial 24 h following peritoneal injury. Granulocyte-mediated tissue phago-cytosis and bacteriostasis is directed by macrophage-derived factors. At this juncture granulocytes may play a beneficial role by combating bacterial in-fection. However, high local concentrations of granulocyte chemotactic and activating factors may evoke enhanced PMN demargination and migration to the site of injury, resulting in granulocyte hyperactivation and extensive phagocytic injury to viable peritoneal surfaces. Activated macrophages may likewise contribute to tissue injury through the production of toxic oxygen radicals and proteolytic enzymes.

Excessive inflammatory cell activation may impact on adhesion formation via two mechanisms. Net tissue injury may be increased as a consequence of phagocytic injury to undamaged mesothelium by overly active phagocytes. Of perhaps greater importance is the influence of phagocytic and ischemic tissue injury on fibrinolysis. Buckmann [5a] has shown that the principal determinate of the efficiency of fibrinolysis is the extent to which tPA production by peritoneal surfaces is inhibited by phagocytic injury suffered during the acute postinjury phase of healing. Incomplete fibrinolysis provides a framework of clot matrices for cellularization by fibroblasts and neovascular elements, leading to the formation of dense fibrotic adhesions encasing viscera. Hence an excessive inflammatory response to surgical injury may lead to impaired fi-brinolysis and cellularization of fibrinous adhesions.

Platelet Activation

Platelet activation plays an essential role in the dynamics of posttraumatic peritoneal injury. Excessive platelet activation may exacerbate mesothelial injury through increased local thrombosis, vascular endothelial cell damage, and microvascular shunting of perfusion away from the wound. Chemotactic and inflammatory mediators released from platelets may accentuate peritoneal injury by activated granulocytes and macrophages.

Excessive release of growth factors as a consequence of platelet activation during the acute postinjury phase may influence the course of mesothelial repair and adhesion formation. Activated platelets release a plethora of growth stimulating factors into the wound environment that may affect the kinetics of reperitonealization. Platelet derived growth factor (PDGF), platelet factor 4, connective tissue activating peptide III, β-thromboglobulin, and epidermal growth factor (EGF) are potent fibroblast chemotactins and stimulants of fi-broblast proliferation and collagen deposition. Excessive growth factor release following platelet activation may provide an aberrant stimulus for fibroblast proliferation into fibrin matrices. This process may lead to cellularization of fibrinous adhesions binding adjacent intraperitoneal structures and the for-mation of dense cellular intraperitoneal adhesions.

Perfusion-Reperfusion Injury

Cytokine and platelet factor-mediated activation of PMNs stimulates increased endothelial cell adhesiveness and aggregation. Granulocytes undergo marked alterations in their hemorheologic properties. Activated granulocytes entering terminal capillary beds are too large and adhesive to transit the system, and thus cause capillary plugging and microvascular ischemia [15]. Primed granulocytes are also known to effect direct microvascular injury to endothelial cells. Subsequent reperfusion injury may result in a degree of injury out of proportion to the macrosurgically evident trauma.

Vasoactive Mediators and Fibrin Deposition

Histamine release following traumatic tissue injury promotes transudation of fibrin rich plasma as substrate for clot formation. Secretion of tumor necrosis factor (TNF) by activated macrophages increases microvascular permeability, augmenting histamine-induced fibrin deposition.

Growth Factors and Reperitonealization

The final stage of repair, reperitonealization, is initiated 4–7 days after injury by the proliferation of subperitoneal mesenchymal cells arising from the base of the wound. This process is influenced by acute postinjury phase events through the secretion of growth factors and cytokines by macrophages and platelets. Under optimal circumstances macrophage-directed repair yields mesothelial surfaces indistinguishable from native mesothelium.

Severe tissue injury and ischemia alter this sequence of events. Secretion of macrophage-derived mediators may be augmented to promote the ingrowth of neovascular elements and fibroblasts into fibrinous matrices in an attempt to restore perfusion to damaged structures [6, 7]. Interleukin-1 (IL-1) [16], macrophage-derived growth factor and angiogenesis factor [12] have been implicated in this process. Excessive secretion of growth factors (PDGF, transforming growth factor-β) by platelets may accentuate fibrosis. The precise contribution of these factors, their sequence of production, and the effect of macrophage activation on mediator production remain to be elucidated.

Pharmacologic Modulation of the Acute Postinjury Phase

Early attempts at the design of pharmacologic adhesion prevention strategies were based on a perception of the inflammatory process in the acute postinjury stage wound as an "all or nothing" event. Consequently investigators sought to obliterate the inflammatory response to surgical injury through the use of potent anti-inflammatory agents. Unfortunately the clinical experience with this approach was not impressive. While early reports suggested that high dose glucocorticoid treatment might be efficacious, this finding has not been duplicated by other investigators.

Our evolving understanding of the physiology of mesothelial wound repair has led to a reassessment of this strategy. It is increasingly clear that inflammatory and immunocompetent cells are essential contributors to normal mesothelial healing. The active participation of macrophages appears to be necessary to direct the cellular elements participating in reperitonealization. Aberrant wound healing, in contrast, is in part a sequela of excessive inflammatory cell activation. Thus the goal of surgeons should be to modulate the activity of immune cells in such a way as to influence the progression of healing towards restoration of normal mesothelial continuity.

In the following section we will review the results of animal experiments examining the influence of several "immunomodulatory" drugs on posttraumatic peritoneal repair.

Pentoxifylline

Pentoxifylline is a methylxanthine derivative commonly used for the treatment of peripheral vascular disease. While pentoxifylline is not commonly regarded as a classic "anti-inflammatory" agent, this drug exhibits a variety of unique effects on immunocompetent cells that suggested it might be an effective modulator of acute postinjury phase events impacting on mesothelial repair. These properties are summarized below.

Inflammatory Mediator Production

In vitro studies of pentoxifylline demonstrate a selective modulation of cytokine production [14, 23]. Production of TNF, interleukin-2 (IL-2), IL-8, and interferon-γ are inhibited by pentoxifylline. In contrast, production of IL-6 appears to be stimulated by pentoxifylline while production of IL-1β and interferon-α appears to be unaffected.

Inflammatory Cell Activation

Pentoxifylline acts for the most part to blunt the activation of granulocytes and macrophages. Pentoxifylline inhibits the inflammatory action of TNF and IL-1 on granulocytes in vitro [22]. Effects of pentoxifylline on granulocytes include modulation of directed chemotaxis [21], reduced oxidative burst and neutrophil degranulation [3, 17], inhibition of cytokine-induced granulocyte adherence to endothelium [4], and decreased neutrophil cytotoxicity for endothelial cells [24]. Data from animal models of infectious [21] and noninfectious organ [5] insults suggest that pentoxifylline may prevent injury by reducing the inflammatory activities of granulocytes without affecting their bactericidal capability.

Pentoxifylline has been shown to exert significant influence on macrophage and lymphocyte activation. Pentoxifylline blocks the activation of macrophages by TNF. Cytotoxic T lymphocyte generation and natural killer activity are inhibited by pentoxifylline [23]. This activity is mediated in part by down-regulation of the IL-2 receptor [13].

Microvascular Perfusion

Pentoxifylline appears to enhance perfusion to traumatized tissues via several mechanisms. Inhibition of granulocyte activation prevents capillary plugging by granulocytes, thus avoiding perfusion/reperfusion injury. Platelet aggregation is inhibited by pentoxifylline [25].

Fibrinolysis

Knox has shown that pentoxifylline enhances in vitro macrophage penetration into clots and production of plasminogen activator [8]. Corresponding in vivo activity may result in increased fibrinolysis and release of bound viscera prior to fibroblast proliferation and reperitonealization.

Fibrosis and Healing

Recent data suggest that pentoxifylline may modulate the influence of growth factors on mesothelial repair. Pentoxifylline inhibits PDGF and IL-1 driven fibroproliferation [1]. Emerging data suggests that pentoxifylline may act as a competitive antagonist for PDGF receptor [11]. TNF-stimulated collagen synthesis [2] and glycosaminoglycan synthesis are inhibited by pentoxifylline [1]. Of interest, pentoxifylline has been shown to reduce fibrosis in animal models [11].

Taken as a whole, these in vitro and experimental data suggest that pentoxifylline acts to ameliorate inflammatory processes without compromising the organism's ability to fight infection. Given these properties and the fact that pentoxifylline is a nontoxic, well tolerated drug, we studied the influence of this agent on peritoneal wound repair in animal models.

Our initial experiments were performed in the hamster uterine horn primary injury model for fallopian tubal surgery [18]. Perisurgical treatment with pentoxifylline at doses of 0.1–10 mg/kg administered subcutaneously at 12 h intervals provided significant protection against posttraumatic adhesion formation. A majority of animals demonstrated no gross adhesion formation. In those animals that formed adhesions, bands were generally limited to the uterus, were filmy in nature, and were easily separable. Pentoxifylline treated animals at the extremes of the dose response curve (0.001 and 25 mg/kg 12 h) consistently formed dense adhesions similar to controls. No gross evidence of significant complications such as increased infectious morbidity, bleeding dysfunction, or failure of wound healing was noted.

A most interesting finding was that delaying the initiation of therapy by as much as 72 h did not reduce the efficacy of adhesion prevention. Initiation of therapy at time points beyond 72 h resulted in adhesion formation equivalent to control. In the duration of therapy experiment, administration of three doses was sufficient to effect a significant reduction in adhesion score. Maximal adhesion prevention was observed with seven or more injections.

Consistent findings were obtained in the rabbit adhesion reformation model [19]. New Zealand White rabbits were randomized to treatment with vehicle (n =12) vs subcutaneous pentoxifylline 2.5 mg/kg/q12h for six doses (n=12) immediately following lysis of established adhesions. Seven days later rabbits were killed and evaluated in a blind manner to quantify adhesion reformation (postscore). Using a scoring scale of 0=no adhesions, 4+= most severe, the prescore was not different for pentoxifylline and control (3.8 vs 3.9, respectively); however, postscore (0.7 vs 3.7) was markedly reduced by pentoxifylline ($p < 0.001$).

Data from the dose- and time-response experiments in the primary injury model suggest that pentoxifylline-mediated adhesion prevention is the result of interventions at multiple sites along the adhesion formation cascade. Significant adhesion reduction was observed with administration of three perioperative injections (24 h of therapy). This finding is consistent with a modulation of acute postinjury inflammatory events. Results of the initiation of therapy experiment demonstrate that a delay in administration of the drug by as much as 72 h had no significant effect on adhesion reduction. These data are consistent with an effect of pentoxifylline on later aspects of mesothelial repair.

Iloprost

Platelet activation, platelet-endothelial cell interaction, and thrombosis are critical events in the pathogenesis of adhesion formation. We hypothesized that modulation of these events might offer a mechanism to influence the course of peritoneal repair.

Prostacyclin (PGI), a product of the cyclooxygenase pathway of prostaglandin synthesis, is an essential regulator of vascular tone, platelet function, and thrombosis following vascular injury. Platelet activation in response to most known stimulants is dramatically inhibited by PGI in vivo. Vascular elaboration of PGI may reduce nonspecific phagocytic tissue injury by inhibiting the production of inflammatory cell chemotactic and activating factors and by ameliorating inflammatory cell activation. PGI has been suggested to have "cytoprotective" properties in a variety of organ injury states, postulated to be the result of cell membrane protection from free radical production.

Given the impact of PGI on platelet-endothelial interactions and fibrinolysis, we theorized that PGI analogs might be useful as a modulator of posttraumatic peritoneal healing. Iloprost, a long lasting PGI analog, shares many properties of the parent compound. Vasodilatory, platelet suppressant, fibrinolytic, and "cytoprotective" activities of iloprost equal or exceed that of PGI [10].

Data obtained in the hamster uterine horn primary injury model demonstrate preoperatively administered iloprost to be a potent inhibitor of primary adhesion formation [20]. This activity occurred in a dose dependent manner with maximal adhesion reduction observed at a dose of 4 mg/kg. The therapeutic index of iloprost in this indication was fairly broad, with significant adhesion prevention occurring over two orders of magnitude. Perioperative administration of iloprost did not lead to increased infectious morbidity, failure of wound healing, or obvious bleeding disorders.

Summary

Prevention of postsurgical adhesion formation requires attention to each aspect of the adhesion formation cascade. Given that the events of the acute postinjury phase exert a marked influence on fibrinolysis and macrophage-directed reperitonealization, it is evident that pharmacologic interventions at this stage of healing have the potential to favorably influence the ultimate outcome of surgical interventions.

Our understanding of the role of inflammatory cells in the regulation of the adhesion formation cascade provides a rational basis for the design of pharmacological adjuvants for adhesion prevention. Our objective as surgeons is to restrain inflammatory cell activation to the level needed to maintain wound homeostasis. Adjuvant pharmacologic therapies should be directed at preventing nonspecific tissue injury as a consequence of excessive inflammation. Data from our laboratory demonstrates the potential for the use of immunomodulatory drugs to limit inflammatory cell activation and reduce adhesion formation. Carefully controlled trials are needed to establish the utility of this approach in the clinical setting.

References

1. Berman B, Duncan MR (1989) Pentoxifylline inhibits normal human dermal fibroblast in vitro proliferation, collagen, glycosaminoglycan, and fibronectin production and increases collagenase activity. J Invest Dermatol 92: 605–610
2. Berman B, Wietzerbin J, Sanceau M, Merlin G, Duncan MR (1992) Pentoxifylline inhibits certain constitutive and tumor necrosis factor induced activities of normal dermal fibroblasts. J Invest Dermatol 98: 706–712
3. Bessler H, Gigal R, Djaldetti M, Zahavi I (1986) Effect of pentoxifylline on the phagocytic activity, cAMP levels, and superoxide anion production by monocytes and polymorphonuclear cells. J Leukocyte Biol 40: 747–754
4. Berticchi F, Proserpio P, Lampugnani MG, Dejana E (1988) The effect of pentoxifylline on polymorphonuclear cell adhesion to cultured endothelial cells, a preliminary report. In: Mandell GL, Novick WJ Jr (eds) Pentoxifylline and leukocyte function. Proc Pentoxifylline Symposium, Key Biscayne. Hoechst-Roussel Pharmaceuticals, Somerville, p 68
5. Bjornson AB, Kippenberg RW, Bjornson HS (1988) Effects of pentoxifylline on inflammatory and immunological responses in a guinea pig model of thermal injury. In: Mandell GL, Novick WJ Jr (eds) Pentoxifylline and leukocyte function. Proc Pentoxifylline Symposium, Key Biscayne. Hoechst-Roussel Pharmaceuticals, Somerville, pp 154–156

5a. Buckman RF, Buckman TD, Hufnagel H, Gervin AS (1976) A physiologic basis for the adhesion free healing of deperitonealized services. Surg Res 21: 67–76
6. Knighton DR, Silver IA, Hunt TK (1981) Regulation of wound-healing angiogenesis- Effect of oxygen gradients and inspired oxygen concentration. Surgery 90: 262–270
7. Knighton DR, Hunt TK, Scheuenstuhl H, Halliday BJ, Werb Z, Banda MJ (1983) Oxygen tension regulates the expression of angiogenesis factor by macrophages. Science 221: 1283–1285
8. Knox P (1988) Leukocyte-mediated activation of the fibrinolytic pathway and the effects of pentoxifylline. In: Mandell GL, Novick WJ Jr (eds) Pentoxifylline and leukocyte function. Proc Pentoxifylline Symposium, Key Biscayne. Hoechst-Roussel Pharmaceuticals, Somerville, p 96
9. Leibvoich SJ, Ross R (1976) A macrophage-dependent factor that stimulates the proliferation of fibroblasts in vitro. Am J Pathol 84: 501–513
10. Musail J, Wilczynska M, Sladek K, Cierniawski CS, Nizankowski R, Szczeklik A (1986) Fibrinolytic activity of prostacyclin and iloprost in patients with peripheral vascular disease. Prostaglandins 31: 61–70
11. Peterson TC (1993) Pentoxifylline prevents fibrosis in an animal model and inhibits platelet-derived growth factor-driven proliferation of fibroblasts. Hepatology 17: 486-493
12. Polverni PJ, Cotran RS, Gimbrone MA, Unanue ER (1977) Activated macrophages induce vascular proliferation. Nature (Lond) 269: 804–806
13. Rao KMK, Currie MS, Mc Cachren SS, Cohen HJ (1991) Pentoxifylline and other methylxanthines inhibit interleukin-2 receptor expression in human lymphocytes. Cell Immunol 35: 314
14. Rieneck K, Diamant M, Haahr P-M, Schönharting M, Bendtzen K (1993) In vitro immunomodulatory effects of pentoxifylline. Immunol Lett 37: 131–138
15. Schmid-Schönbein GW (1987) Capillary plugging by granulocytes and the no-reflow phenomenon in the microcirculation. Fed Proc 46: 2397–2401
16. Schmidt JA, Oliver CN, Lepe-Zuniga JL, Green I, Gery I (1984) Silica-stimulated monocytes release fibroblast proliferation factors identical to interleukin-1. J Clin Invest 79: 1462–1472
17. Slater K, Wiseman MS, Shale DJ, Fletcher J (1988) The effect of pentoxifylline on neutrophil function in vitro and ex vivo in human volunteers. In: Mandell GL, Novick WJ Jr (eds) Pentoxifylline and leukocyte function. Proc Pentoxifylline Symposium, Key Biscayne. Hoechst-Roussel Pharmaceuticals, Somerville, p 115
18. Steinleitner A, Lambert H, Kazensky C, Danks P, Roy S (1989) Use of pentoxifylline as an adjuvant to prevent postsurgical adhesion formation: preliminary investigations in a rodent model. J Gynecol Surg 5: 367–373
19. Steinleitner A, Lambert H, Kazensky C, Danks P, Roy S (1990) Pentoxifylline, a methylxanthine derivative, prevents postsurgical adhesion reformation in rabbits. Obstet Gynecol 75: 926–928
20. Steinleitner A, Lambert H, Suarez M, Serpa N, Robin B (1991) Reduction of primary posttraumatic adhesion formation with the prostacyclin analog iloprost in an animal model. Am J Obstet Gynecol 165: 1817–1820
21. Sullivan GW, Patselas TN, Redick JA, Mandell GL (1984) Enhancement of chemotaxis and protection of mice from infection. Trans Assoc Am Physicians 97: 337–345
22. Sullivan GW, Carper HT, Novick WJ, Mandell GL (1988) Inhibition of the inflammatory action of interleukin-1 and tumor necrosis factor (alpha) on neutrophil function by pentoxifylline. Infect Immun 56: 1722–1729
23. Tilg H, Eibl B, Pichl M et al. (1993) Immune response modulation by pentoxifylline in vitro. Transplantation 56: 196–201
24. Till GO, Warren JS, Gannon DE et al. (1988) Effects of pentoxifylline on phagocyte responses in vitro and acute and chronic inflammatory responses in vivo. In: Mandell GL, Novick WJ Jr (eds) Pentoxifylline and leukocyte function. Proc Pentoxifylline Symposium, Key Biscayne. Hoechst-Roussel Pharmaceuticals, Somerville, pp 124–137
25. Weithmann KU (1983) Reduced platelet aggregation by effects of pentoxifylline on vascular prostacyclin isomerase and platelet cyclic AMP. Gen Pharmacol 14: 161–162

10.5 Prevention of Adhesions in Rabbits by Intraabdominal Application of Lipid Compounds

K.-H. Treutner, P. Bertram, M. Klimaszewski, and V. Schumpelick

Introduction

Peritoneal adhesions account for significant morbidity and mortality. They can impair intestinal motility resulting in intermittent abdominal pain or even complete intestinal obstruction. Adhesions make repeated abdominal approaches by laparotomy or laparoscopy, which have been increasing, both time-consuming and hazardous. Adhesions are also an important cause of female infertility and failure of refertilization procedures.

In a postmortem study (n=752) adhesions were found in 67% of patients after abdominal surgery, but only in 28% of patients who had not undergone prior operations of the peritoneal cavity. Following minor surgery, e.g. appendectomy, the rate was 51% and increased to 93% after multiple celiotomies [29]. Another study of patients with intestinal obstruction caused by adhesions and bands (n=1477) confirms these data. In this group 86% had a history of abdominal surgery, mostly minor procedures including appendectomies (38%) or gynecologic operations (28%) [17]. Peritoneal adhesions are the leading cause of intestinal obstruction, with an overall rate of 20%–41% increasing to 54%–74% for those patients with small bowel obstruction. A history of previous approaches to the peritoneal cavity is found in up to 92% of these cases. Strangulation of the small intestine is caused by adhesions and bands in 29% [3, 5, 11, 12, 15].

About 1% of all admissions and 3% of all laparotomies in general surgery are due to complications from peritoneal adhesions [13, 24]. The recurrence rate after division of adhesions is 11%–21% [12]. Questionnaire surveys in the United Kingdom and in Germany revealed that currently there are no measures to control the formation and reformation of peritoneal adhesions which have proved their efficacy or gained widespread acceptance among general surgeons [18, 24].

Adhesions are caused by a trauma of the peritoneal membrane. Additionally, foreign body reactions, e.g. from glove dusting powder, can lead to the formation of adhesions. The layer of mesothelial cells can be damaged by infection and ischemia and by a surgical trauma. The latter consists not only of the necessary wounds from approach and resection of a diseased organ, but also of minor traumas from tissue handling and retraction, use of swabs and towels, and drying out of the delicate serous membrane. These injuries result in the release of fibrinous exudate and the formation of potentially transient adhesions. The fibrinolytic activity of the traumatized peritoneum, however, is decreased. The fibrin deposits are not completely resolved but infiltrated by fibroblasts and capillary vessels. Consequently, the areas of adhesions are transformed into permanent collagen strands [2, 9, 28].

A large number of agents have been screened in both experimental and clinical settings for their efficacy in preventing or controlling the formation of peritoneal adhesions [4]. However, there is a paucity of standardized trials with substances acceptable for routine usage. The agent of choice should be a fluid in order to cover not only the sites of a visible surgical trauma, but also to protect from incidental lesions of the peritoneum. Furthermore it should be free from adverse side effects to allow routine application after every surgical procedure. Design of an experimental study must guarantee a standardized, reproducible method of inducing adhesions and an objective, quantitative measurement of the adhesions for statistical evaluation.

Animal Experiments

A series of animal experiments was performed to establish a model for the induction and measurement of peritoneal adhesions and to find a substance capable of reducing the formation of primary adhesions, readhesions after adhesiolysis, and adhesions from general peritonitis.

Induction and Assessment of Adhesions

We developed special instruments to induce peritoneal adhesions by controlled abrasion of defined areas of the visceral and parietal peritoneum. A stamp consisting of two cylinders with a spring in their hollow lumen was calibrated to a pressure of 400 pcm^{-2}. Very fine-grained emery paper was mounted to the curved plate at the tip of the stamp. A bench was constructed, based on the size of the experimental animal, to serve as a firm abutment without traction on the mesenteric vessels. By these means the peritoneum of the abdominal wall, the tip of the appendix and the ileum was abraded within a total area of 10 cm^2.

The resulting areas of adhesions were measured after excision of the affected tissues and subtle dissection of all adhesions. The gut was cut open along the mesenteric attachment. Afterwards all specimens could be placed on the plane surface of a digitizer board connected to a standard personal computer. Custom-made software allowed for definition of every single area by up to 500 points, computing of the total area per animal, and storage of the data on a hard disk. The process of planimetry could be visually controlled on the monitor to avoid input failures.

After preliminary trials this setup was succesfully used in our first series of experiments on rats. The standardized induction resulted in reproducible areas of adhesions and the computer-aided measurement delivered precise data for statistical analysis [27]. Therefore we used this study design for the following studies on rabbits.

Prevention of Primary Adhesions

A total of 100 female Chinchilla rabbits underwent median laparotomy and standardized peritoneal abrasion, as described above, under general anesthesia with xylazine and ketamine i.v. The procedure was completed by continuous mass closure of the abdominal wall and interrupted polyglycolic acid skin sutures. Whereas the animals of the control group received no medication, the rabbits of the other groups were treated by single intraabdominal application of four different solutions in a constant volume of 10 ml/kg body weight prior to the final closure of the peritoneal cavity. The substances and dosages are given in Table 1. Phosphatidylcholine (PC) was obtained as Lipostabil N iv from Rhône-Poulenc Rorer (Cologne, Germany), sphingolipid (SL) and galactolipid (GL) as trial substances from Scotia LipidTeknik (Stockholm, Sweden).

After an interval of 10 days, the animals were killed by intraveneous injection of an overdose of pentobarbital. The abdominal cavity was approached via paramedian incision. Thereby neither the previously abraded area nor the peritoneal suture line, both probable sites of adhesions, was affected. The adhesions were dissected and the areas of the adhesions were measured by planimetry, as described above, by an investigator unaware of the identity of the trial group. The results are given in Fig. 1. Statistical evaluation by the Wilcoxon test showed significant differences ($p < 0.01$) of the mean adhesion areas between the control group (C) and the animals that received normal saline (NaCl) compared to the rabbits treated with the three different lipid compounds (PC, SL, GL) (26).

Prevention of Readhesions After Adhesiolysis

In the next step we wanted to know whether those lipid compounds which efficiently reduced formation of primary adhesions in the previous experiment would display the same action after dissection of adhesions. Since the reduction of adhesions by the lipid compounds in the last study was highly significant compared not only to the controls but also to the normal saline group, in the subsequent studies the animals receiving the NaCl solution served as controls. Furthermore statistical analysis revealed that the number of animals could probably be reduced to ten per group.

Table 1. Substances and dosages of the five trial groups

Group	n	Substance	Dosage/kg body weight
C	20	–	–
NaCl	20	NaCl 0.9%	10 ml
PC	20	Phosphatidylcholine	70 mg
SL	20	Sphingolipid	70 mg
GL	20	Galactolipid	70 mg

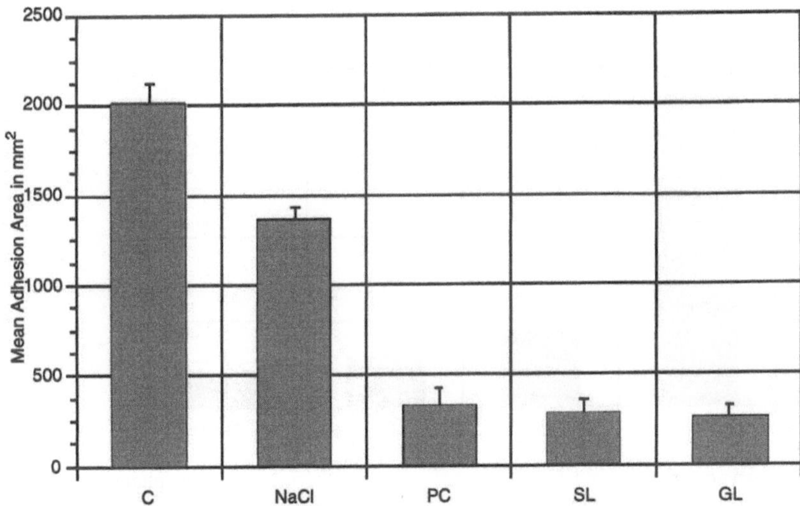

Fig. 1. Mean adhesion areas ± SEM after peritoneal abrasion. *C*, control; *PC*, phosphatidylcholine; *SL*, sphingolipid; *GL*, galactolipid

A total of 40 female Chinchilla rabbits underwent laparotomy and induction of peritoneal adhesions, as described above. After an interval of 10 days all animals were relaparotomized for subtle dissection of all adhesions. Assigned to four groups the animals received either NaCl, PC, SL, or GL intraperitoneally in a volume of 10 ml/kg body weight prior to closure of the abdominal cavity. The dosages of the respective substances equaled those of the previous experiment (Table 1).

After another interval of 10 days the animals were killed by intravenous pentobarbital injection and the adhesion areas were assessed by computer-aided planimetry, as described above. The results are shown in Fig. 2. The extent of readhesion formation was significantly reduced ($p < 0.01$, Wilcoxon test) in all three groups treated by lipid compounds (PC, SL, GL) compared to the NaCl controls [25].

Prevention of Adhesions from Peritonitis

Encouraged by the efficacy of the lipid compounds in prevention of the formation and reformation of adhesions based on the mechanical trauma of peritoneal abrasion, we initiated a study on adhesions from peritonitis. For this purpose we used a modification of the standard CLP (cecal ligation and puncture) model [30].

A total of 40 female of Chinchilla rabbits underwent median laparotomy and ligation of the 15 mm long tip of the appendix. Furthermore, the ligated appendix tip was perforated by an 18-gauge injection cannula to induce direct leakage of the bowel contents. The abdomen was closed by running absorbable

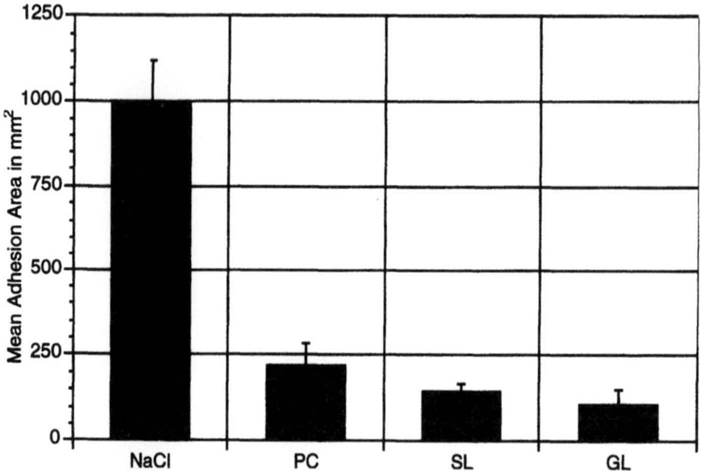

Fig. 2. Mean adhesion areas ± SEM after dissection of adhesions. *PC*, phosphatidylcholine; *SL*, sphingolipid; *GL*, galactolipid

sutures and reopened after an interval of 12 h. After this period of time the animals had developed a macroscopically visible necrosis of the ligated tip of the appendix and a general peritonitis with purulent secretion. These findings were supported by light microscopy of histologic specimens and microbiological cultures of swabs.

The necrotic tip of the appendix was resected and the lumen was closed by a running polyglycolic acid suture. The peritoneal cavity was rinsed with 10 ml of normal saline. Additionally, all animals received a single shot of cefoxitin i.v. (40 mg/kg body weight). As in the previous experiment the rabbits were randomly assigned to four different groups for intraperitoneal treatment with either normal saline NaCl, PC, SL, or GL. Again, the volume was 10 ml/kg body weight and the dosages also remained the same (Table 1).

After an interval of 10 days the animals were sacrificed and the adhesion areas were measured by the same technique used for the other studies. The mean adhesion area in the NaCl group was smaller than those of the comparable group after peritoneal abrasion. However, statistical analysis by the Wilcoxon test again showed a significant reduction (p < 0.01) of adhesion formation after administration of the lipid compounds (PC, SL, GL). The results are shown in Fig. 3 [22].

Results

The intraabdominal application of lipid compounds resulted in a significant reduction of the mean adhesion area compared to treatment with normal saline in all three experimental settings. We did not observe any adverse side effects such as bleeding or healing disorders. Light microscopic studies of specimens stained with sirius red and fast green for specific staining of collagen and

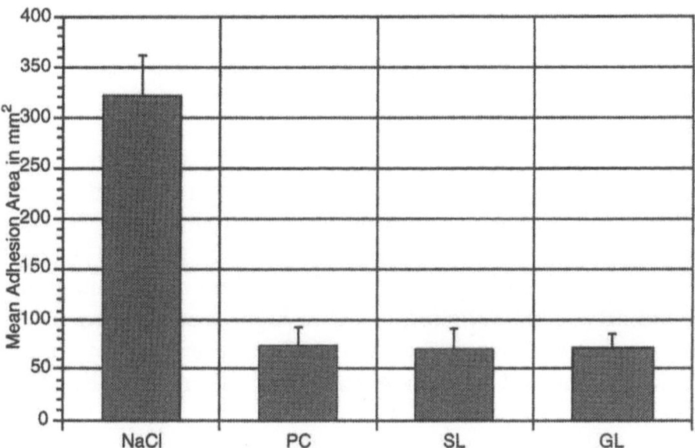

Fig. 3. Mean adhesion areas ± SEM after general peritonitis. *PC*, phosphatidylcholine; *SL*, sphingolipid; *GL*, galactolipid

noncollagenous protein demonstrated thicker adhesive bridges in the control group and the normal saline groups than in those animals of the lipid groups. The latter observations, however, were not quantified.

Discussion

Adhesions develop from peritoneal lesions by abrasion, ischemia, foreign bodies, and infection. The resulting complaints and complications account for a significant clinical workload and a major socioeconomic impact [7]. Current measures of restricting the surgical trauma to a minimum and of prophylaxis and control of infections are neither sufficient nor reliable to solve the problem. Even subtle preparation via a laparoscopic approach, so-called minimally invasive surgery, is followed by adhesion formation [21].

The finding of a reduced posttraumatic fibrinolytic activity prompted studies on the prevention of postoperative adhesions by fibrinolytic agents, especially tissue plasminogen activator (rt-PA). Although these substances proved their efficacy in animals studies their widespread routine usage is not anticipated because of the potential hazard of bleeding and healing disorders [8, 10]. The use of barriers such as oxidized, regenerated cellulose (Interceed TC7) or polytetrafluoroethylene (Gore-Tex) proved to be valuable in experimental and clinical settings [6, 7, 14]. The application of these patches, however, must be restricted to circumscript areas of the peritoneum, leaving nonvisible, incidental lesions without protection.

Our above-reported studies demonstrated a significant efficacy of three different lipid compounds (PC, GL, SL) in reducing the areas of adhesions after primary serosal abrasion, peritoneal lesions from adhesiolysis and bacterial infection. Additional data from our laboratory demonstrate the superior effect of these lipid compounds over a number of other substances for intraabdominal application [23]. Postoperative hemorrhage or healing disorders, even of the stump of the appendix in the peritonitis model, comparable to an intestinal anastomosis, was not observed.

These polar lipids are surface-active materials that coat the peritoneum with a hydrophilic lubricant layer. It is presumed that the serous membrane is thereby protected during the healing process. Other studies using PC could also demonstrate the beneficial effect of a single intraabdominal dose [1, 16, 19, 20]. In one trial using rats, an impairment of the healing of intestinal anastomoses was found after administration of PC in high concentrations of 160 and 240 mg/kg body weight. These increased doses, however, did not improve adhesion prevention compared to the application of 80 mg/kg body weight [19].

In conclusion, our data indicate that lipid compounds may be potential agents for routine prevention of postoperative adhesions. All peritoneal lesions could possibly be protected by a single intraabdominal application. Further studies may qualify these lipid compounds for clinical trials.

References

1. Ar'Rajab A, Ahren B, Rozga J, Bengmark S (1991) Phosphatidylcholine prevents postoperative peritoneal adhesions: an experimental study in the rat. J Surg Res 50: 212–215
2. Buckman RF, Woods M, Sargent L, Gervin AS (1976) A unifying pathogenetic mechanism in the etiology of intraperitoneal adhesions. J Surg Res 20: 1–5
3. Cheadle WG, Garr EE, Richardson JD (1988) The importance of early diagnosis of small bowel obstruction. Am Surg 54: 565–569
4. Christen D, Buchmann P (1991) Peritoneal adhesions after laparotomy: prophylactic measures. Hepatogastroenterology 38: 283–286
5. Deutsch AA, Eviatar E, Gutman H, Reiss R (1989) Small bowel obstruction: a review of 264 cases and suggestions for management. Postgrad Med J 65: 463–467
6. Diamond MP, Wiseman DM, Linsky C (1994) Interceed (TC7) absorbable adhesion barrier. Inf Reproduct Med Clin North Am 5: 485–508
7. diZerega GS (1994) Contemporary adhesion prevention. Fertil Steril 61: 219–235
8. Dunn RC, Mohler M (1993) Effect of varying days of tissue plasminogen activator therapy on the prevention of postsurgical adhesions in a rabbit model. J Surg Res 54: 242–245
9. Ellis H (1990) The hazards of surgical glove dusting powders. Surg Gynecol Obstet 171: 521–527
10. Evans DM, McAree K, Guyton DP, Hawkins N, Stakleff K (1993) Dose dependency and wound healing aspects of the use of tissue plasminogen activator in the prevention of intra-abdominal adhesions. Am J Surg 165: 229–232
11. McEntee G, Pender D, Mulvin D, McCullough M (1987) Current spectrum of intestinal obstruction. Br J Surg 74: 976–980
12. Menzies D (1992) Peritoneal adhesions – incidence, cause, and prevention. Surg Annu 24: 27–45
13. Menzies D, Ellis H (1990) Intestinal obstruction from adhesions – how big is the problem? Ann R Coll Surg Engl 72: 60–63
14. Montz FJ, Monk BJ, Lacy SM (1992) The Gore-Tex surgical membrane: effectiveness as a barrier to inhibit postradical pelvic surgery adhesions in a porcine model. Gynecol Oncol 45: 290–293

15. Mucha P (1987) Small intestinal obstruction. Surg Clin North Am 67: 597–620
16. Rozga J, Andersson R, Srinivas U, Ahren B, Bengmark S (1990) Influence of phosphatidylcholine on intra-abdominal adhesion formation and peritoneal macrophages. Nephron 54: 134–138
17. Räf LE (1969) Causes of abdominal adhesions in cases of intestinal obstruction. Acta Chir Scand 135: 73–76
18. Scott Coombes DM, Vipond MN, Thompson JN (1993) General surgeons' attitudes to the treatment and prevention of abdominal adhesions. Ann R Coll Surg Engl 75: 123–128
19. Snoj M, Ar'Rajab A, Ahren B, Bengmark S (1992) Effect of phosphatidylcholine on postoperative adhesions after small bowel anastomosis in the rat. Br J Surg 79: 427–429
20. Snoj M, Ar'Rajab A, Ahren B, Larsson K, Bengmark S (1993) Phospholipase-resistant phosphatidylcholine reduces intra-abdominal adhesions induced by bacterial peritonitis. Res Exp Med Berl 193: 117–122
21. Tittel A, Schippers E, Treutner K-H, Anuroff M, Polivoda M, Öttinger A, Schumpelick V (1994) Laparoskopie versus Laparotomie – Eine tierexperimentelle Studie zum Vergleich der Adhäsionsbildung im Hund. Langenbecks Arch Chir 379: 95–98
22. Treutner K-H, Bertram P, Klimaszewski M, Winkeltau G, Schumpelick V (1995) Prevention of adhesions from ruptured appendicitis by intraabdominal lipid compounds in rabbits. Eur Surg Res 27 Suppl 1: 89
23. Treutner K-H, Bertram P, Lerch MM, Klimaszewski M, Sobesky J, Winkeltau G, Schumpelick V (1995) Prevention of postoperative adhesions by single intraperitoneal medication. J Surg Res 59: 764–771
24. Treutner K-H, Bertram P, Löser S, Winkeltau G, Schumpelick V (1995) Prophylaxe und Therapie intraabdomineller Adhäsionen – Eine Umfrage an 1200 Kliniken in Deutschland. Chirurg 66: 398–403
25. Treutner K-H, Bertram P, Pfeiffer E, Schumpelick V (1995) Rezidivprophylaxe von Verwachsungen nach Adhäsiolyse. Langenbecks Arch Chir, Springer, Berlin Heidelberg New York, pp 673–675
26. Treutner K-H, Klimaszewski M, Bertram P, Schumpelick V (1994) Adhäsionsprophylaxe mit Lipidverbindungen. Langenbecks Arch Chir (Suppl), Springer, Berlin Heidelberg New York, pp 45–48
27. Treutner K-H, Winkeltau G, Lerch MM, Stadel R, Schumpelick V (1989) Postoperative, intraabdominelle Adhäsionen – Ein neues standardisiertes und objektiviertes Tiermodell und Testung von Substanzen zur Adhäsionprophylaxe. Langenbecks Arch Chir 374: 99–104
28. Vipond MN, Whawell SA, Thompson JN, Dudley HA (1990) Peritoneal fibrinolytic activity and intra-abdominal adhesions. Lancet 335: 1120–1122
29. Weibel M-A, Majno G (1973) Peritoneal adhesions and their relation to abdominal surgery – a postmortem study. Am J Surg 126: 345–353
30. Wichterman KA, Baue AE, Chaudry IH (1980) Sepsis and septic shock – A review of laboratory models and a proposal. J Surg Res 29: 189–201

10.6 Two-Phase In Vivo Comparison Studies of the Tissue Response to Polypropylene, Polyester, and Expanded Polytetrafluoroethylene Grafts Used in the Repair of Abdominal Wall Defects

K.A. LeBlanc

Introduction

The choice of biomaterial for repair of abdominal wall defects is of considerable importance because the prosthesis is often placed directly on the abdominal viscera (intraperitoneal approach). If the prosthetic material used tends to adhere to the serosa of the viscera, serious complications can occur, including erosion into the bowel, fistula formation, infection, technical problems if reoperation is necessary, and bowel obstruction [8]. Thus, many studies of biomaterials employed in hernia surgery have focused on adhesion formation.

I previously studied [7] biologic tissue response and adhesion formation in rabbits in which monofilament, woven polypropylene mesh (Marlex, C.R. Bard, Murray Hill, New Jersey), multifilament, knitted polypropylene mesh (Surgipro, United States Surgical Corp., Norwalk, Connecticut), and expanded polytetrafluoroethylene (ePTFE) (Gore-Tex Soft Tissue Patch [STP], W.L. Gore & Associates, Flagstaff, Arizona) had been implanted with use of an onlay technique. As compared with the two mesh materials, the ePTFE patch produced fewer, less dense adhesions and a decreased inflammatory tissue response. Here, a more comprehensive comparative investigation of the tissue response to prosthetic materials in the same animal model is described. A total of seven prosthetic devices used in hernia repairs were studied, including three types of ePTFE grafts.

Methods

Two study protocols were used, each of which was divided into two phases. Adult New Zealand White rabbits were used in both protocols. The animals were cared for in accordance with the "Guide for the Care and Use of Laboratory Animals" (NIH publication no. 86-23, revised 1985). The first protocol compared ePTFE and Marlex mesh in phase 1 and ePTFE and Surgipro mesh in phase 2. The second compared ePTFE and Prolene mesh in phase 1 and ePTFE and Mersilene mesh in phase 2.

In each phase of both protocols, a 3.75 cm disk of ePTFE material (Gore-Tex STP, DualMesh Biomaterial, or MycroMesh Biomaterial) and a 3.75 cm disk of a mesh material were implanted intraabdominally, directly adjacent to the viscera, through an incision in the linea alba, with one disk placed on each side of the rabbit. A continuous suture was used to secure the material. After implantation, the animals had free access to water and standard laboratory food. Their conditions were recorded weekly by a veterinarian or animal technician.

The rabbits were killed at 7, 15, or 90 days after biomaterial implantation and specimens obtained for gross and histologic analysis. Each disk and 2 cm of surrounding tissue was removed and placed in 10% buffered, neutral formalin. If adhesions were present, they were transected, leaving any attached tissue intact.

In the specimens evaluated 7 or 15 days after implantation, only histologic observations were performed. In the specimens explanted at 90 days, the percentage of specimens of each material having adhesions was recorded, and the adhesions were scored by two different observers with use of a modified Diamond scale [3], which evaluates both extent and tenacity. Extent scores ranged from 0 (no adhesions) to 4 (adhesions to > 75% of the implant). Tenacity scores were 1 (adhesions easily separated from tissue), 2 (adhesions separable by blunt dissection), or 3 (adhesions separable only by sharp dissection). The scores assigned by the two observers were averaged and compiled to calculate an overall adhesion score for each prosthetic material studied.

For the histologic studies, each specimen was embedded in paraffin, sectioned, and stained with hematoxylin and eosin or Milligan's trichrome for evaluations of tissue response, cellular migration and collagen deposition into the interstices and around the material (tissue incorporation), and inflammation.

Results

Figure 1 shows the percentage of specimens obtained at 90 days after implantation having adhesions to the abdominal viscera, according to the type of prosthetic material. Figure 2 shows the adhesion scores for all the materials, based on observation of specimens obtained 90 days after implantation. The ePTFE patches uniformly had the lowest frequency of adhesions and the least dense adhesions. No adhesions at all were observed with the DualMesh Biomaterial patches (25 specimens). Of the non-ePTFE materials, Surgipro had the fewest and least dense adhesions.

Representative gross and histologic findings at 90 days are shown in Figs. 3–12. In general, adhesions to the mesh materials were larger, more numerous, and more firmly attached than those to the ePTFE patches. The foreign body reaction with polypropylene and polyester was more intense than that with ePTFE at 7 and 15 days but had tapered off by 90 days to become similar to the mild reaction observed with ePTFE throughout the study period. In general, the specimens with the ePTFE patches showed a more normal healing response, with good ingrowth and reperitonealization and mild inflammation.

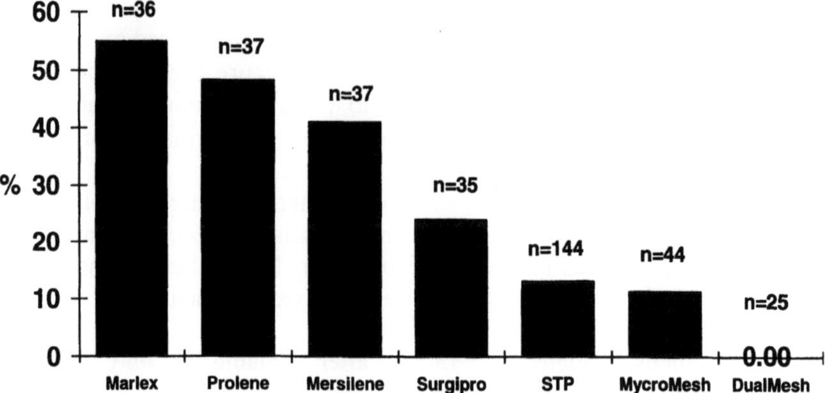

Fig. 1. Percentage of biomaterial implants having adhesions to the abdominal viscera at 90 days after implantation

Discussion

Pathogenesis of Adhesion Formation

Diamond and DeCherney [3] have characterized peritoneal adhesion formation as resulting from "the normal healing process gone awry." The peritoneum heals by means of metaplasia of the mesenchymal tissue underlying the injury [3], with new mesothelium developing from islands of epithelial cells that attach throughout the surface of the wound and proliferate [4]. Inflammation produces exudates containing large amounts of fibrinogen. These coagulate, causing intraperitoneal structures to be connected by fibrinous material [1]. This network is then infiltrated by fibroblasts, macrophages, and plasma cells. Granulation tissue forms, and in a healthy peritoneum, the fibrinous mass is

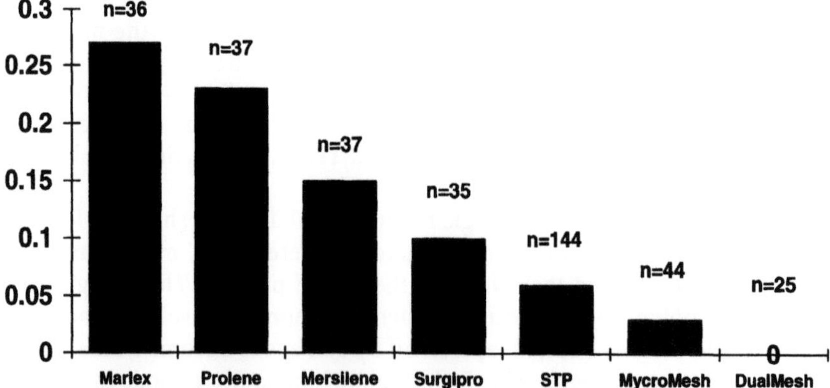

Fig. 2. Adhesion scores, based on the extent and tenacity of adhesions to the abdominal viscera, for biomaterials implanted for 90 days

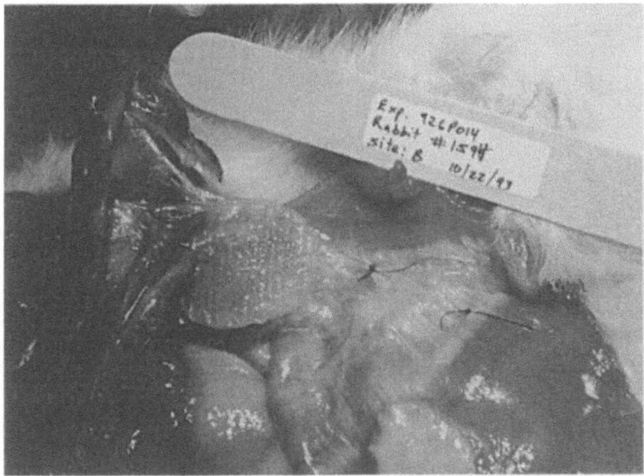

Fig. 3. Specimen of Prolene mesh explanted at 90 days. The serosa of the large and small bowel (*left*) is firmly adherent to the mesh

absorbed through the action of plasminogen activator [1]. With resolution of the mass, fibroblast proliferation produces healing of the defect without adhesion formation [3].

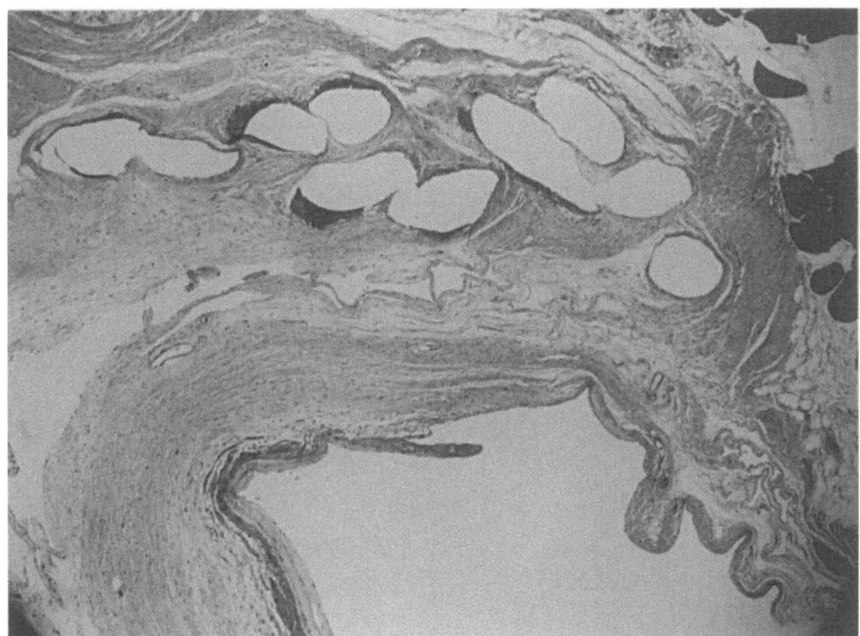

Fig. 4. Histologic study of Prolene mesh shows the serosa of the small bowel (*bottom*) adherent to the fibrosis encapsulating the mesh (empty vacuoles), Milligan's trichrome, × 10

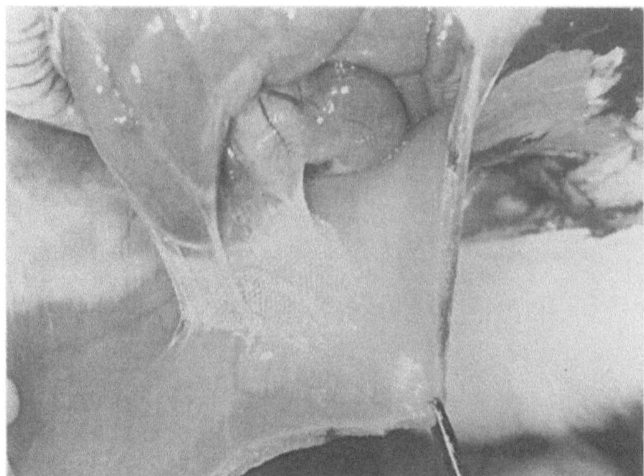

Fig. 5. Specimen of Mersilene mesh explanted at 90 days. Anteriorly, the serosal surface of the bowel is firmly adherent to the mesh. A large wrinkle extends the entire length of the mesh

Adhesions occur when fibrinolytic activity is suppressed and the fibrinous mass is not dissolved. The development of adhesions has been associated with mechanical trauma, chemical agents, drying of the serosa in combination with bleeding, ischemia, infection, and the presence of a foreign body [5]. Im-

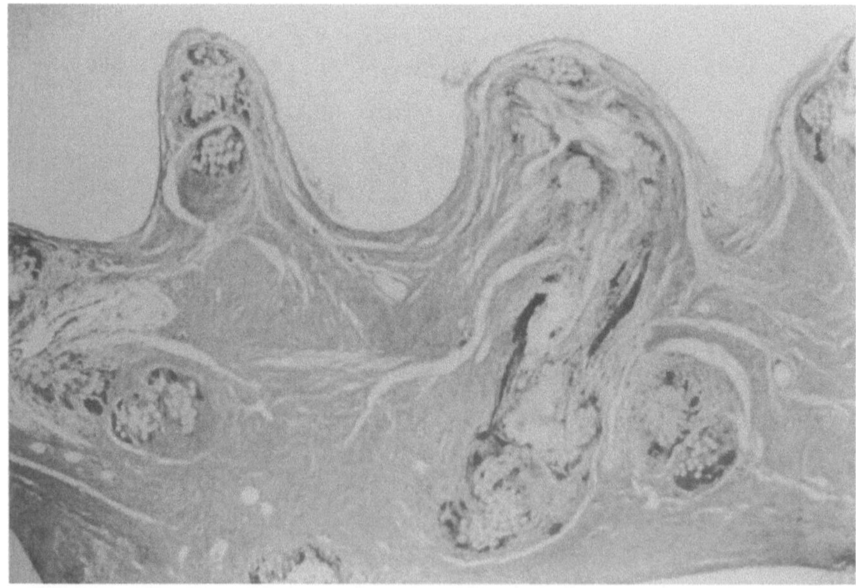

Fig. 6. Histologic study shows extensive wrinkling of Mersilene mesh, which is completely encapsulated by dense scar tissue, Milligan's trichrome, × 10

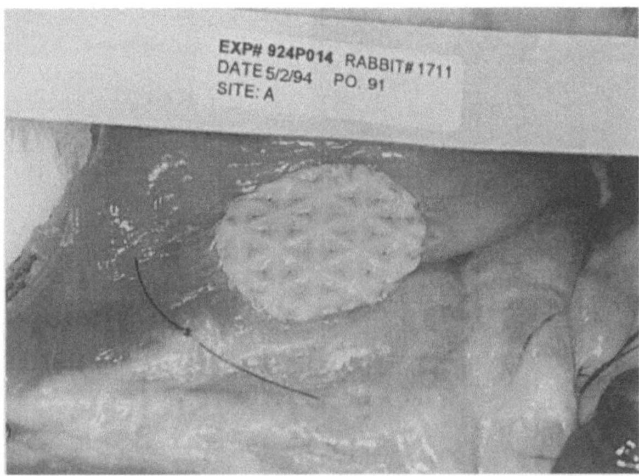

Fig. 7. Specimen of MycroMesh explanted at 90 days. The macropores are completely filled in with a thin filmy membrane resembling neomesothelium. The surrounding soft tissue is unremarkable, and there is no evidence of adhesions

plantation of prosthetic materials impairs fibrolytic activity principally by producing ischemia due to tight suturing or decreasing the proliferation of mesothelial cells [1], but other mechanisms may also be involved.

Although the formation of adhesions between a prosthesis used in a hernia repair and the abdominal viscera is undesirable, host tissue infiltration and ingrowth into the prosthesis is important to the success of the repair. Such tissue incorporation prevents distortion and migration of the material and reinforces the repair [1].

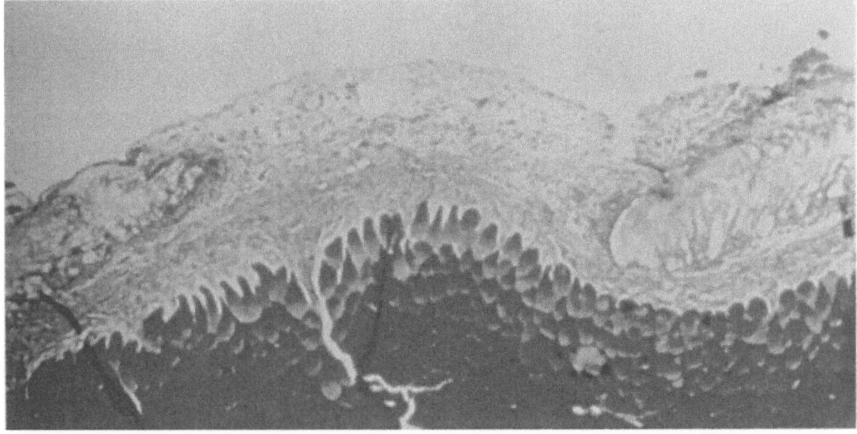

Fig. 8. Histologic study shows the macropore of MycroMesh completely filled in with numerous endothelial cells, fibroblasts, and histiocytes. A monolayer of cells covers the macropore, resembling neomesothelium. Milligan's trichrome, × 2.5

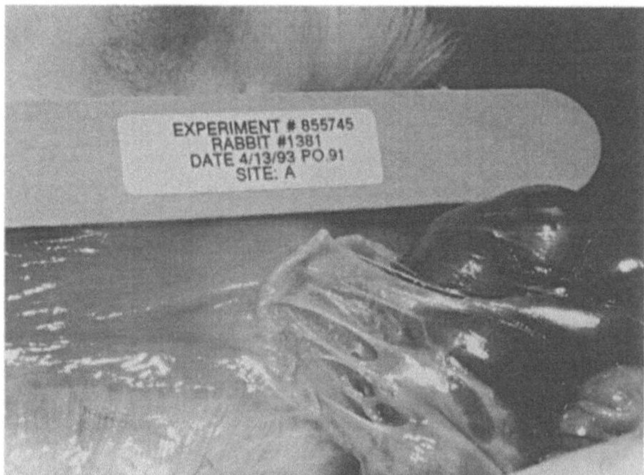

Fig. 9. Specimen of Surgipro mesh explanted at 90 days. The serosal surface of the large bowel is firmly adherent to the visceral surface of the mesh

Previous Experimental Studies of Adhesion Formation

Several investigations in animals have compared prosthetic material with respect to adhesion formation; most have studied Marlex and STP.

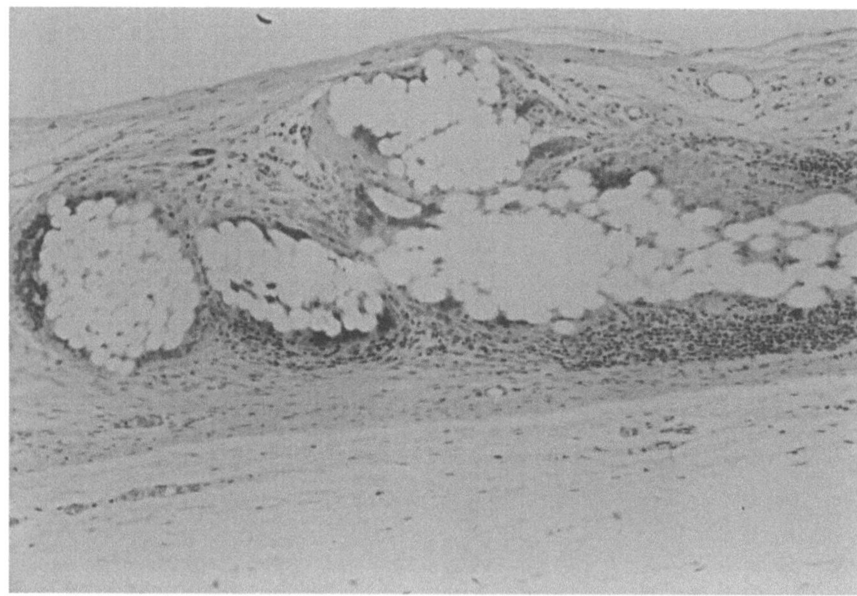

Fig. 10. Histologic study shows a hypercellular (histiocytic and lymphocytic) reaction around the Surgipro mesh filaments. Hematoxylin and eosin, × 10

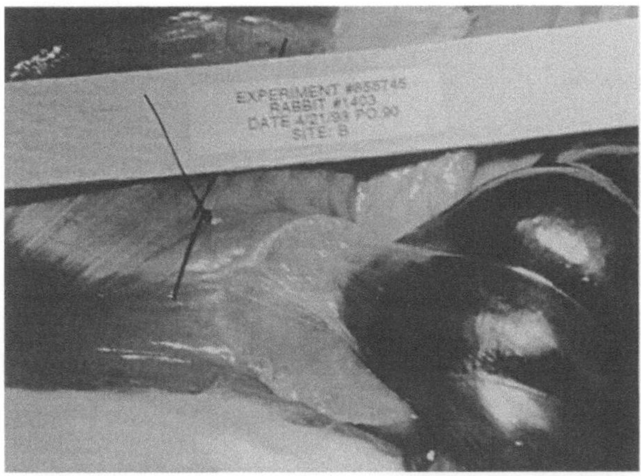

Fig. 11. Specimen of Marlex mesh explanted at 90 days. The entire surface of the mesh is adherent to the large bowel. The serosal surface of the large bowel is firmly adherent to the mesh toward the posterior edge, and fibrous bands connect the serosa of the rest of the bowel to the mesh

Law and Ellis [6] created abdominal wall defects in rats and repaired them with either Marlex mesh, an ePTFE patch, or polyglycolic acid mesh by using an onlay technique. The rats were killed at 1, 2, 4, 8 or 22 weeks after implantation, and the abdominal wall was opened to expose the implanted material and the adhesions on the surface of the peritoneum. The density of adhesions was graded on a scale similar to that used in the current study.

The grade of the adhesions to ePTFE was significantly lower than that of the adhesions to Marlex at from 1 to 8 weeks after implantation, although there was no difference at 22 weeks. In addition, the grade of the adhesions to ePTFE was significantly lower than that of the adhesions to polyglycolic acid mesh at from 2 to 22 weeks after implantation, although there was no difference at one week. Histologic studies showed that the Marlex specimens were incorporated by dense collagen fibers in the presence of a mild foreign body reaction, that omental adhesions had enveloped the fibers of the mesh and become firmly attached to it, and that mesothelial cells were present in an irregular pattern. In contrast, collagen had penetrated the interstices of the ePTFE patches in a regular pattern, and mesothelial cells had appeared in a continuous layer on the peritoneal surface. The polyglycolic acid mesh did not induce a strong fibrous response, and the fibrous tissue that did develop did not adequately support the abdomen.

In discussing their findings, Law and Ellis [6] observed that adhesion formation is inversely related to the number of mesothelial cells on the peritoneal surface. They also theorized that the rigidity and abrasive surface of Marlex may have been responsible for the adhesions with that material.

In a study by Murphy et al. [8], either Marlex or STP was used to repair full thickness abdominal wall defects in rats. The animals were killed 107–140 days after implantation, and the adhesions between the prosthetic materials

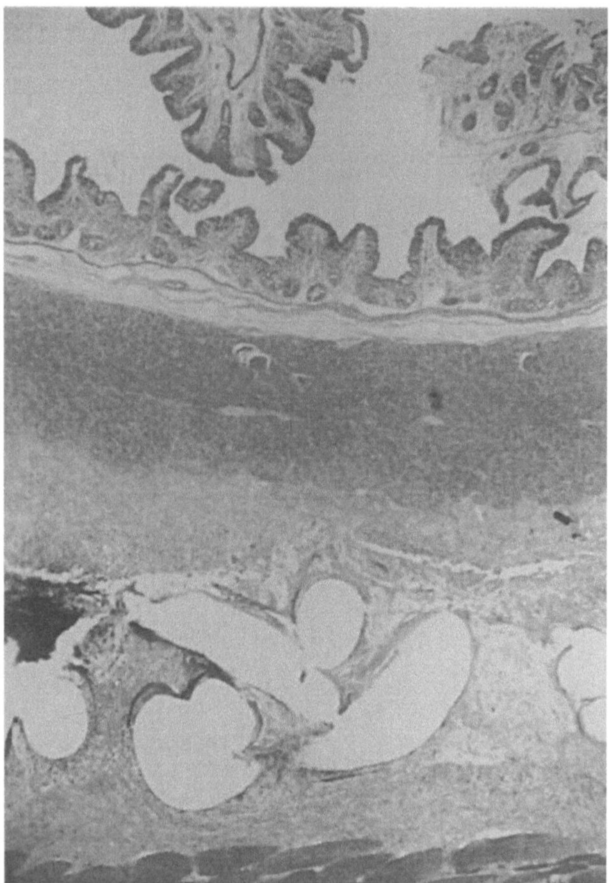

Fig. 12. Histologic study shows the serosa of the small bowel (*top*) adherent to granulation tissue and a prolific cellular response around Marlex mesh. Milligan's trichrome, × 10

and the abdominal viscera were graded. The resulting adhesion indices were 1.37 ± 0.12 (mean ± SD) in the STP group and 2.62 ± 0.12 in the Marlex group ($p < 0.005$). Histologic studies showed chronic inflammatory cells, fibroblasts, and rare giant cells in the Marlex specimens, as well as collagen fibers encircling the prosthetic material. The STP specimens had a focal reaction of mostly giant cells, with fewer fibroblasts and less collagen than was observed in the Marlex samples. Murphy et al. [8] suggested that ePTFE would be the best prosthesis to use in cases in which the viscera and prosthetic material must be in apposition because of a lack of protective omentum.

Brown and colleagues [2] studied adhesion formation after abdominal wall reconstruction with either Marlex or STP in guinea pigs with control wounds, contaminated wounds, or experimental peritonitis. The animals were killed 5 days after implantation and the adhesions graded on a scale of 1 (no adhesions) to 4 (dense adhesions). In all instances, STP produced fewer adhesions than did Marlex mesh, and those that developed were easier to remove. Histologic investigations showed no differences between the materials with respect to tissue incorporation, although the authors commented that this may have been related to the short sampling time.

Simmermacher and coworkers [9] used either STP or Marlex to repair full-thickness abdominal wall defects created in rats. The animals were killed 8 weeks after implantation of the prosthetic material. Adhesions between the material and the viscera were graded on the same scale used by Law and Ellis [6].

The omental-adhesion grade in the Marlex group was significantly higher than that in the STP group. In addition, intestinal adhesions occurred more often in the Marlex group. In contrast to other experimental investigations, the histologic evaluation in this study found no ingrowth of tissue in the STP. The Marlex prosthesis was fully incorporated with fibrocollagenous tissue [9].

In my previous study [7], Marlex, Surgipro, and STP were implanted in New Zealand White rabbits, with each animal receiving two different prosthetic materials, which were placed directly adjacent to the viscera. The rabbits were killed at 7, 14, and 90 days, and the adhesions scored according to the same criteria used in the current study.

At 7 days, 100% of the Marlex specimens, 75% of the Surgipro specimens, and 16% of the STP specimens had adhesions. The adhesion scores for those materials were 0.57, 0.42, and 0.09, respectively. These results were essentially unchanged at 14 days. At 90 days, 59% of the Marlex, 28% of the Surgipro, and 9% of the STP specimens had adhesions, and the adhesion scores were 0.3, 0.11, and 0.04, respectively.

Histologic studies of the STP at 7 days showed a continuous mesothelial layer, with cellular migration into the interstices of the material by histiocytes and fibroblasts. At 14 days, there was collagen deposition in the interstices; by 90 days, this had increased, with no evidence of encapsulation. Inflammation was not observed, although occasional foreign body cells appeared on the interface between the patch and the tissue.

The Marlex mesh had a concentric alignment of collagen fibers around individual mesh filaments, which increased until a dense, hypertrophic scar was observed at 90 days. Mesothelialization was patchy. The Surgipro specimens also had dense, unorganized collagen fibers and irregular mesothelialization. Inflammation was evident with both meshes. Numerous foreign body giant cells were observed at 7 days, and lymphocytes and plasma cells were seen at 90 days.

The current study used the same animal model and similar protocols, except that it included two additional mesh materials (Prolene and Mersilene) and two new types of ePTFE patches. One of them, DualMesh Biomaterial, has two distinct surfaces; one is very smooth (micropores < 3 μmm), whereas the other is similar to STP (micropores ~ 22 μmm). DualMesh is designed to be implanted with the smooth surface against the tissue or viscera to which minimal tissue attachment is desired and the other surface against the surface where tissue incorporation is desired. The other new ePTFE patch, MycroMesh

Biomaterial, has macropores to facilitate tissue incorporation and visualization of structures beneath the material during laparoscopic surgery.

Conclusions

This comprehensive comparative study of seven biomaterials (including three types of ePTFE grafts) in a rabbit model, as well as previous investigations in animals, suggests that ePTFE patch material is the most appropriate biomaterial to use in intraperitoneal repairs of abdominal wall defects, in which the graft is placed directly against the abdominal viscera. Experimental studies have consistently documented an increased likelihood of adhesion formation with macroporous meshes. The development of adhesions in patients who have undergone hernia repair increases the risk of several complications, the most serious of which is bowel obstruction. The long-term clinical effects of placing macroporous meshes directly on vascular structures and the vas deferens, as in, for example, laparoscopic hernia repair, are unknown but may have serious consequences.

References

1. Annibali R, Fitzgibbons RJ Jr (1994) Prosthetic materials and adhesion formation. In: Arregui ME, Nagan RF (eds) Inguinal hernia: advances or controversies? Radcliffe Medical Press, Oxford, p 115
2. Brown GL, Richardson JD, Malangoni MA, Tobin GR, Ackerman D, Polk HC Jr (1985) Comparison of prosthetic materials for abdominal wall reconstruction in the presence of contamination and infection. Ann Surg 210: 705–711
3. Diamond MP, DeCherney AH (1987) Pathogenesis of adhesion formation/reformation: application to reproductive pelvic surgery. Microsurgery 8: 103–107
4. diZerega GS (1994) Contemporary adhesion prevention. Fertil Steril 61: 219–235
5. Holmdale L, Al-Jabreen M, Risberg B (1994) Experimental models for quantitative studies on adhesion formation in rats and rabbits. Eur Surg Res 24: 248–256
6. Law NW, Ellis H (1988) Adhesion formation and peritoneal healing on prosthetic materials. Clin Materials 3: 95–101
7. LeBlanc KA (1994) Two-phase in vivo comparison study of adhesion formation of the Gore-Tex Soft Tissue Patch, Marlex Mesh and Surgipro using a rabbit model. In: Arregui ME, Nagan RF (eds) Inguinal hernia: advances or controversies? Radcliffe Medical Press, Oxford, p 501
8. Murphy JL, Freeman JB, Dionne PG (1989) Comparison of Marlex and Gore-Tex to repair abdominal wall defects in the rat. Can J Surg 32: 244–247
9. Simmermacher RKJ, Schakenraad JM, Bleichrodt RP (1994) Reherniation after repair of the abdominal wall with expanded polytetrafluoroethylene. J Am Coll Surg 178: 613–616

10.7 Evaluation of Seprafilm Bioresorbable Membrane in a Rat Cecal Abrasion Model

J.M. Burns, M.J. Colt, R.L. Carver, L. Burgess, and K.C. Skinner

Introduction

A number of methods and agents to prevent postsurgical adhesions have been investigated in animal surgery models and in human clinical studies. These methods include pharmacologic agents, such as fibrinolytics which disrupt early fibrin matrix formation [1, 2] viscous solutions, such as Dextran, and carboxymethylcellulose, which separate tissues after injury via hydroflotation [3, 4]; surgical tissue lubricants that reduce tissue damage during surgery [5]; and barrier membranes, which mechanically separate injured serosal surfaces until remesothelialization occurs [6, 7].

Barrier membranes are intended to prevent adhesions at specific sites of tissue injury where adhesions are likely to form, such as along incisions or deperitonealized surfaces. An ideal adhesion barrier should be biocompatible, separate injured tissues during the critical early stages of adhesion development, require minimal effort for placement, and be useful in a number of clinical situations. Seprafilm (HAL-F) Bioresorbable Membrane, composed of sodium hyaluronate and carboxymethylcellose, has recently been developed to meet these criteria. This membrane is intended to provide a temporary physical barrier between serosal tissue surfaces during the early phases of surgical wound repair when adhesions may form, generally within 3–7 days following tissue injury [8, 9]. To this end, the components of Seprafilm membrane have been chemically modified to produce a barrier membrane with reduced solubility and an increased in vivo residence time compared to the native polymers. In a recent preclinical study, Seprafilm Bioresorbable Membrane significantly reduced adhesion formation in a canine pericardial adhesion model [10]. The ability of the Seprafilm membrane to reduce adhesion formation in humans has recently been reported. Seprafilm membranes were placed over the viscera and under the anterior abdominal incision line prior to closing the fascia following cholectomy in an ileo-anal pull-through procedure [11]. Upon laparoscopic examination of the incision line following the ileostomy take-down (8-12 weeks following the cholectomy), only 6% of the non-treatment control patients had no midline adhesions, compared to 51% of the Seprafilm patients. Seprafilm also significantly reduced adhesions to the anterior and posterior uterus following myomectomy surgery in a recently reported prospective, multicenter, randomized clinical trial [12]. Prior to initiating these human clinical trials we wished to examine the potential adhesion prevention effectiveness of Seprafilm membrane in an experimental model of peritoneal injury. Because surgeons may use more than one membrane to ensure adequate coverage of damaged tissue, we also examined the effectiveness of multiple membrane layers.

Materials and Methods

All surgical procedures were conducted according to the guidelines specified in the NIH "Guide for the Care and Use of Laboratory Animals" [13] (U.S Patent No. 4, 937, 270, 1990; U.S Patent No. 5, 017, 229, 1991). Female Sprague-Dawley rats (approximately 250 g each, Charles River Breeding Labs, Wilmington, MA) were weighed and anesthetized with a single intramuscular injection of ketamine hydrochloride (85 mg/kg) and xylazine hydrochloride (6 mg/kg). The abdomen of each animal was shaved and scrubbed with alcohol and a betadine solution. A 4-cm midline skin incision was made with a no. 10 scalpel blade, beginning approximately 2 cm caudal to the xyphoid process. A no. 11 scalpel blade was used to pierce the linea alba and to extend the laparotomy opening.

Seprafilm membrane (Genzyme, Cambridge, MA) was provided in sterile 12×15 cm sheets that were cut into 5×5 cm pieces immediately prior to use.

In one study, the ceca of 80 animals were subjected to a gauze abrasion injury following laparotomy. The cecum of each rat was externalized with the aid of sterile cotton-tipped swabs. The contents of the cecum were expressed manually into the ascending colon. A constant force, constant area, rotary gauze abrasion device was employed to induce an operator independent abrasion injury known to cause cecal adhesions in 70%–100% of control animals [5]. The abrasion device utilized a motor-driven rotating spline shaft that delivered a controlled 70-g abrasive force to the cecum. A 1.5-cm-diameter flat surface of type VII surgical gauze (Johnson and Johnson Medical, Arlington, TX) was secured to the end of the rotating shaft by a rubber septum.

The cecum was immobilized during the abrasion procedure by a flexible holder with a single 1.5-cm-diameter opening, which exposed only the defined amount of tissue surface to be abraded. Each cecum was abraded for 60 revolutions of the gauze-tipped shaft at four sites: (1) the distal portion of the anterior surface, (2) the proximal portion of the anterior surface, (3) the distal portion of the posterior surface, and (4) the proximal portion of the posterior surface.

Following the abrasion procedure, animals were randomly assigned to one of two groups. In the treatment group, 40 animals received approximately 5×5 cm Seprafilm Bioresorbable Membrane. The membrane was folded over the cecum so that the organ was covered completely, and the cecum was returned to the abdominal cavity. The control group consisted of 40 animals which received no further treatment following cecal abrasion. The laparotomy incision was closed in two layers as described for the sidewall model, and animals were allowed to recover completely in an incubator. Thereafter they were maintained in groups with food and water ad libitum. Seven days post

Table 1. Adhesion scoring system for cecal injury model

Description	Adhesion score
No adhesions	0
Filmy adhesion with easily identifiable plane of attachment	1
Mild adhesion with difficult dissection of plane of attachment	2
Moderate adhesion with difficult dissection of plane of attachment	3
Dense adhesion with non-dissectable plane of attachment	4

surgery, all of the animals were killed by CO_2 asphyxiation. A researcher who was unaware of the animals' group assignments evaluated cecal adhesions according to a predetermined scale (Table 1).

In a second study, 40 female Sprague Dawley rats had a laparotomy performed and ceca abraded as described above. Following cecal abrasion, animals were randomized into one of the following groups: (1) a single Seprafilm Bioresorbable Membrane was placed such that it completely covered the abraded cecum; (2) two overlapping membranes were placed over the cecum; (3) three overlapping membranes were placed over the cecum; (4) a non-treatment control group. The cecum was returned to the abdominal cavity. The muscle was closed in a simple continuous pattern with 3-O Dexon suture. The skin and attendant fascia were closed with 9-mm stainless steel staples. Following recovery, animals were maintained in groups with free access to food and water. After 7 days, animals were killed via CO_2 asphyxiation. Adhesions were evaluated according to the scoring system in Table 1 by a researcher who was unaware of group assignment. The mean incidence of adhesions, the percentage of animals with no adhesions, and the percentage of animals with significant adhesions were recorded.

Statistical Analysis

The percentage of each group of animals with at least one significant adhesion (grade 2 or higher), as well as the percentage of animals in each group with no adhesions, were compared by chi-square analysis. The mean numbers of cecal adhesions ($\pm$SEM) of all grades for treatment and control groups were compared using the Tukey-Kramer method of multiple comparison analysis. A p value of less than 0.05 was considered statistically significant for both tests.

Results

One animal in the rat cecal injury control group died of unknown causes.

In the first study, employing a single membrane, the mean number of cecal adhesions in the Seprafilm membrane group decreased 89% from 1.9 $\pm$ 0.4 in the control group to 0.2 $\pm$ 0.1 in the Seprafilm group ($p < 0.001$) (Table 2). The percentage of animals with at least one cecal adhesion of grade 2 or higher was significantly lower in the membrane group than in the control group (20% vs.

Table 2. Rat cecal abrasion model

Group	Mean number ± SEM	% Animals with no adhesions	% Animals with adhesion ≥ grade 2
Control	1.9 ± 0.4[a]	18% (4/39)[b]	92% (36/39)[b]
Seprafilm	0.2 ± 0.1	80% (32/40)	20% (8/40)[b]

[a]$P < 0.001$ (Tukey-Kramer)
[b]$P < 0.001$ (chi-square)

92%, $p < 0.001$). Finally, the percentage of animals with no cecal adhesions increased 4.4 times from 18% in the control group to 80% in the Seprafilm group ($p < 0.001$).

In the multiple membrane study, 20% of the animals in the control group (no treatment) had no cecal adhesions, compared to 90%, 80%, and 80% for the single, double, and triple layer groups respectively (Fig. 1a). The mean number of cecal adhesions was significantly lower in each of the membrane groups than in the control group (Fig. 1b), as was the percentage of animals with adhesions of grade 2 or higher (Fig. 1c). There were no differences in adhesion scores between any of the membrane treatment groups.

Discussion

Seprafilm Bioresorbable Membrane is composed of the naturally occurring biopolymer sodium hyaluronate (HA) and carboxymethylcellulose (CMC). Native hyaluronate, which is found throughout mammalian soft tissues, clears rapidly from the peritoneal cavity and does not have sufficient residence time to act as a significant adhesion prevention barrier. For example, Grainger et al. [14] showed that a chemically modified HA slab prevented adhesion in a rabbit ovarian surgery model, while non-modified HA did not. CMC has shown some promise in animal studies when used as a hydroflotation solution [3, 4], but it has not been tested in human clinical trials. We have chemically modified the HA and CMC in Seprafilm Bioresorbable Membrane to render it insoluble and less susceptible to enzymatic and free radical degradation in vivo. The chemical modification involves reaction of HA and CMC with the water-soluble carbodiimide 1-(3-demethylaminopropyl)-3-ethylcarbodiimide hydrochloride (EDC). This reaction converts a portion of the carboxylate groups on the HA and CMC to cationic N-acylurea (Fig. 2). This chemical modification prolongs the persistence of the Seprafilm Bioresorbable Membrane so that it clears from the peritoneum in about 7 days, the ideal residence time during early wound repair for an adhesion prevention barrier.

In the current studies, the adhesion scores for the control groups in these two separate studies were very consistent, indicating the reproducibility of this method to induce tissue trauma and adhesion formation. Seprafilm Bioresorbable Membrane prevented adhesions in a highly significant number of animals when compared to surgical controls in a rat cecal abrasion model for

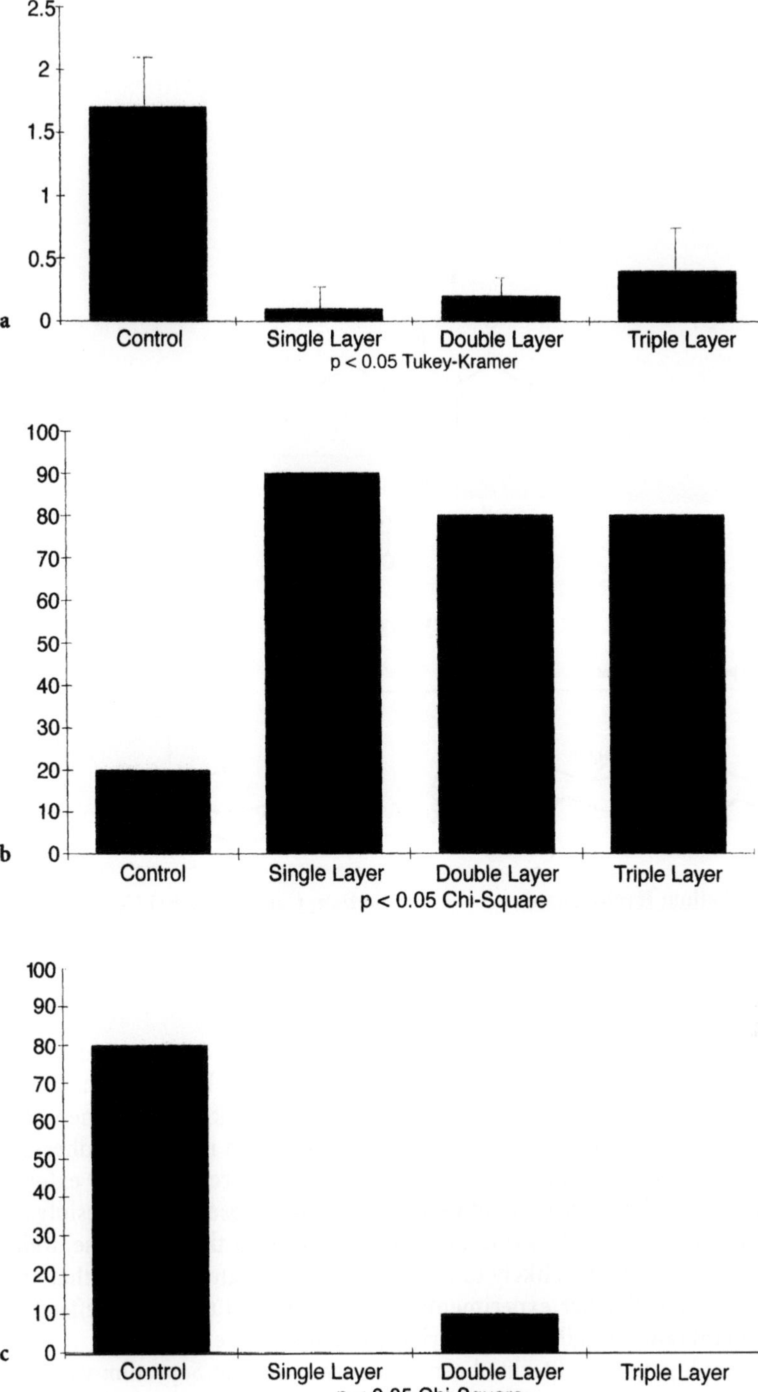

Fig. 1a–c. Multiple layer study; **a** mean number of adhesions; **b** percentage of animals with no adhesions; **c** percentage of animals with adhesions $\geq$ grade 2

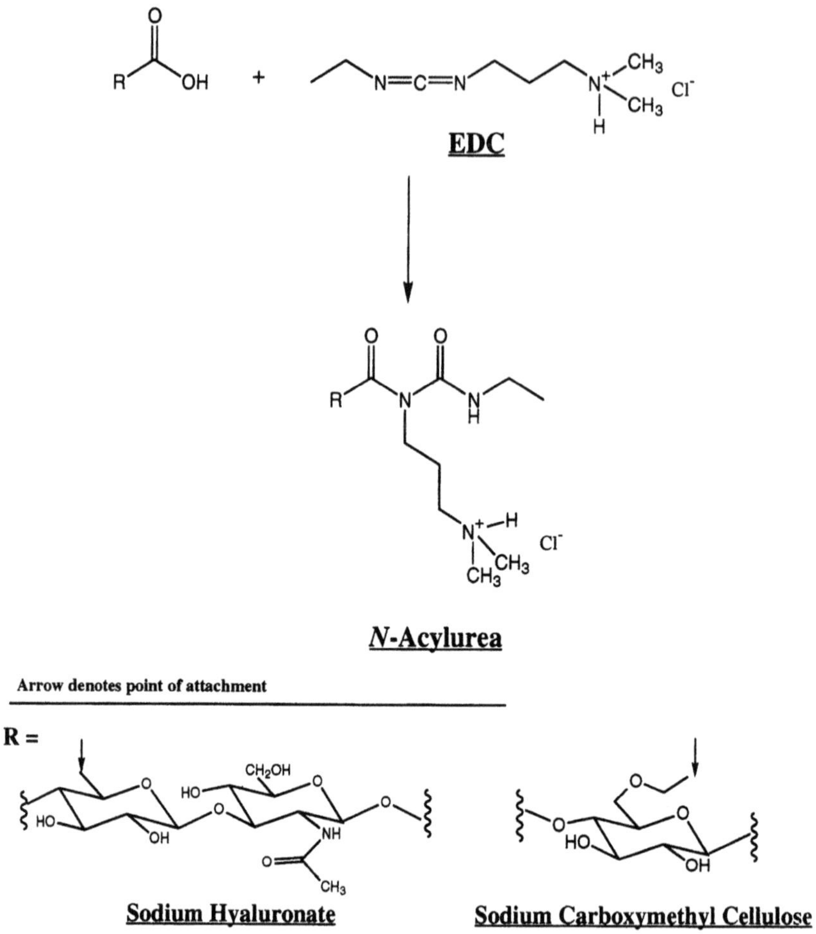

EDC

N-**Acylurea**

Arrow denotes point of attachment

R =

CH$_2$OH

Sodium Hyaluronate

Sodium Carboxymethyl Cellulose

Fig. 2. Chemical structures

adhesion formation. Additionally, the severity of adhesions, as measured at day 7 after injury, was lower in the Seprafilm treatment group. Because adhesions, once formed, may continue to organize for a time, it is not known whether, at a later time, membrane and control groups would differ with respect to adhesion severity. It is most desirable to prevent adhesions or reduce their extent; however, reducing the severity of adhesions will make subsequent adhesiolysis easier for the surgeon and less traumatic to the tissue. In the latter case, mild filmy adhesion might be less likely to reform after lysis than adhesions that are dense and vascular. Further experimentation is warranted to test the effect of Seprafilm membrane on adhesion severity and adhesion reformation.

A study employing a rat uterine horn model showed that Seprafilm was not effective [15] because the membrane did not stay on the small uterine horn. This was most likely because the horn did not provide sufficient surface area for membrane adherence. Clinical trials using the membrane in myomectomy surgery and major abdominal surgery therefore employed sheets large enough to ensure coverage of the site of tissue injury even if the membrane moved slightly. To ensure adequate coverage of surfaces at risk for adhesion formation, surgeons will sometimes use multiple and overlapping membranes. Our multiple layering study was, therefore, conducted to assess whether additional product reduces adhesion prevention efficacy. The results demonstrate that Seprafilm membrane does not lose efficacy with multiple layering. Future studies will investigate whether multiple layers of Seprafilm improve its efficacy in more severe adhesion models.

References

1. Doody KJ, Dunn RC, Buttram VC (1989) Recombinant tissue plasminogen activator reduces adhesion formation. Fertil Steril 51: 509–512
2. Menzies D, Ellis H (1991) The role of plasminogen activator in adhesion prevention. Surg Gynecol Obstet 172: 362–368
3. Diamond MP, DeCherney AH, Linsky CB, Cunningham T, Constantine B (1988) Adhesion re-formation in the rabbit uterine horn model. Int J Fertil 33: 372–375
4. Diamond MP, DeCherney AH, Linsky CB, Cunningham T, Constantine B (1988) Assessment of carboxymethylcellulose and 32% dextran 70 for prevention of adhesions. Int J Fertil 33: 278–282
5. Burns JW, Skinner K, Colt J et al. (1995) Prevention of tissue injury and post-surgical adhesions by precoating tissues with hyaluronic acid solutions. J Surg Res 59: 644–652
6. Interceed (TC7) Adhesions Barrier Study Group (1989) Prevention of postsurgical adhesions by Interceed (TC7), an absorbable adhesion barrier. Fertil Steril 51: 933–938
7. Haney AF, Hesla J, Hurst BS, Kettel LM et al. (1995) Expanded polytetrafluoroethylene (Gore-Tex Surgical Membrane) is superior to oxidized regenerated cellulose (Interceed TC7 +) in preventing adhesions. Fertil Steril 63: 1021–1026
8. Raftery AT (1973) Regeneration of parietal and visceral peritoneum. Br J Cell Biol 60: 293–299
9. Raftery AT (1973) Regeneration of parietal and visceral peritoneum. J Anat 115: 375–392
10. Mitchell JD, Lee R, Neya K, Vlahakes GJ (1994) Reduction in experimental pericardial adhesions using a hyaluronic acid bioabsorbable membrane. Eur J Cardiothorac Surg 8: 149–152
11. Becker JM, Dayton MT, Fazio VW et al. (1996) Seprafilm bioresorbable membrane in the prevention of postoperative abdominal adhesions: a prospective, randomized, double-blinded multicenter study. The 3rd International Congress on Pelvic Surgery and Adhesion Prevention, 29 Feb-2 March 1996, San Diego
12. Diamond MP, Bieber E, Coddington C, Franklin R, Brunert G et al. (1996) Reduction of adhesions after uterine myomectomy by Seprafilm Membrane, a blinded, prospective, randomized, multicenter clinical study. The 3rd International Congress on Pelvic Surgery and Adhesion Prevention, 29 Feb-2 March 1996, San Diego
13. U.S. Department of Health and Human Services (1986) Guide for the care and use of laboratory animals. National Institutes of Health, Revised 1985. NIH publication no. 86–23
14. Grainger DA, Meyer W, DeCherney A, Diamond M (1991) The use of hyaluronic acid polymers to reduce postoperative adhesions. J Gynecol Surg 7: 97–100
15. Yarali H, Zahradka BFH, Gomel V (1994) Hyaluronic membrane for reducing adhesion formation and reformation in the rat uterine horn. J Reprod Med 39: 667–670
16. Johnson & Johnson (1994) Interceed (TC7) absorbable adhesion barrier: directions for use. JJM, Arlington, USA
17. Pagidas K, Tulandi T (1992) Effects of Ringer's Lactate, Interceed (TC7) and Gore-Tex Surgical Membrane on postsurgical adhesion formation. Fertil Steril 57: 199–201

10.8 Use of Adhesion Prevention Barriers in Gynecological Surgery

M.H. Thornton, J.D. Campeau, and G.S. diZerega

Introduction

A large amount of research has recently been dedicated to the reduction of adhesion formation, due to the morbidity associated with postoperative adhesions as well as a recent emphasis on cost containment in health care. The incidence of adhesions following laparotomy has been well documented [1–4]. Recently Menzies and Ellis, in a prospective analysis, found that patients with one or more abdominal operations had a 93% incidence of intra-abdominal adhesions compared to 10% of patients undergoing laparotomy for the first time [5]. Adhesions are associated with a major economic burden. A recent survey of general surgeons by Scott-Coombes reported an estimated incidence of 12 000–14 000 cases per year of adhesion related admissions in the United Kingdom [6]. When considering only hospital cost and surgeon fees, adhesiolysis in the United States was $1179 million in 1988 [7]. However, if outpatient medical costs were included, this would substantially increase the economic burden of abdominal adhesive disease. A multidisciplinary resurgence in the interest of peritoneal repair has increased awareness and led to an improved understanding of adhesion formation. Physical barriers that prevent adhesion formation by limiting tissue apposition during the critical stages of mesothelial repair have become available for all intra-abdominal surgical subspecialities. This review will discuss traditional adhesion prevention adjutants; provide an overview of studies for adhesion prevention barriers, including a perspective for their use; and, finally, discuss the future of adhesion prevention.

Complications from Intraperitoneal Adhesions

Intestinal Obstruction

The most serious complication of intraperitoneal adhesions is intestinal obstruction. Intestinal obstruction requires immediate surgical correction and can be fatal. In the majority of patients with intestinal obstruction secondary to postoperative adhesion formation, the presenting symptoms occur long after surgery. Intestinal mobility may lead to entrapment of a loop of bowel by a preexisting adhesion many years after that adhesion had formed. Menzies and Ellis demonstrated that the incidence of intestinal obstruction was 1% within the first postoperative year. Thus, the presence of intra-abdominal adhesions may become clinically manifest even many years after the surgical procedure [5]. A recent report demonstrated a significant contribution of gynecologic surgery, especially hysterectomy, to postoperative bowel obstruction [8].

Chronic Pelvic Pain

Peritoneal adhesions are one of the major causes of chronic or recurrent pelvic pain in 13%–26% of women [9–13]. Stout reported 79% of patients with pelvic pain had either endometriosis and/or adhesions and that the adhesion scores correlated with the pain assessment [11]. However, the presence of adhesions is often difficult to associate with the degree and location of the pelvic pain. It was suggested that chronic pain arises as a result of the restriction of movement of pelvic organs due to adhesions [11–14]. Since both sensory and vasomotor nerves supply the peritoneum, most of the parietal peritoneum is sensitive to pain. Pain fibers have not been clearly demonstrated for visceral peritoneum. The recent immunohistochemical identification of nerve fibers in pelvic adhesions from women may provide an anatomical basis for further studies of pain associated with adhesions [15]. From a clinical point of view, the relationship between pelvic pain and adhesions is often less clear. Many gynecologists observe patients with a few adhesions who report significant pain, whereas other patients who are found to have significant adhesions may not describe pain symptoms. The only significant predictor of adhesions in patients with pelvic pain is prior pelvic surgery, while the significant physical findings which predict adhesions are an adnexal mass and decrease in uterine mobility [11, 13, 14].

Removal of adhesions in patients with pelvic pain usually leads to relief of symptoms [11–14, 16–19]. In 1985, Chan and Wood reported a clear reduction in pain after lysis of adhesions involving the tubes and ovary [14]. More recent studies have confirmed these findings. Steege and Stout reported a reduction of pelvic pain in women with chronic pain following laparoscopic lysis of adhesions [16]. Prognosis was not related to the extent of adhesions. However, about 25% of their patients returned with pain within 3–5 months presumably due to reformation of the adhesions. Daniell reported on 42 patients with significant prior surgical histories and adhesions as the suspected source of the patients' pain [17]. Following laparoscopic adhesiolysis, 67% of the patients noted improvement of pain at 4 months follow-up. Similarly, in a retrospective review, Sutton reported that 81% of patients experienced pain relief after laparoscopic laser adhesiolysis [18]. These results were confirmed by Peters, who showed in a controlled study that lysis of adhesions reduced pelvic pain in patients with severe adhesions [19]. However, there may also be no improvement in pelvic pain after laparoscopic lysis of adhesions.

Residual Ovarian Pain

The presence of pain, a pelvic mass and dyspareunia represent the three most common findings in the 1%–3% of post-hysterectomy patients who subsequently return to their gynecologist with "residual ovarian syndrome" [20–23]. Among 122 patients who required subsequent removal of their ovaries after previous hysterectomy (10.3%), Grogan found the most common presenting symptom to be pelvic pain due to adhesions involving the ovary [21]. Adhesions and peri-oophoritis as well as a retroperitoneal location of the ovary may prevent follicular rupture into the peritoneal cavity and give rise to an expanding polycystic mass [22, 23].

Secondary Sterility in Females

Adhesion formation is well-recognized as a major cause of infertility in women. Drake and Grunert reported that, of 38 infertile females with otherwise normal outpatient evaluations, 31% had adhesions upon diagnostic laparoscopy [24]. DeCherney and Mezer found that approximately 75% of the 61 infertile females who had undergone prior salpingostomy had adhesions at follow-up laparoscopy [25]. Trimbos-Kemper et al. observed a similar incidence of periadnexal adhesions among the 188 infertile female patients they studied [26].

Surgical Techniques to Reduce Adhesion Formation

Peritoneal Closure

Adhesions, delayed healing, and wound breakdown are often attributed to failure of peritoneal suturing or the presence of deperitonealized areas within the abdomen. To reconstruct the pelvis after removal of viscera and parietal peritoneum seems a logical procedure. However, when reviewing the physiology of peritoneal re-epithelialization it is known that peritoneal healing differs from that of skin [4]. When a defect is made in the peritoneum the entire surface becomes epithelialized simultaneously and not gradually from the borders, as in epidermalization of skin wounds. Although multiplication and migration of mesothelial cells from the margin of the wound contribute to the regenerative process, they do not play major roles. New mesothelium develops predominately from islands of epithelial cells that attach throughout the wound surface and then proliferate [10, 11]. Consequently, large peritoneal wounds re-epithelialize about as quickly as small peritoneal wounds. Examination of data indicates that approximation of peritoneum by sutures to cover vascularized areas denuded by the previous dissection may not facilitate peritoneal repair. A wide variety of animal studies demonstrated enhanced adhesion formation to suture lines when peritoneum is closed over denuded tissue. All experimental evidence indicates that areas of denuded peritoneum will heal satisfactorily and that the suturing of peritoneum actually increases the incidence of adhesions [27]. Clinical reports after oncological surgery and/ or gastrointestinal resection demonstrated normal healing of unsutured peritoneum. No instances of bowel obstruction occurred and the surgical sites were covered by a smooth glistening peritoneal surface [27]. Strickler found that, in patients who had peritoneal closure in the original operation, the adhesions causing the obstruction were always to the site of reperitonealization. In patients with intestinal obstruction in whom the peritoneum was left open, the adhesions causing obstruction were remote from the site of spontaneous reperitonealization adhesions [8].

The value of peritoneal closure at the time of cesarean birth was evaluated prospectively. Hull and Varner [28] as well as Pietrantoni et al. [29] compared the clinical outcome of post-cesarean section patients who did or did not undergo peritoneal closure. Closure of the peritoneum extended the duration of the surgical procedure by 5 min. There were no differences between the groups in the postoperative incidence of wound infection, dehiscence, endometritis, ileus, or length of hospital stay. Nonclosure of the visceral and parietal peritoneum after low transverse cesarean section had no adverse effects on recovery and decreased the operating time. Tulandi et al. showed no difference in adhesions to the previous laparotomy incision after closure with or without peritoneal suturing [30].

Laparoscopy

Although many clinicians assume that laparoscopic surgery will reduce and often eliminate postoperative adhesion formation, the data to support this assumption are not compelling. Diamond et al. reported a 96% incidence of adhesions in 51 patients after laparoscopic adhesiolysis and only a 50% decrease in adhesion scores [31]. To follow-up, Diamond et al. performed a prospective multicenter study using early (8–79 days, mean 35 days after initial laparoscopic surgery) second-look laparoscopy [32]. Of the areas where adhesions were lysed, 67% contained adhesions at second-look. However, de novo adhesion formation was substantially reduced by laparoscopic surgery. In 16% of the patients and in 25% of the anatomical sites in those patients new adhesions were noted. In only four patients did the adhesion score remain the same or decrease. Although laparoscopic surgical techniques reduce de novo adhesion formation, adhesion reformation continues to be a major concern.

Use of Drugs to Reduce Adhesions

Recently, Larsson and the Nordic Adhesion Prevention Study Group preliminarily reported on the failure of intraperitoneal corticosteroids (Solu Medrol 500 mg ip) to reduce adhesion scores in infertility patients [33]. Jansen demonstrated that intraperitoneal use of heparin in women was also not effective in preventing adhesions [34]. The question arises as to why pharmacological agents that work in the test tube or in animal models do not work in patients? Evidence points to a fundamental limitation in drug delivery. The mesothelium of the peritoneum contains a rich vascular supply. Any drug going to the peritoneum goes through the vascular system. Surgeons clamp, cut, tie, and burn, producing avascular, ischemic areas. The resulting ischemia allows for persistence of fibrin and the formation of adhesions. Fibrin is going to persist at these ischemic sites, as there is no vascular supply to provide oxygen to the tissues; thus, there is reduced fibrinolytic activity [35]. Pharmaceutical approaches to adhesion prevention therefore await technology which will deliver drugs to the site of potential adhesion formation for the duration necessary to achieve clinical benefit.

Use of Liquid Devices to Reduce Adhesions

Intraperitoneal adhesion formation can be prevented by eliminating the formation of fibrin bridges between healing tissues. Devices commonly used in an effort to separate tissue surfaces during postsurgical repair include both liquids and barriers. Liquids currently in use include dextran and crystalloid.

Dextran

Dextran is a water-soluble glucose polymer originally used as a plasma expander. It can be manufactured in a variety of molecular weights; however most of the research in adhesion prevention has focused on a 32% solution of dextran 70 (average molecular weight of 70 000 daltons) suspended in 10% dextrose (Hyskon, Pharmacia, Uppsala, Sweden).

Two prospective, controlled clinical studies using infertility surgery reported a significant beneficial effect of Hyskon on the prevention of adhesion formation. In one study patients undergoing surgery for distal tubal disease, endometriosis, or pelvic adhesions had 250 ml of Hyskon or saline instilled into the peritoneal cavity prior to closure [36]. Adhesions occurred more frequently in control patients than in Hyskon-treated patients. In a second study by Rosenberg and Board, patients were randomized to receive 200 ml of Hyskon or 200 ml of Ringer's lactate intraperitoneally prior to closure [37]. Adhesion scores tended to worsen in patients who received Ringer's lactate, while the scores improved in patients who received Hyskon. Both studies noted that the adhesion reduction effects were largely limited to "dependent" portions of the pelvis. Not all clinical evaluations found a beneficial effect of Hyskon on adhesion formation. Hyskon was evaluated in a prospective, randomized, multicenter study in Scandinavia and Finland [38]. Following operations for fertility, 250 ml of Hyskon or 250 ml of 0.9% saline was instilled into the pelvic cavity. Follow-up laparoscopy revealed no difference between the two treatment groups. Jansen also reported no benefit from the addition of 100–200 ml Hyskon on adhesion scores at follow-up laparoscopy performed 12 days after infertility surgery [39]. Due to the relative lack of efficacy, the Pharmacia company withdrew their submission to the FDA for Hyskon as a device to reduce intraperitoneal adhesion formation.

The clinical use of Hyskon may be associated with important side effects [40]. Anaphylactic shock or allergic symptoms occur in a small percentage of patients given Hyskon intraperitoneally. Transient weight gain and ascites are commonly observed; the most common clinical complication is vulvar edema, which may occur in 2% of patients. Administration of Hyskon into the peritoneal cavity may produce a transient increase in the postoperative serum transaminase levels. Edema of the leg, pleural effusion, and coagulopathy occur less frequently. All of these side effects resolved either spontaneously or with supportive therapy. Since intravenous administration of dextran can prolong coagulation time, dextran-treated patients undergoing anticoagulation therapy should be carefully monitored.

Crystalloid Solutions

The most commonly used adjuvant to reduce adhesion formation is crystalloid solution, such as lactated Ringer's solution, phosphate buffered saline, or normal saline, which is administered as an instillate at the end of the surgical procedure. Absorption of water and electrolytes from the peritoneal cavity is rapid, with up to 500 ml of physiologic saline absorbed in less than 24 h [41]. Thus, 200 ml volume of Ringer's lactate would be absorbed in 6 h. Since it takes 5-8 days for the peritoneal surface to remesothelialize, crystalloid would theoretically be absorbed well before the process of fibrin deposition and adhesion formation was completed [42]. From a theoretical point of view intraperitoneal crystalloid would thus not be expected to prevent adhesion formation.

A substantial body of clinical data is available to assess the benefit of crystalloid instillate in adhesion prevention. During the early 1980s, four clinical studies were published which compared dextran to crystalloid used as instillates to prevent adhesion formation [36-39]. A combination of these studies showed an adhesion reformation rate of approximately 80% in patients who received crystalloid instillates. Many of these crystalloid treated patients had more adhesions at the time of second-look than prior to the initial procedure. This high rate of adhesion formation with the use of intraperitoneal instillates was confirmed by Fayez and Schneider [43]. More recently, reports have appeared describing the use of crystalloid solutions to reduce adhesion formation after laparoscopic ovarian surgery. Naether and Fischer instilled 300-500 ml of saline into the peritoneal cavity after laparoscopic coagulation of the ovarian surface in patients with polycystic ovarian disease [44]. When compared to a previous series treated in a similar fashion by these authors without the crystalloid instillation, they found no difference in the incidence of adhesions (17% vs 19%, respectively). Gurgan et al. instilled 150 ml of Ringer's lactate into the pelvis after laparoscopic electrocautery or Nd: YAG laser vaporization of the ovarian surface in polycystic ovarian disease patients: 82% were found to have adhesions to the ovarian surface at second-look laparoscopy [45]. Tulandi initiated a pilot study evaluating the efficacy of crystalloid solutions for post-myomectomy adhesion prevention. The study was terminated due to lack of benefit for his patients.

Use of Barriers to Reduce Adhesions

Many natural and synthetic materials have been tested which mechanically separate adjacent surfaces during reperitonealization and thereby diminish adhesion formation. However, the majority of these products were either ineffective or actually enhanced formations. Recently, the FDA has approved two prevention barriers, Interceed and Preclude, for adhesion use. These are described below.

An Absorbable Barrier: Oxidized Regenerated Cellulose (Interceed)

Ideally, a physical barrier for adhesion prevention should not effect healing, persist during the critical stages of re-epithelialization and then undergo absorption. Oxidized regenerated cellulose barriers appear to satisfy these criteria (Interceed absorbable adhesion barrier, Johnson & Johnson, Arlington, TX). In addition, oxidized regenerated cellulose does not support bacterial growth; rather this material exhibits antibacterial properties in vivo.

Ovarian Surgery

Efficacy of Interceed after ovarian surgery has been evaluated in five clinical studies (Table 1). Franklin et al. conducted a prospective, multicenter, randomized study to assess the efficacy of Interceed as a barrier to the reformation of ovarian adhesions after surgery involving the ovaries [46]. A total of 52 patients with bilateral ovarian disease were treated at initial laparotomy. At the end of the procedure, one ovary was wrapped with Interceed (Fig. 1), the other was left uncovered. Treatment with Interceed eliminated the formation of adhesions in nearly twice as many ovaries compared to surgery alone (control ovaries), as determined by second-look laparoscopy. This difference represents an 86% improvement over control in preventing adhesion formation or reformation.

Larsson studied 66 women with infertility due, at least in part, to bilateral adnexal adhesions [47]. Adhesiolysis was performed through laparotomy with microsurgical techniques. Interceed was applied to one ovary while the contralateral ovary served as the untreated control. The results indicated that microsurgical techniques alone resulted in a significant reduction of postoperative adhesions to the adnexa (Fig. 2). Further, the number of ovaries without adhesions at the time of second-look laparoscopy was significantly increased, by approximately two-fold, when the ovaries were covered with Interceed. When combined with microsurgical techniques, Interceed reduced adhesion reformation scores by 70%.

Table 1. Clinical studies with barriers confirm efficacy

Laparotomy	Barrier	Patients (n)	Reference
Ovarian surgery			
Cystectomy	Interceed	66	[47]
	Interceed	52	[46]
	Interceed	20	[48]
	Interceed	31	[68]
Pelvic sidewall			
Adhesiolysis	Interceed	74	[50]
	Interceed	134	[52]
	Interceed	63	[53]
	Interceed	35	[55]
	Interceed	28	[54]
	Preclude/Interceed	32	[57]
Tubal surgery			
Adhesiolysis	Interceed	66	[47]
Salpingostomy	Interceed	21	[57]
Myomectomy	Preclude	16	[64]
	Interceed	50	[69]
Endometriosis			
Resection stage III-IV	Interceed	28	[53]
Endometrioma	Interceed	14	[46]
Severe disease	Interceed	32	[70]
Pelvic surgery	Preclude	18	[63]
	Preclude/Interceed	57	[71]
Laparoscopy			
Ovarian cystectomy	Interceed	17	[49]
Ovarian drilling	Interceed	20	[72]
Endometriosis	Interceed	32	[69]

Van Geldorp evaluated the use of Interceed as an ovarian wrap [48] (Fig. 1). Some 20 patients underwent bilateral ovarian surgery, including cystectomy, removal of endometriosis and endometriomas as well as adhesiolysis via laparotomy. At the end of the procedure one ovary was chosen on a randomized basis for wrapping with Interceed while the other served as an unwrapped control. Estimation of the ovarian surface with adhesions (damaged area left after adhesiolysis) was made at laparoscopy 4–8 weeks later. There were 11 treatment (55%) and three control (15%) ovaries which had no adhesions. Overall, 17 of the treatment (85%) and only five (25%) of the control ovaries had a reduction in the size of the initial area of injury at second-look. Ten of the other control ovaries had an increase in area involved in adhesions compared with only one of the Interceed treated ovaries. Wrapping the ovary with Interceed after ovarian surgery significantly reduced the area involved with adhesions to the ovary as well as the adjacent attachment sites from which adhesions had been removed.

Keckstein et al. evaluated the efficacy of Interceed in 17 patients following laparoscopic removal of 16 cysts and 22 endometriomas. At second-look laparoscopy 13 of the 17 Interceed-treated ovaries (76%) and six of the 17 control ovaries (35%) were free of adhesions [49].

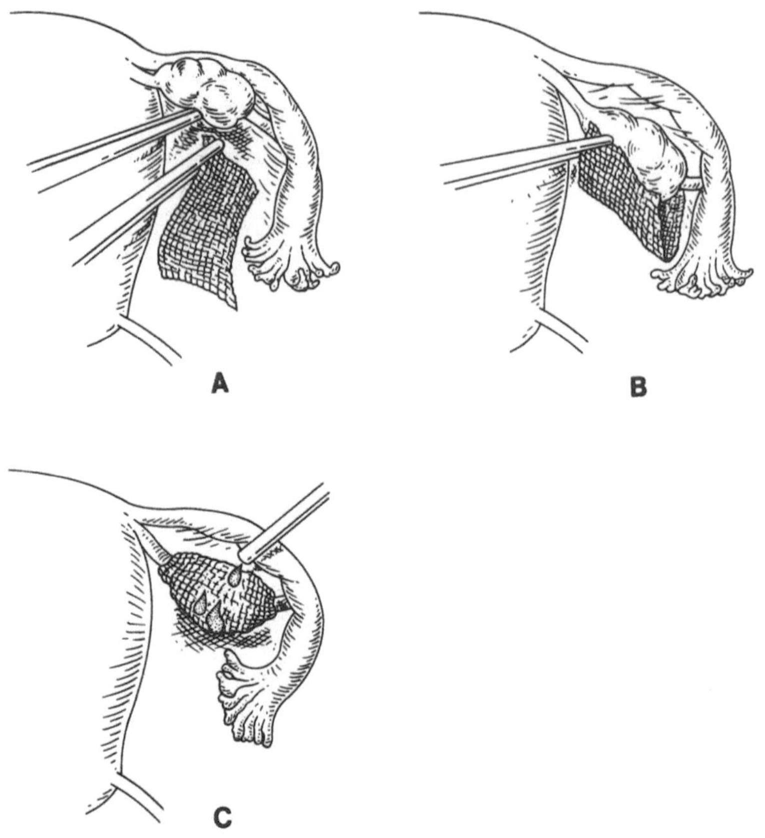

Fig. 1A–C. The ovary is completely wrapped with Interceed; **A** by lifting the ovary away from the ovarian fossa and placing a corner of Interceed (1/2 piece) up into the fossa; **B** allowing the ovary to return to normal position thereby holding the Interceed in place; **C** moistening with a few drops of irrigating solution to insure adherence of the barrier to the ovary

Tubal Surgery

Larsson and coworkers evaluated the efficacy of Interceed as an adjuvant in the prevention of postoperative adhesion reformation to the fallopian tube and fimbria [47, 50]. Adhesiolysis was performed in infertility patients (n=66) with bilateral adhesions attached to both fallopian tubes. The side of Interceed application was randomly assigned. Follow-up laparoscopy after 4–10 weeks indicated that twice as many fallopian tubes were free of adhesions after the use of Interceed compared to microsurgery alone (Fig. 2). Curto et al. reported a 100% incidence of adhesion-free fimbria when Interceed was used to cover the fimbria after salpingostomy [51]; however, their series was uncontrolled and reported results in only 21 of their 54 patients.

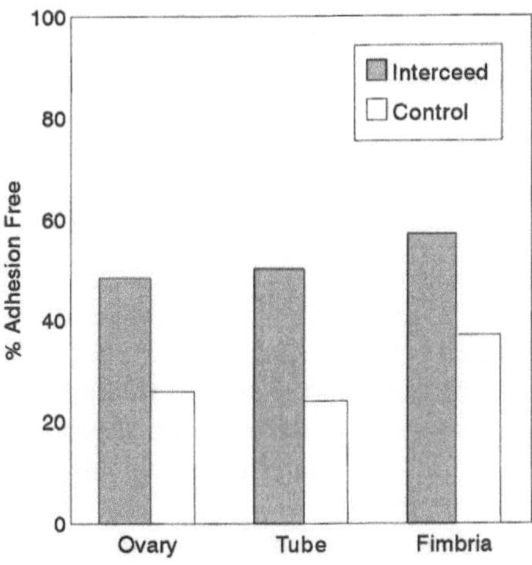

Fig. 2. Bilateral adnexal surgery was performed on infertility patients (n=66) including removal of adhesions from ovaries, fimbria, and the fallopian tube. Interceed use on the surgical site prevented adhesion reformation compared to surgery only control. Ovary: 47% vs 26%, $p<0.02$; fimbria: 50% vs 24%, $p<0.01$; fallopian tube 58% vs 38%, $p<0.05$. (From [47])

Adhesiolysis

The initial clinical evaluation of Interceed was conducted in fertility patients who underwent lysis of bilateral pelvic sidewall adhesions [50, 52]. Following adhesiolysis, the area of the deperitonealized surface was measured. Interceed was applied in an amount sufficient to completely cover deperitonealized surfaces on the sidewall; the contralateral sidewall was left uncovered, thereby serving as control. At second-look laparoscopy, Interceed was found to significantly reduce the incidence, extent, and severity of postoperative adhesions. Confirmatory studies were published by Sekiba et al. (n=63 patients) [53], Li and Cooke ($n = 27$ patients) [54], as well as Reid et al. ($n = 35$ patients) [55].

Similar demonstrations of Interceed efficacy at the pelvic sidewall after adhesiolysis were reported in two clinical studies in which Preclude was used as a comparison on the contralateral sidewall. Both the Adhesion Barriers Study Group [56] and Haney et al. [57] reported a significant reduction of sidewall adhesions with Interceed use in 29 and 19 patients, respectively. Importantly, none of these studies nor any other clinical study reported any adverse reaction of surrounding organs or tissues attributable to Interceed or the permanent barrier Preclude (see below) use when used in women. This is in direct contrast to reports by some investigators when Interceed was used in murine mouse models [58, 59] but not in rabbit models [60–62].

Endometriosis

Interceed was also effective in preventing adhesion formation after removal of severe endometriosis in 28 patients (American Fertility Society endometriosis grade IV: 25 patients, grade III: 3 patients) [53]. After completion of all operative procedures, including lysis of pelvic sidewall adhesions, one side was randomly assigned coverage with Interceed. In 28 patients with severe endometriosis, significantly fewer Interceed-treated sidewalls contained adhesions than on the control side, as determined by second-look laparoscopy.

A Permanent Barrier: Polytetrafluoroethylene (Preclude)

Preclude (W.L. Gore Co., Flagstaff, AZ) is a thin sheet (0.1 mm) of expanded polytetrafluoroethylene which is used as a substitute for the pericardium. Preclude has a small pore size (≤ 1 μm) that retards cellular penetration. The membrane must be fixed in place within the body and is nonabsorbable. It is antithrombogenic, nonreactive, and easy to handle at laparotomy. Experience in cardiovascular surgery has shown use of PTFE to result in minimal adhesion formation when used as a pericardial substitute.

A multicenter, noncontrolled study evaluated Preclude in patients treated for one of the following conditions: (1) moderate to severe pelvic adhesive disease, (2) significant deperitonealization, or (3) leiomyomata (Table 1) [63]. Adhesions were lysed and/or a myomectomy was performed. The area covered by the Preclude had significantly lower scores than prior to surgery. There was no morbidity (i.e., infection, inflammation) attributable to the use of the PTFE barrier. At second-look, all of the Preclude was removed by cutting the sutures and withdrawing the barrier through an operating trocar. Histological analysis of the retrieved barrier showed no tissue adherence to the material and mild to no foreign body response. Third-look laparoscopy of a single sidewall site showed no adhesion formation subsequent to Preclude removal.

Myomectomy

Tulandi and coworkers performed myomectomies in 28 patients via laparotomy [64]. All patients had two uterine incisions located on the fundus and posterior uterus. All incisions were sutured closed and randomly assigned coverage with Preclude (Fig. 3) or left as uncovered control. Suturing of the Preclude was performed with 7-0 nylon or polypropylene. The number of adhesion-free sites covered by Preclude was significantly greater than in the control (Fig. 4), as determined by second-look laparoscopy. Adhesions to the Preclude sites were found mainly at the edges of the barriers. In situ the PTFE was covered by a thin layer of tissue that readily separated during removal of the material. The surgical membrane was easily removed by cutting the sutures and applying gentle traction. Histologic examination of the barrier revealed no tissue attachment to the material. The interstices were filled with proteinaceous fluid, and the surface occasionally showed the presence of fibroblasts, histocytes, erythrocytes, and mesothelial cells.

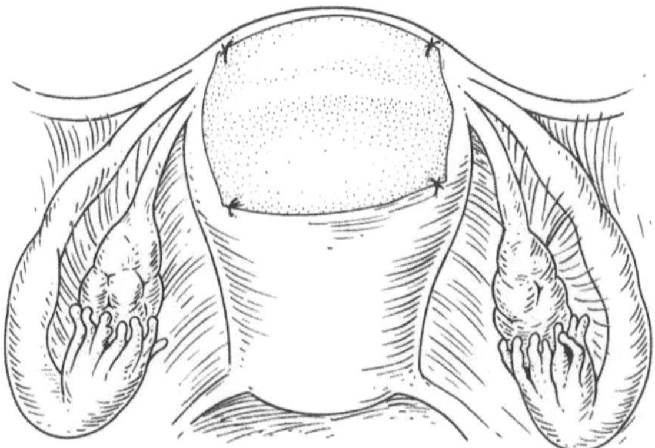

Fig. 3. Application of Preclude is shown over a myomectomy incision. Permanent sutures are used to insure positioning of barrier which was cut to cover the entire area at risk for adhesion formation

Summary

While both solid barriers were shown to be safe and effective in all human clinical trials, their use did not eliminate adhesions in all patients. The use of adhesion prevention barriers have become routine in many clinical practices. It is important to emphasize that the use of these adjuvants is not a substitute for established surgical techniques [16, 22, 65–67]. Efficacy of the barriers is limited to surgical situations in which the area in question can be completely

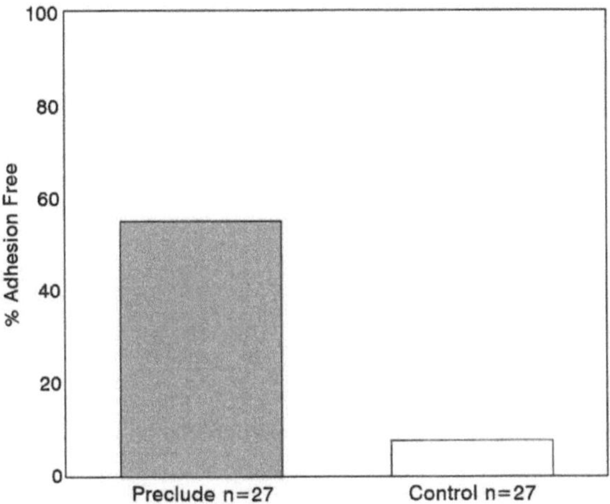

Fig. 4. Prevention of adhesion formation with the use of Preclude to cover suture sites after myomectomy (55.6% adhesion-free sites) compared to suture-only site. Control, 7.4%, $p<0.01$. (Adapted from [64])

Table 2. Careful attention to the technical details of Interceed application is needed to maximize efficacy

1. Apply at the end of the procedure.
2. Complete hemostasis must be achieved before application.
3. Remove all irrigation fluid and instillates from peritoneal cavity. If Trendelenburg positioning is used then place patient in reverse Trendelenburg and remove as much of the irrigation fluid as possible from the cul-de-sac
4. Cut to size to allow at least a 5 mm margin around area at risk.
5. Apply Interceed. If Interceed becomes black upon application, then blood is present and may reduce efficacy:
   - Remove Interceed and achieve hemostasis.
   - Apply new piece of Interceed Barrier as specified below.
6. Apply Interceed dry and in a single layer. If more than one piece is required, allow the pieces to overlap by a margin of 3–5 mm to ensure contiguous coverage of the area at risk.
7. No sutures needed.
8. Moisten with up to 2 ml of irrigant per 3" × 4" piece.

Table 3. Careful attention to the details of Preclude application is needed to maximize efficacy

1. Cutting to proper size is essential: Ensure that the repair site is completely covered by the Preclude, including overlap of the edges of the repair site. If the Preclude is cut too small, excessive stress may be placed on the tissue by Preclude and sutures may pull out. If the Preclude is sized too large, excessive wrinkling may occur, possibly resulting in undesired tissue attachment.
2. In suturing, use nonabsorbable suture with a tapered, piercing point, or reverse cutting needle of appropriate size to anchor the material. Absorbable sutures can be used once the material is adequately anchored. If *ONLY* absorbable sutures are used with Preclude, the repair may fail, possibly resulting in detachment from the implant site. Thus, it is essential not to use only absorbable sutures to anchor the Preclude.
   For best results, use monofilament sutures and use the minimum number of sutures required to maintain adequate anchoring of the Preclude. Do not use a conventional cutting needle. Do not allow excessive wrinkles in the Preclude.
3. In cases in which Preclude is to be left in the patient, consideration should be given to the patient signing an informed consent for the retention of a nonabsorbable device.

covered. Physician acceptance is constrained by technical difficulties including the need for hemostasis and removal of excess peritoneal fluid (Interceed: Table 2) as well as fixation techniques and concerns regarding subsequent removal of the barrier (Preclude: Table 3).

References

1. Damario MA, Rock JA (1995) Methods to prevent postoperative adhesion formation in gynecologic surgery. J Gynecol Technol 1: 77
2. Sutton C, Diamond MP (1993) Endoscopic Surgery for Gynaecologists. W.B. Saunders, Philadelphia
3. Diamond MP, Daniell JF, Feste J et al. (1987) Adhesion reformation and de novo adhesion formation after reproductive pelvic surgery. Fertil Steril 47: 864–866
4. diZerega GS, Rodgers KE (1992) The peritoneum. Springer, New York Berlin Heidelberg

5. Menzies D, Ellis H (1990) Intestinal obstruction from adhesions-how big is the problem? Ann Royal Coll Surg Engl 72: 60–63
6. Scott-Coombes DM, Vipond MN, Thompson JN (1993) General surgeons' attitudes to the treatment and prevention of abdominal adhesions. Ann R Coll Surg Engl 75: 123–128
7. Ray NF, Larsen JW Jr, Stillman RJ, Jacobs RJ (1993) Economic impact of hospitalizations for lower abdominal adhesiolysis in the United States in 1988. Surg Gynecol Obstet 176: 271–276
8. Strickler B, Blanco J, Fox HE (1994) The gynecologic contribution to intestinal obstruction in females. J Am Coll Surg 178: 617–620
9. Lundberg WI, Wall JE, Mathers JE (1973) Laparoscopy in evaluation of pelvic pain. Obstet Gynecol 42: 872–876
10. Kresch AJ, Seifer DB, Sachs LB et al. (1984) Laparoscopy in 100 women with chronic pelvic pain. Obstet Gynecol 64: 672–674
11. Stout AL, Steege JF, Dodson WC, Hughes CL (1991) Relationship of laparoscopic findings to self-report of pelvic pain. Am J Obstet Gynecol 146: 73–79
12. Howard FM (1993) The role of laparoscopy in chronic pelvic pain: Promise and pitfalls. Obstet Gynecol Surv 48: 357–358
13. Steege JF, Stout AL, Somkuti SG (1993) Chronic pelvic pain in women: toward an integrative model. Obstet Gynecol Surv 48: 95–110
14. Chan CLK, Wood C (1985) Pelvic adhesiolysis-the assessment of symptom relief by 100 patients. Aust NZJ Obstet Gynaecol 25: 295–299
15. Kligman I, Drachenberg C, Papadimitriou J, Katz E (1993) Immunohistochemical demonstration of nerve fibers in pelvic adhesions. Obstet Gynecol 82: 566–568
16. Steege JF, Stout AL (1991) Resolution of chronic pelvic pain after laparoscopic lysis of adhesions. Am J Obstet Gynecol 165: 278–283
17. Daniell JF (1989) Laparoscopic enterolysis of chronic abdominal pain. J Gynecol Surg 5: 61–66
18. Sutton C, MacDonald R (1990) Laser laparoscopic adhesiolysis. J Gynecol Surg 6: 155–159
19. Peters AAW, Trimbos-Kemper GCM, Admiral C et al. (1992) A randomized clinical trial on the benefit of adhesiolysis in patients with intraperitoneal adhesions and chronic pelvic pain. Br J Obstet Gynaecol 99: 59–62
20. Christ JE, Lotze EC (1975) The residual ovary syndrome. Obstet Gynecol 46: 551–556
21. Grogan RH (1967) Reappraisal of residual ovaries. Am J Obstet Gynecol 97: 124–129
22. Parker G (1991) Ovarian remnant and residual ovary syndromes. In: Nichols D (ed) Reproductive gynecologic surgery. Mosby Year Book, St. Louis, pp 295–310
23. Bukovsky I, Liftshitz Y et al. (1988) Ovarian residual syndrome. Surg Gynecol Obstet 167: 132–134
24. Drake TS, Grunert GM (1980) The unsuspected pelvic factor in the infertility investigation. Fertil Steril 34: 27–31
25. DeCherney AH, Mezer HC (1984) The nature of posttuboplasty pelvic adhesions determined by early and late laparoscopy. Fertil Steril 41: 643–666
26. Trimbos-Kemper TCM, Trimbos JB, van Hall EV (1985) Adhesion formation after tubal surgery: results of the eight-day laparoscopy in 188 patients. Fertil Steril 43: 396–400
27. Duffy DM, diZerega GS (1994) Is peritoneal closure necessary? Obstet Gynecol Surv 49: 817–822
28. Hull DB, Varner MW (1991) A randomized study of closure of the peritoneum at Cesarean delivery. Obstet Gynecol 77: 818–821
29. Pietrantoni M, Parsons MT, O'Brien WF et al. (1992) Peritoneal closure or non-closure at Cesarean section. Obstet Gynecol 77: 293–296
30. Tulandi T, Hum GS, Gelfand MM (1988) Closure of laparotomy incisions with or without peritoneal suturing and second-look laparoscopy. Am J Obstet Gynecol 158: 536–537
31. Diamond MP (1992) Adhesion prevention. In: Gershenson DM, DeCherney AH, Curry SL (eds) Operative gynecology. WB Saunders, Philadelphia
32. Operative Laparoscopy Study Group (1991) Postoperative adhesion development after operative laparoscopy: evaluation at early second-look procedures. Fertil Steril 55: 700–704

33. Larsson B (1994) Clinical experiences with corticosteroids, 32% Dextran 70 and Interceed (TC7) as adjuvant therapy for postoperative adhesion prevention in fertility surgery. 29th Congress of the Federation of Scandinavian Societies of Obstetrics and Gynecology. Oulu, Finland 1994, Abst SP97

34. Jansen RPS (1988) Failure of peritoneal irrigation with heparin during pelvic operations upon young women to reduce adhesions. Surg Gynecol Obstet 166: 154–160

35. diZerega GS (1994) Contemporary adhesion prevention. Fertil Steril 61: 219–235

36. Adhesion Study Group (1983) Reduction of postoperative pelvic adhesions with intraperitoneal 32% dextran 70: a prospective, randomized clinical trial. Fertil Steril 40: 612–619

37. Rosenberg SM, Board JA (1984) High-molecular weight dextran in human infertility surgery. Am J Obstet Gynecol 148: 380–385

38. Larsson B (1985) Effect of intraperitoneal instillation of 32% dextran 70 on postoperative adhesion formation after tubal surgery. Acta Obstet Gynecol Scand 64: 437–441

39. Jansen RPS (1985) Failure of intraperitoneal adjuncts to improve the outcome of pelvic operations in young women. Am J Obstet Gynecol 153: 363–371

40. diZerega GS, Campeau JD (1994) Use of instillates to prevent intraperitoneal adhesions: Crystalloid and Dextran. Infertil and Reprod Med Clin of North American 5: 463–478

41. Shear L, Swartz C, Shinaberger J et al. (1965) Kinetics of peritoneal fluid absorption in adult man. N Engl J Med 272: 123–127

42. Duffy DM, diZerega GS (1996) Adhesion controversies: pelvic pain as a cause of adhesions, crystalloids in preventing them. J Repro Med 41: 19–26

43. Fayez JA, Schneider PJ (1987) Prevention of pelvic adhesion formation by different modalities of treatment. Am J Obstet Gynecol 157: 1184–1188

44. Naether OGJ, Fischer R (1993) Adhesion formation after laparoscopic electrocoagulation of the ovarian surface in polycystic ovary patients. Fertil Steril 60: 95–98

45. Gurgan T, Kisnisci H, Yarali H et al. (1991) Evaluation of adhesion formation after laparoscopic treatment of polycystic ovarian disease. Fertil Steril 56: 1176–1178

46. Franklin RR, Malinak RL, Larsson B, Jansen RPS et al. (1995) Reduction of ovarian adhesions by the use of Interceed. Obstet Gynecol 86: 335–338

47. Nordic Adhesion Prevention Study Group (1995) The efficacy of Interceed (TC7) for prevention of reformation of postoperative adhesions on ovaries, fallopian tubes and fimbriae in microsurgical operations for fertility: a multicenter study. Fertil Steril 63: 709–714

48. Van Geldorp H (1994) Interceed absorbable adhesion barrier reduces the formation of postsurgical adhesions after ovarian surgery. Fertil Steril 62: (Abst) 273

49. Keckstein J, Karageorgieva E, Roth A, Sasse V, Tuttlies F, Ulrich U (1996) Reduction of postoperative adhesion formation after laparoscopic ovarian cystectomy. Hum Reprod 11: 579–582

50. Interceed (TC7) Adhesion Barrier Study Group (1989) Prevention of postsurgical adhesions by Interceed (TC7), an absorbable adhesion barrier: a prospective randomized multicenter clinical study. Fertil Steril 51: 933–938

51. Curto JM, Bentolia D, Villois G, Torresgarsa G, Etchegaray M, Ba J (1992) Use of Interceed (TC7) absorbable adhesion barrier to reduce postoperative adhesion reformation in infertility and endometriosis surgery. World Cong Fertil Steril Abst 46

52. Azziz R, and INTERCEED (TC7) Adhesion Barrier Study Group II (1993) Microsurgery alone or with INTERCEED absorbable adhesion barrier for pelvic sidewall adhesion reformation. Surg Gynecol Obstet 177: 135–139

53. Sekiba K, and The Obstetrics and Gynecology Adhesion Prevention Committee (1992) Use of Interceed (TC7) absorbable adhesion barrier to reduce postoperative adhesion reformation in infertility and endometriosis surgery. Obstet Gynecol 79: 518–522

54. Li TC, Cooke ID (1994) The value of an absorbable adhesion barrier, Interceed, in the prevention of adhesion reformation following microsurgical adhesiolysis. Br J Obstet Gynecol 101: 281–286

55. Reid RL, Lie K, Spence JE, Tulandi T, Yuzpe A (1993) Clinical evaluation of the efficacy of heparin-saturated Interceed for prevention of adhesion reformation in the pelvic sidewall of the human. Prog Clin Biol Res 381: 261–264

56. Adhesion Barriers Study Group (1992) Prevention of pelvic sidewall adhesions using barrier methods: ePTFE (Gore-Tex Surgical Membrane) and Oxidized Regenerated Cellulose (Interceed TC7): Preliminary report. 48th Annual Meeting American Fertility Society. Abst 0-059
57. Haney AF, Hesla J, Hurst BS et al (1995) Expanded polytetrafluoroethylene (Gore-Tex Surgical Membrane) is superior to oxidized regenerated cellulose (Interceed TC7) in preventing adhesions. Fertil Steril 63: 1021-1024
58. Haney AF, Doty E (1993) Expanded polytetrafluoroethylene but not oxidized regenerated cellulose prevents adhesion formation and reformation in a mouse uterine horn model of surgical injury. Fertil Steril 60: 550-558
59. Haney AF, Doty E (1992) Murine peritoneal injury and de novo adhesion formation caused by oxidized-regenerated cellulose (Interceed TC7) but not expanded polytetrafluoroethylene (Gore-Tex Surgical Membrane). Fertil Steril 57: 202-208
60. Linsky CB, Diamond MP, Cunningham T et al (1987) Adhesion reduction in the rabbit uterine horn model using an absorbable barrier, TC7. J Reprod Med 32: 17-20
61. Diamond MP, Cunningham T, Linsky CB et al. (1990) Interceed (TC7) An adjuvant for adhesion reduction: animal studies. Prog Clin Biol Res 358: 131-143
62. Steinleitner A, Lopez G, Suarez M et al. (1992) An evaluation of Flowgel as an intraperitoneal barrier material for the prevention of postsurgical adhesion reformation. Fertil Steril 57: 305-308
63. Surgical Membrane Study Group (1992) Prophylaxis of pelvic sidewall adhesion formation with Gore-Tex Surgical Membrane: a multicenter clinical investigation. Fertil Steril 57: 921-932
64. Myomectomy Adhesion Multicenter Study Group (1995) An expanded polytetrafluoroethylene barrier (Gore-Tex Surgical Membrane) reduces post-myomectomy adhesion formation. Fertil Steril 63: 491-493
65. Liu CY (1992) Laparoscopic hysterectomy: a review of 72 cases. J Reprod Med 37: 351-355
66. Dlugi AM, Saleh WA, Jacobsen G (1992) KTP/532 laser laparoscopy in the treatment of endometriosis-associated infertility. Fertil Steril 57: 1186-1193
67. Pados G, Camus M, DeMunch L, DeVroey P (1992) Laparoscopic application of Interceed (TC7). Hum Reprod 8: 1141-1143
68. Reid R, Spence J, Tulandi T, Yuzpe A (1993) Clinical experience of Interceed (TC7) absorbable adhesion barrier and heparin. Fertil Steril 60: (Abst) 160
69. Mais V, Ajossa S, Piras B, Guerriero S, Marongiu D (1995) Prevention of de-novo adhesion formation after laparoscopic myomectomy: a randomized trial to evaluate the effectiveness of an oxidized regenerated cellulose absorbable barrier. Hum Reprod 10: 3133-3135
70. Mais V, Ajossa S, Marongiu D, Peiretti R, Guerriero S, Benedetto G (1995) Reduction of adhesion reformation after laparoscopic endometriosis surgery: a randomized trial with an oxidized regenerated cellulose absorbable barrier. Obstet Gynecol 86: 512-515
71. Korell M (1995) Möglichkeiten der Adhasionsprophylaxe Medifact, Landsberg, pp 103-121
72. Giannacodimos G, Douligeris N, Lappas K (1992) Prevention of postsurgical adhesions by Interceed (TC7) in polycystic ovary syndrome treated by CO_2 laser vaporization laparoscopy. Proceedings of the Eighth Annual Meeting of the European Society of Human Reproduction and Embryology, The Netherlands, Abst 61

Springer-Verlag
and the Environment

We at Springer-Verlag firmly believe that an international science publisher has a special obligation to the environment, and our corporate policies consistently reflect this conviction.

We also expect our business partners – paper mills, printers, packaging manufacturers, etc. – to commit themselves to using environmentally friendly materials and production processes.

The paper in this book is made from low- or no-chlorine pulp and is acid free, in conformance with international standards for paper permanency.